Depression in Later Life

Medical Psychiatry

1. Handbook of Depression and Anxiety: A Biological Approach, *edited by Johan A. den Boer and J. M. Ad Sitsen*
2. Anticonvulsants in Mood Disorders, *edited by Russell T. Joffe and Joseph R. Calabrese*
3. Serotonin in Antipsychotic Treatment: Mechanisms and Clinical Practice, *edited by John M. Kane, H.-J. Möller, and Frans Awouters*
4. Handbook of Functional Gastrointestinal Disorders, *edited by Kevin W. Olden*
5. Clinical Management of Anxiety, *edited by Johan A. den Boer*
6. Obsessive-Compulsive Disorders: Diagnosis • Etiology • Treatment, *edited by Eric Hollander and Dan J. Stein*
7. Bipolar Disorder: Biological Models and Their Clinical Application, *edited by L. Trevor Young and Russell T. Joffe*
8. Dual Diagnosis and Treatment: Substance Abuse and Comorbid Medical and Psychiatric Disorders, *edited by Henry R. Kranzler and Bruce J. Rounsaville*
9. Geriatric Psychopharmacology, *edited by J. Craig Nelson*
10. Panic Disorder and Its Treatment, *edited by Jerrold F. Rosenbaum and Mark H. Pollack*
11. Comorbidity in Affective Disorders, *edited by Mauricio Tohen*
12. Practical Management of the Side Effects of Psychotropic Drugs, *edited by Richard Balon*

13. Psychiatric Treatment of the Medically Ill, *edited by Robert G. Robinson and William R. Yates*
14. Medical Management of the Violent Patient: Clinical Assessment and Therapy, *edited by Kenneth Tardiff*
15. Bipolar Disorders: Basic Mechanisms and Therapeutic Implications, *edited by Jair C. Soares and Samuel Gershon*
16. Schizophrenia: A New Guide for Clinicians, *edited by John G. Csernansky*
17. Polypharmacy in Psychiatry, *edited by S. Nassir Ghaemi*
18. Pharmacotherapy for Child and Adolescent Psychiatric Disorders: Second Edition, Revised and Expanded, *David R. Rosenberg, Pablo A. Davanzo, and Samuel Gershon*
19. Brain Imaging in Affective Disorders, *edited by Jair C. Soares*
20. Handbook of Medical Psychiatry, *edited by Jair C. Soares and Samuel Gershon*
21. Handbook of Depression and Anxiety: Second Edition, Revised and Expanded, *edited by Siegfried Kasper, Johan A. den Boer, and J. M. Ad Sitsen*
22. Aggression: Psychiatric Assessment and Treatment, *edited by Emil F. Coccaro*
23. Depression in Later Life: A Multidisciplinary Psychiatric Approach, *edited by James M. Ellison and Sumer Verma*
24. Autism Spectrum Disorders, *edited by Eric Hollander*

ADDITIONAL VOLUMES IN PREPARATION

Handbook of Chronic Depression: Diagnosis and Therapeutic Management, *edited by Maurizio Fava and Jonathan Alpert*

Depression in Later Life

A Multidisciplinary Psychiatric Approach

edited by

James M. Ellison

McLean Hospital
Belmont, and
Harvard Medical School
Boston, Massachusetts, U.S.A.

Sumer Verma

McLean Hospital
Belmont, and
Boston University School of Medicine
Boston, Massachusetts, U.S.A.

MARCEL DEKKER, INC. NEW YORK • BASEL

ISBN: 0-8247-4246-X

This book is printed on acid-free paper.

Headquarters
Marcel Dekker, Inc.
270 Madison Avenue, New York, NY 10016
tel: 212-696-9000; fax: 212-685-4540

Eastern Hemisphere Distribution
Marcel Dekker AG
Hutgasse 4, Postfach 812, CH-4001 Basel, Switzerland
tel: 41-61-260-6300; fax: 41-61-260-6333

World Wide Web
http://www.dekker.com

The publisher offers discounts on this book when ordered in bulk quantities. For more information, write to Special Sales/Professional Marketing at the headquarters address above.

Current printing (last digit):
10 9 8 7 6 5 4 3 2 1

PRINTED IN THE UNITED STATES OF AMERICA

Series Introduction

During Sigmund Freud's long career, he got many things right. These included his early recognition of the means of distinguishing conversion from the organic paralyses, the importance of subconscious motivations on our conscious behavior, and the impact of early experience on the developing personality.

However, he also got some important things wrong. The most widely publicized of these have been his views on female development and sexuality. Another error, which for many years hobbled our advances, was the notion that people over 50 were less able to benefit from psychotherapy. Time and experience have clearly proven this view to be an egregious error.

Increasing longevity—the result of better nutrition, cleaner water, and advances in medicine—has resulted in a larger and aging population. The aged and their problems have necessarily attracted the attention of the medical specialties to their care. Unfortunately, the illnesses afflicting the elderly are myriad, and often many are present in a single individual. This presents us with difficulties in diagnosis and in planning appropriate treatment. Is the patient's apathy the result of occult infection, dementia, depression, or some combination of these? If it is depression, is it a primary depression, or is it a reaction to illness or life circumstance? It is essential that the careful clinician untangle these threads, and then treat each effectively while keeping in focus the potential interactions of medications and other interventions, both good (as is often true of the combination of medication and psychotherapy) and bad. When properly treated, the elderly get better and are capable of learning. Although our brains age, they remain able to make new synapses. Even old dogs can learn new tricks.

Depression, while common in all stages of life, seems particularly debilitating in the aged. Perhaps this is because we accumulate losses of all sorts—of people important to us, of bodily function, of social status. Our brains age and lose neurons, particularly in the absence of stimulation. All physicians, family doctors, specialists, and mental health professionals need to recognize depression as well as its causes in the individual patient, and must be able to respond with the proper treatments. Ellison and Verma have brought together a distinguished group of contributors to lead us through this labyrinth.

William A. Frosch

Foreword

Do we all inevitably become depressed in old age? Certainly there is much to be depressed about—loss of loved ones and friends as well as loss of health and function are expected changes at this stage of life. It is also the time when one reflects on one's life and perhaps dwells on the difficulties and disappointments along the way. Any one of these factors alone would be catalyst enough to engender a state of depression. It is no surprise, then, that many of us try to avoid getting old by enlisting help—ranging from pills, herbs, and diets to fanatical exercise and surgery.

Counterbalancing this obsession and fear about aging has been the mushrooming of scientific data about the aging process and the emotional disturbances that may accompany the late phases of life. It turns out that depression is *not* more common in old age. On the contrary, the onset of a first depressive episode is less common after the age of 60 than it is before 60. There is also growing research that focuses on the relationship between medical illnesses and depression, the link between changes in life circumstances and the onset and worsening of depression, and the role of medications in contributing to depression. Armed with better understanding, we can now diagnose depression more accurately, link its onset with medical illness, and treat the symptoms accordingly.

If one looks at the latest research data in their entirety, it becomes clear that it is not depression itself that is a problem in old age; it is that the word "depression" has been used indistinctly to describe all the unpleasant life experiences of the aged. It is therefore imperative that we distinguish between unhappiness (and its symptoms) as an accompaniment to the many losses of late life and depression as a clinical entity requiring treatment. Unhappiness does not require psychiatric treatment! Grief, for example, is a normal healthy response to the losses that occur in late life. Although some grief may progress to a true clinical depression, it can simply resolve over time.

A related concept, which was first put forth by Erik Erikson, can help us understand the emergence of depression or demoralization in late life. The last of the eight stages of human psychological development—that of old age—has a specific psychological task. As described by Erikson, it is to reflect on one's past life and to integrate it in a realistic way with one's sense of self. In this last phase of life, there can be a sense of achievement and fulfillment as well as feelings of depression over losses and failures. The danger lies in not recognizing the often subtle difference between ordinary late-life depression and the true clinical condition. The former may or may not require therapeutic intervention, but the latter should almost always be treated.

Despite a growing body of knowledge, as illustrated in this volume, there is invariably a failure in the medical community to accurately diagnose true late-life clinical depression. It may be due to "ageism"—the biased, incorrect belief that an older person's depression is "normal for their age"—or a simple lack of understanding. A typical example occurs following the death of a spouse. The surviving elderly individual may harbor thoughts of death, too. Such desire is not necessarily a sign of depression and is certainly understandable. However, research and clinical experience have shown that the wish may also be a manifestation of clinical depression; that person will likely respond to antidepressant medication.

Late-life depression has also been consistently underdiagnosed when it is associated with serious medical illness. The same incorrect medical reasoning applied to the death wish is often applied to elderly patients who have a serious medical illness. The clinician (and, often, family members) assumes that the elderly person with a serious illness is too ill or frail to be treated with psychotropic medication. In fact, depression associated with medical illness is often helped by antidepressants. Research has shown that antidepressant treatment initiated following a stroke or a heart attack is highly effective.

These successes in treating the many forms of depressive states in the elderly illustrate the importance of informed and timely therapeutic intervention. As reflected in this volume, many therapeutic techniques are now available for treating the elderly. Psychopharmacological approaches, in particular, have grown in number, as well as in effectiveness. It is no longer appropriate for a clinician who treats older individuals to be ignorant of the latest antidepressants—as well as established effective medications—or afraid to use them.

Therein lies the importance of up-to-date volumes such as *Depression in Later Life*. More than ever, it is essential for clinicians to have available a comprehensive volume on the diagnosis, prevalence, and treatment of late-life depression. Let us hope that as this information grows and is disseminated, older patients' suffering will be more readily recognized and alleviated.

Carl Salzman, M.D.
Massachusetts Mental Health Center
and Harvard Medical School
Boston, Massachusetts, U.S.A.

Preface

The high prevalence, frequent recurrence, and serious consequences of depressive disorders in young and middle-aged adults are well recognized. The effects of depression on the elderly population, however, have been less widely appreciated. Although demographic studies indicate a low rate of major depressive disorder among community-dwelling elderly Americans, the prevalence approaches 15% when nonmajor depressive disorders are included. Studies among the medically ill or institutionalized elderly, furthermore, reveal very high rates of major depression. In long-term care facilities, where late-life depression is most rampant, more than 40% of residents show significant depressive symptoms. These are alarming numbers, because the presence of depression in later life has dire health consequences: excess suffering and functional limitation, increased morbidity from medical causes, and accelerated mortality as a result of concurrent medical illnesses or suicide. In the highest risk group for suicide—depressed white males 85 years of age and older—the suicide rate is more than five times that of the general population.

Given the aging of the American population and the enhanced survival of the infirm elderly, it is increasingly important that clinicians know how to diagnose and treat late-life depression. At present, however, even recognition of this disorder is too limited. Affected seniors may minimize their psychological distress and focus more directly on somatic or cognitive concerns, inadvertently obscuring the correct diagnosis. Primary care clinicians—the health care providers likely to see the greatest number of depressed elderly individuals and therefore most in need of awareness—frequently miss the correct diagnosis. Even when the proper diagnosis is made, elderly patients who present depressive symptoms to a primary care physician are less likely than younger ones to receive adequate antidepressant treatment, psychotherapy, adequately intensive follow-up care, or referral to a mental health specialist. Mental health specialists, too, have shown limited recognition of depression among older patients. The need is apparent, therefore, for greater awareness of geriatric depression in its varied manifestations and for further education of all clinicians and the public, including family members and caregivers of depressed elders.

The literature on treatment of late-life depression includes numerous studies of pharmacotherapy and a smaller number of psychotherapy studies, but our therapeutic approach still contains many areas of uncertainty. Treatments for depression among the oldest old, the medically ill, and the demented elderly, for example, have received much less attention than treatment of younger, medically healthier late-life depressives. Beyond effects on symptom alleviation, we still know too little about how treatment affects quality of life. Furthermore, we need to better understand how to integrate somatic therapies with psychotherapeutic approaches, which are now recommended by experts as an important treatment component for late-life depression but still too infrequently applied in practice.

With invaluable contribution from noted experts, we have tried to present herein a comprehensive picture of late-life depression and to identify the areas in need of further investigation. This volume is intended for use by all clinicians who evaluate and treat depressed elderly individuals. Psychiatrists and other mental health specialists, as well as primary care clinicians, should find information that is both up to date and practical. In addition, we, along with the chapter authors, have attempted to present this important illness and its treatment in a larger context, highlighting its multifaceted manifestations and effects as well as the currently available range of treatments. It is our earnest hope that the publication of this book will increase professional and public awareness of late-life depression, disseminate the most current knowledge, help identify areas for further inquiry, and contribute to a growing body of literature dedicated to improving quality of life in the later years.

James M. Ellison
Sumer Verma

Acknowledgments

Edited books, at their best, incorporate expert contributions on a given topic into a broader view than any individual could achieve alone. Sometimes this breadth is achieved at the expense of ambiguities and stylistic inconsistencies introduced by a writing process that relies on individual contributors who separately shape and supply their portions of the final product. In the case of this book, however, we were fortunate to be working with a group of collaborators who in many cases not only contributed their own chapters but also generously advised us regarding the overall goals of the book. The resulting volume, we hope, has enhanced the quality and value of each author's work. For their own chapters and their help in improving the entire book, we wish to express our gratitude to each of our contributing authors. Working with them has been a rewarding experience. In addition, two research assistants offered far more time and energy than we ever expected, each reviewing and helping to prepare multiple chapters. We expect their contributions here to be the first of many publications from this scholarly pair: Yosef Berlow and Noah Meyers.

The patients and staff of the McLean Hospital Geriatric Psychiatry Program, where we are privileged to work, also deserve our grateful recognition. They have helped us to understand both the devastating consequences of depression and the remarkable benefits possible with effective treatment. Our rich clinical experiences at McLean Hospital have grounded this book clinically so as to increase its practical value to practitioners treating older adults.

Two editors from Marcel Dekker, Inc., deserve our praise for sticking with us during the occasionally frustrating process of this book's completion. Jinnie Kim acquired this book and supported our efforts throughout with apparently unfailing faith, and Michael Deters made certain that production progressed in as timely and flawless a manner as humanly possible. We unreservedly thank these two for their good humor, expertise, and helpful coaching.

Finally, we wish to thank our families. One never appreciates in advance the commitment of time that will be required to complete a project such as this; it is always beyond any initial estimate. Our spouses and children have made a silent but absolutely necessary contribution to our work by sharing our conviction of its importance and by encouraging our continued writing even at times when they would have preferred our presence. For their love and their support of this book, as in so many other areas of our lives, we wish to dedicate our work to them.

Contents

Contributors

Francesca Cannavo Antognini, Ph.D. Geriatric Psychiatry Program, McLean Hospital, Belmont, and Department of Psychiatry, Harvard Medical School, Boston, Massachusetts, U.S.A.

Yosef Berlow Memory Diagnostic Clinic, McLean Hospital, Belmont, Massachusetts, U.S.A.

Ashok J. Bharucha, M.D. University of Pittsburgh School of Medicine, Pittsburgh, Pennsylvania, U.S.A.

Donald Davidoff, Ph.D. Neuropsychological and Psychodiagnostic Testing Service, McLean Hospital, Belmont, and Department of Psychology, Harvard Medical School, Boston, Massachusetts, U.S.A.

Dale A. D'Mello, M.D. Department of Psychiatry, Michigan State University, East Lansing, and St. Lawrence Hospital, Lansing, Michigan, U.S.A.

P. Murali Doraiswamy, M.D. Departments of Psychiatry and Medicine, Duke University Medical Center, Durham, North Carolina, U.S.A.

James M. Ellison, M.D., M.P.H. Geriatric Psychiatry Program, McLean Hospital, Belmont, and Department of Psychiatry, Harvard Medical School, Boston, Massachusetts, U.S.A.

Martin Goldstein, M.D. Department of Neurology, Weill Medical College of Cornell University, New York, New York, U.S.A.

Gary L. Gottlieb, M.D. Department of Psychiatry, Harvard Medical School, and Brigham and Women's Hospital, Boston, Massachusetts, U.S.A.

Kelly Harless Department of Psychiatry, University of California, San Diego, La Jolla, California, U.S.A.

Michael E. Henry, M.D. Affective Disorders Laboratories and Brain Imaging Center, McLean Hospital, Belmont, and Department of Psychiatry, Harvard Medical School, Boston, Massachusetts, U.S.A.

Helen H. Kyomen, M.D. McLean Hospital, Belmont, and Harvard Medical School, Boston, Massachusetts, U.S.A.

Janet Lawrence, M.D. Memory Diagnostic Clinic, McLean Hospital, Belmont, and Department of Psychiatry, Harvard Medical School, Boston, Massachusetts, U.S.A.

Noah M. Meyers* University of Pittsburgh School of Medicine, Pittsburgh, Pennsylvania, U.S.A.

James G. O'Brien, M.D. Department of Family and Community Medicine, University of Louisville, Louisville, Kentucky, U.S.A.

Abi V. Rayner, M.D. Department of Family and Community Medicine, University of Louisville, Louisville, Kentucky, U.S.A.

Charles F. Reynolds III, M.D. Intervention Research Center for Late-Life Mood Disorders, Department of Psychiatry, University of Pittsburgh School of Medicine, Pittsburgh, Pennsylvania, U.S.A.

Stephen Seiner, M.D. McLean Hospital, Belmont, and Harvard Medical School, Boston, Massachusetts, U.S.A.

**Current affiliation*: Cornell University, Ithaca, New York, U.S.A.

Yvette Sheline, M.D. Departments of Psychiatry, Neurology, and Radiology, Washington University, St. Louis, Missouri, U.S.A.

Fred Silverstone McLean Hospital, Belmont, Massachusetts, U.S.A.

E. Yusuf Sivrioglu, M.D. Department of Psychiatry, Uludag University Medical School, Bursa, Turkey, and Geriatric Psychiatry Program, McLean Hospital, Belmont, Massachusetts, U.S.A.

Rein Tideiksaar, Ph.D. ElderCare Companies, Inc., Philadelphia, Pennsylvania, U.S.A.

Sumer Verma, M.D. Geriatric Psychiatry Fellowship and Education, McLean Hospital, Belmont, Department of Psychiatry, Harvard Medical School, and Department of Psychiatry, Boston University School of Medicine, Boston, Massachusetts, U.S.A.

Nava Vogel Belmont Council on Aging, Belmont, Massachusetts, U.S.A.

Jennifer L. Woehr, Psy.D. Department of Neuropsychology, McLean Hospital, Belmont, and Department of Psychiatry, Harvard Medical School, Boston, Massachusetts, U.S.A.

Sidney Zisook, M.D. Department of Psychiatry, University of California, San Diego, La Jolla, and Veterans Affairs San Diego Healthcare System, San Diego, California, U.S.A.

Depression in Later Life

1

Epidemiology of Late-Life Depression

Dale A. D'Mello
Michigan State University, East Lansing, and St. Lawrence Hospital, Lansing, Michigan, U.S.A.

INTRODUCTION

Demographics of the Elderly

The term *late adulthood* or *old age* usually refers to the stage of the life cycle that begins at the age of 65 years. Gerontologists divide older adults into two groups: the young old (65–74 years), and the old old (>75 years). The elderly comprise the fastest growing segment of the U.S. population (U.S. Census Bureau). This disproportionate rate of growth is expected to accelerate in the decades ahead (see Fig. 1). Between 1980 and 1990, the population over age 85 grew by 40% and the number of centenarians doubled. In fact, centenarians are now the fastest-growing subpopulation of the elderly. And by the year 2050, some 834,000 living Americans will have celebrated their 100th birthday (Schneider, 2002). This number exceeds the present-day population of the state of South Dakota. Two-thirds of all the people in the entire history of the world who have reached the age of 65 are alive today (Smith, 1997)! And by the year 2050, it is projected that there will be more people over than under age 65 years (U.S. Census Bureau). Women live longer than men. The number of men per 100 women drops sharply in the twilight years (Fig. 2). As a result, older women, as opposed to older men, bear a disproportionate burden of caring for their aging spouses (Fig. 3).

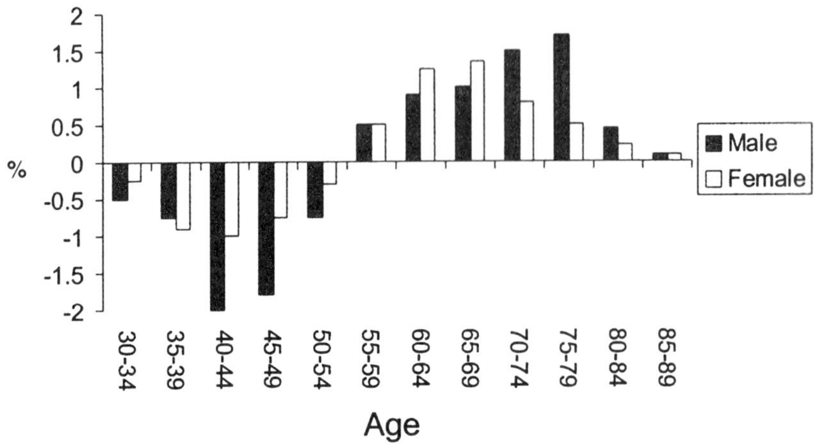

FIGURE 1 Projected demographic changes in the United States, 2000–2025. (From U.S. Census Bureau, 1996).

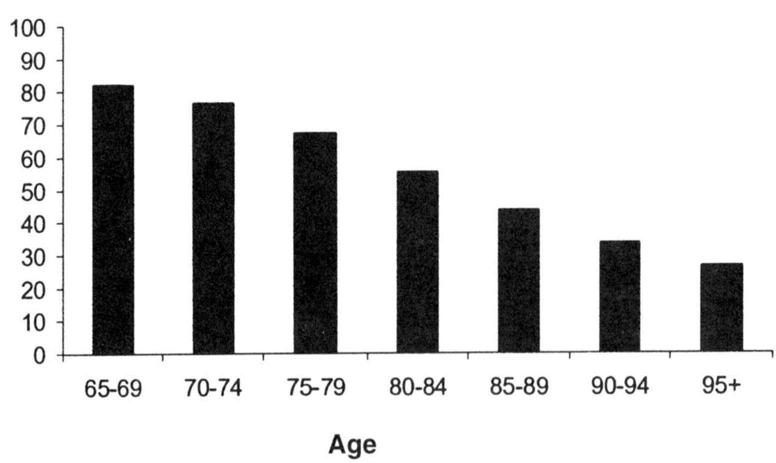

FIGURE 2 Number of men per 100 women by age. (From U.S. Census Bureau, 1996).

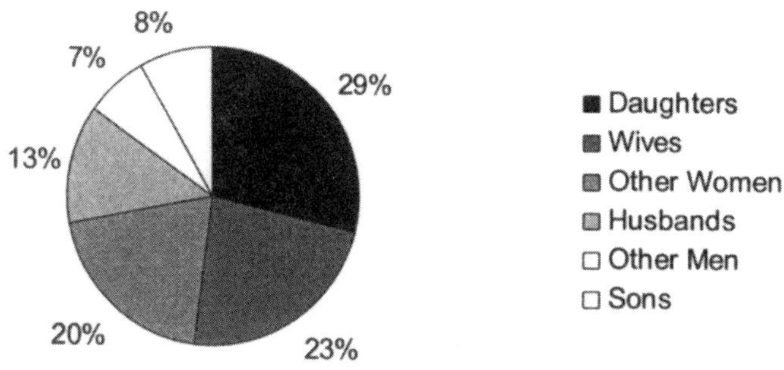

FIGURE 3 Caretakers and their relationship to the elderly care recipient. (From Select Committee on Aging, U.S. House of Representatives, 1987).

Demographics of Depression in the Elderly

Late-life depression is *not* a necessary consequence of normal aging (Roberts et al., 1997). It is a widespread and serious medical disorder. Significant depressive symptoms affect over 5 million of the 35 million people over the age of 65 years in the United States (Colenda et al., 2000). The consequences of this are substantial: impaired compliance with medical treatment, overutilization of health care resources, diminished quality of life, and premature mortality. Nevertheless, depression is frequently underdiagnosed; when properly diagnosed, it is often undertreated (Koenig et al., 1997b). The purpose of this chapter is to illustrate the magnitude of the problem in order to lay the groundwork for discussion of diagnosis and treatment of this condition and its related variants.

PREVALENCE OF LATE-LIFE DEPRESSION

Population-Based Studies

The Epidemiological Catchment Area Study (ECA), completed in the early 1980s, assessed the 6-month prevalence of psychiatric disorders as defined in the *Diagnostic and Statistical Manual of Mental Disorders*, third edition (DSM-III), of the American Psychiatric Association in five U.S. communities. The overall prevalence of major depression in the elderly, estimated at 1% (Weissman et al., 1988; Myers et al., 1984), was lower than in younger individuals. The women sampled had a higher rate of depression (1.4%) than the men (0.4%). Diagnosable mood disorders affected between 2 and 4% of the elderly. The prevalence of major depression among the elderly population in the Cache County (Utah) study was 4.4% in women and 2.7% in men (Steffens et al., 2000). A secondary analysis of the National Health Examination Follow-up Study (Zonderman and Costa, 1991) did not observe an appreciable difference in the prevalence of depressive symptoms across the life span with one possible exception. The oldest old reported a higher number of depressive symptoms than others.

Why Estimates from Population Studies Are Low

Several authorities (Snowdon, 1990; Blazer et al., 1987) have questioned the validity of these large population-based studies. They have argued that the elderly display fewer or masked symptoms, a different spectrum of symptoms, or more typically variant symptoms, such as minor depression. In addition, perhaps the commonly used diagnostic criteria (DSM-IV) and screening tools, such as the National Institute of Mental Health Diagnostic Interview Schedule (DIS), are more applicable for the diagnosis of depression in younger populations. Hence, these instruments may be neither sufficiently sensitive nor applicable for the detection of depression in an older population (Knauper and Wittchen, 1994). Some have suggested that whereas the elderly experience symptoms similar to those of younger people, they do so at a subthreshold level (Blazer et al., 1987). In addition they may be less likely than younger people to label their symptoms as "depressive" (Hasin and Link, 1988).

Furthermore, older individuals experience more physical illness than younger individuals. They may attribute their depressive symptoms to concurrent medical problems: the demoralization and fatigue that accompany physical illness or the effect of prescribed medications (Rabins, 1996). Persons over the age of 65 represent only 12–13% of the population but receive approximately one-third of medications prescribed (Wilcox, 1994). The elderly bear a disproportionate burden of life's vicissitudes: loss, and conflict, physical illness, and disability. For all of these reasons, the prevalence of late-life depression may be routinely underestimated.

The Birth Cohort Effect

Progressive increases have been observed in the prevalence of depression in successively younger birth cohorts throughout the twentieth century (Weissman et al., 1984; Klerman et al., 1985). In addition, each birth cohort appears to have experienced the onset of symptoms at an earlier age than the previous cohort (Fig. 4). Possible causes of the cohort effect include changes in urbanization, the family structure, and the role of women. This is yet another dynamic that is likely to propel the prevalence of depression into stratospheric proportions in the decades ahead.

Inclusive Diagnostic Methods and the Prevalence of Depression

Population studies that employ more inclusive diagnostic approaches (including less severe depressive syndromes than major depressive disorder) tend to arrive

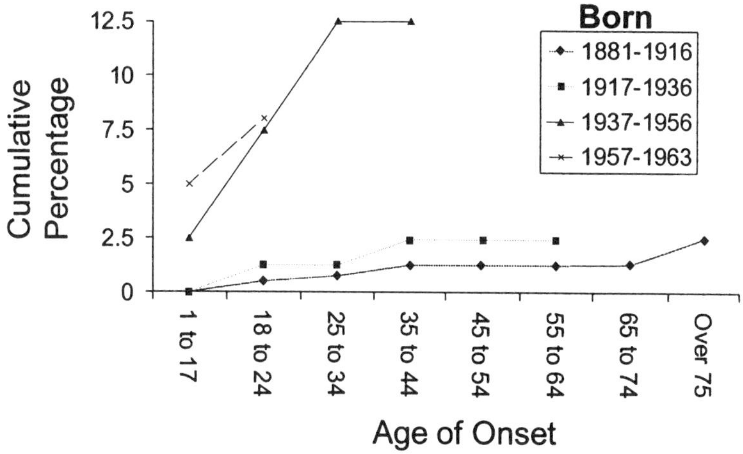

FIGURE 4 Prevalence of major depression for women in the United States by birth cohort. (From Weissman et al., 1984.)

at substantially higher rates of "depression." For instance, Blazer and Williams identified a rate of 10–15% of clinically significant depressive symptoms in the elderly population (Blazer and Williams, 1980). A recent review of the discrepancy as to the prevalence of depression in late life between different studies found that the prevalence of major depression ranged 10-fold, from 5–45% (Koenig and Blazer, 1992), even when the same diagnostic criteria were employed. In older people, depressive symptoms can be caused by physical illness. The difference in prevalence rates has been attributed to varying thresholds among clinicians on when to count symptoms toward the diagnosis of depression and when to attribute them to physical illness. This is an issue of particular importance in determining the prevalence of depressive symptoms in various health care delivery settings, where rates appear to be alarmingly higher (Colenda et al., 2000).

DEPRESSION IN VARIOUS TREATMENT SETTINGS

Primary Care

Unrecognized depression in a medical setting can prolong the length of hospital stay, increase the use of other health resources, and add to the cost of care (Saravay and Lavin, 1994). Depression may decrease motivation to care adequately for an existing medical condition (Fulop et al., 1987). For instance, patients with diabetes and comorbid depression comply poorly with medications (Surridge et al., 1984) and diet and subsequently have more difficulty achieving glycemic control. In addition, they have more ambulatory care visits and significantly higher (fivefold) total health care expenditures than their nondepressed counterparts (Egede et al., 2002). The presence of depression following myocardial infarction is associated with more frequent cardiac arrhythmias, congestive heart failure, and mortality (Frasure-Smith et al., 1993). Depressed patients with coronary artery disease are less likely to adhere to cardiac exercise programs (Blumenthal et al., 1982). Depressed older persons are also significantly more likely to die because of cardiac disease during 50 months of follow-up than nondepressed older persons (Penninx et al., 2001). The risk of cardiac mortality was 1.6 times increased in persons with minor depression and more than 3 times increased in persons with major depression (Penninx et al., 2001).

Prevalence studies of depression in treatment settings report alarmingly higher rates than those observed in community-based surveys. Alexopoulos reported a rate of late-life depression of 17–37% in a primary care setting (Alexopoulos, 1996). Barrett et al. observed that, in a population of elderly patients in a primary care practice, 2.1% of the patients displayed characterological depression, 5.6% had major depression, and as many as 7.9% displayed masked/suspected depression (Barrett et al., 1988). The last group displayed clinical evidence of depression at the interview (e.g., depressed facies and depressive symptoms) but denied feeling depressed. Older people are more likely to seek treatment from primary care physicians than from mental health specialists (German et al., 1985). Hence, the primary setting is an ideal location for the screening, prevention, and management of depression.

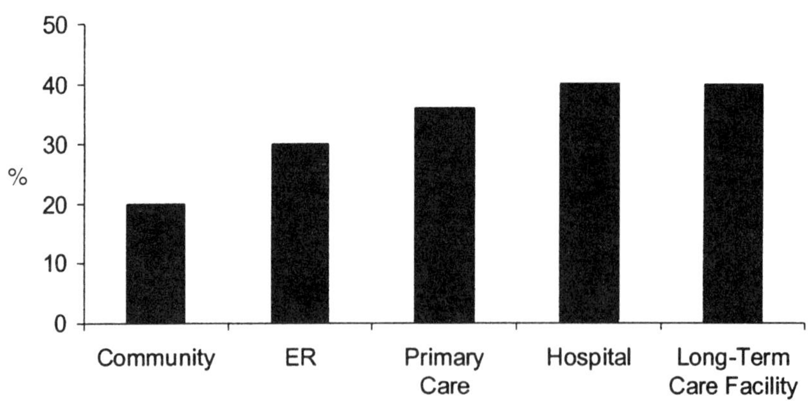

FIGURE 5 Prevalence of depression in later life: percentages represent those with clinically significant depressive symptoms. (From Koenig and Blazer, 1992; Fabacher et al., 2002; Alexopoulos, 1996a; Koenig et al., 1997b; Parmelee et al., 1989.)

Emergency Room

Depressed elders consume more medical resources and present three times more frequently to emergency rooms than those who are not depressed (Katon and Schulberg, 1992). In each of three separate systematic studies (Meldon et al., 1997; Fabacher et al., 2002; Cydulka et al., 1999), one in every three older patients who received treatment in emergency settings displayed clinically significant symptoms of depression. Emergency room physicians failed to identify most of these patients. In yet another study, a positive response to a single screening question (Do you often feel helpless?) yielded a sensitivity of 76% and a specificity of 75% for the diagnosis of depression (Shah et al., 1997).

Medically Ill Hospitalized Populations

In one study cohort, major depression was documented in 11% of patients hospitalized with medical illness. Clinically significant depressive symptoms were documented in 25% of this population. The diagnostic strategy used affected the prevalence rate, with a twofold difference between the extremes (Koenig et al., 1997). A diagnostic strategy that best distinguished a severe and persistent major depression missed 49% of the patients identified with a more inclusive approach. In a university hospital with easy access to psychiatric consultation, the majority of patients with clinically significant depression were not accurately diagnosed (Koenig et al., 1997) and did not receive an antidepressant (Fig. 6). In fact, when an antidepressant was prescribed, the most commonly administered drug was the tricyclic amitriptyline. The dose of amitriptyline prescribed was subtherapeutic: 10–30 mg/day.

Depression is observed in association with almost all known serious medical disorders (McDaniels, 2000). Its prevalence ranges from 50% in conditions such as pancreatic cancer and multiple sclerosis to a low of 5% in end-stage

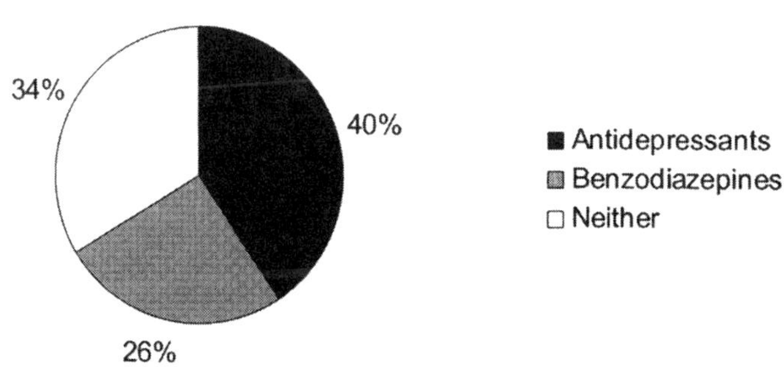

FIGURE 6 Treatment of depression in medically ill hospitalized depressed elderly patients (n = 153). (From Koenig et al., 1997a.)

renal disease. Winokur identified three distinguishing clinical characteristics of depression in the medically ill: older age at onset, cognitive deficits, and absence of suicidal ideation (Winokur, 1990).

Long-Term-Care Facilities

The prevalence of psychiatric illness in general among residents of long-term-care facilities exceeds that observed in the community (Parmalee et al. 1989; Rovner et al., 1986; Tariot et al., 1993). Among randomly selected residents of a public nursing home, 91% met criteria for at least one psychiatric diagnosis; 50% of patients had four or more behavioral problems (Tariot et al., 1993). An alarming one-third of these affected patients had not received psychiatric care since admission. In yet another study 12.4% of residents in a long-term-care facility displayed the symptoms of major depression (Parmalee, et al., 1989). An additional 30.5% experienced less severe but clinically significant depressive symptoms. The presence of depression among the residents of a nursing home was associated with a twofold increased risk of death from any cause in a year of follow-up (Rovner et al., 1991).

DEPRESSION IN THE CONTEXT OF MEDICAL AND NEUROPSYCHIATRIC DISORDERS

Cancer

In one cohort of cancer patients, 25% were diagnosed with major depression or adjustment disorder with depressed mood (Massie and Holland, 1990). The prevalence of depression varies with tumor type, disease stage, severity of pain, and magnitude of disability. The highest rates of depression (50%) appear to occur with cancers that originate in the pancreas and oropharynx (McDaniel et al., 1995). The severity of medical illness, persistence of pain, and inadequacy of social support networks all tend to correlate directly with the emergence of

TABLE 1 Lifetime Prevalence (%) of Major Depression and Dysthymia by Age

Age (years)	Major depression	Dysthymia
18–29	5.0	3.0
30–44	7.5	3.8
45–64	4.0	3.6
>65	1.4	1.7
Total	4.9	3.2

Source: Weissman et al., 1991 (ECA data).

TABLE 2 Center for Epidemiologic Studies Mean Depression Scale (CES-D) Scores by Age from the National Health Examination Follow-Up Study ($N = 9512$)

Age (years)	Men	Women
32–44	6.5	9.1
45–54	6.9	8.9
55–64	7.0	9.1
65–74	7.4	9.2
75–86	9.1	10.6
Mean	7.4	9.4

Source: Zonderman and Costa, 1991.

depression in the patient with cancer (Noyes and Kathol, 1986). Antidepressant medications may be helpful in improving mood and hence morale and compliance with treatment. They may also improve sleep, diminish pain, and alleviate the anorexia caused by the malignant process or chemotherapy.

Coronary Artery Disease

The relationship between depression and coronary artery disease is bidirectional. Coronary artery disease is more common in people with the diagnosis of depression (Glassman and Shapiro, 1998). Depressed people are more likely to smoke, to live sedentary lives, and to comply less well with treatment. Their poor compliance extends equally to the care of concurrent medical conditions such as diabetes, hypertension, and dyslipidemia, which are all common antecedents of coronary heart disease. Furthermore, depression is associated with hyperactivity of the hypothalamic-pituitary-adrenal axis, enhanced platelet activity, increased sympathetic arousal, and decreased heart rate variability (Musselman et al., 1998). Conversely, depression is a common sequel of coronary artery disease; 25% of patients who have experienced acute myocardial infarction develop depression in the subsequent 6-month period. The presence of concurrent depression following myocardial infarction is associated with a more dismal outcome: more frequent cardiac arrhythmias, congestive heart failure, and death (Frasure-Smith et al., 1993). In fact, it has been repeatedly shown that depression is a potential risk factor for subsequent cardiac death (Penninx et al., 2001). The risk for cardiac mortality was 1.6 times increased in persons with minor depression and more than 3 times increased in persons with major depression (Penninx et al., 2001).

Cerebrovascular Disease and Stroke

There is now an enormous literature concerning poststroke depression. Between 25 and 50% of patients will develop depression following a cerebrovascular accident (Astrom et al., 1993; Robinson et al., 1987). Depression is more likely with left-sided and anterior cerebral lesions than with right-sided and posterior lesions. The proximity of the stroke lesion to the left anterior pole correlates more closely with the severity of depression than does the size of the vascular lesion or the severity of subsequent physical disability (Robinson et al., 1983). Additional neuroanatomical correlates of poststroke depression include significant subcortical atrophy and periventricular white matter disease. Depression is more common in those with a family history of depression than in those without such a family history. The clinical expression of poststroke depression resembles depression in other older patients. However, it is often characterized by three clinical symptoms: psychomotor slowing, anxiety, and ideas of reference (Federoff et al., 1991). The presence of depression following a stroke increases mortality 3.4 times in the 10 years following a cerebrovascular accident (Morris et al., 1993).

Dementia

Whereas major depression has been documented in 17–31% of patients with dementia, clinically significant depressive symptoms occur in 50% of patients with dementia (Wragg and Jeste, 1989; Alexopoulos et al., 1991). The prevalence rates for depression in Alzheimer's disease (17–29%) and vascular dementia (19–27%) are about equal (Reifler et al., 1986; Fisher et al., 1990).

Patients with dementia who develop concurrent depression tend to have a genetic vulnerability to depression. The depression is often characterized by self-pity, rejection sensitivity, and anhedonia. However, the classic neurovegetative signs of depression are often less apparent (McGuire and Rabins, 1994). On occasion, elderly patients develop a depressed mood as a prodrome to dementia. In fact, a depressed mood has been associated with a subsequent threefold increase in dementia risk (Devanand et al., 1996).

Parkinson's Disease

After Alzheimer's disease, Parkinson's disease is the most common neurodegenerative disorder of advancing age. Unrecognized early symptoms of the disorder affect as many as 10% of those over 60 years of age (Young, 1999). The hallmark physical signs include the clinical triad of tremor, rigidity, and bradykinesia. In addition, cognitive (dementia) and mood (depression) symptoms are pervasive. Estimates of the prevalence of depression in Parkinson's disease range from 32% in population-based studies to 51% in hospital-based studies (Zesiewicz et al., 1999; Cummings, 1992). The depressive symptoms often precede the onset of motor signs. They are considered to be an expression of neuropathological changes rather than an emotional response to the disorder and are directly related to the degenerative changes in the basal ganglia. The depression of Parkinson's disease is characterized by less self-blame and guilt but more dysphoria, anxiety, and suicidal ideation (Zesiewicz et al., 1999).

Chronic Pain

About 43% of patients experiencing chronic pain suffer from depression (Katon et al., 1985). The wide variability in estimates of major depressive disorder in samples of patients with chronic back pain range from 16% to as high as 73% (Gallagher et al., 1995). Rates of depression in community populations of people with chronic pain are lower than those in clinical samples. Fishbain et al. observed that 16 of 28 general chronic pain patients visiting a pain clinic met the DSM-III criteria for major depression (Fishbain et al., 1986). Breslau et al., in a large-scale epidemiological survey, established that the lifetime prevalence of major depression was approximately three times higher in persons with migraine and other severe headaches than in control subjects (Breslau et al., 2000). Patients with chronic pain syndromes and concurrent depression are at greater risk for the development of prescription opioid dependence. Furthermore, denial of depression and masking of symptoms with benzodiazepines and opioid analgesics may obscure the diagnosis of depression (Bouckoms, 1996). Chronic pain has been identified as a risk factor for suicide (Breibart, 1993). Not surprisingly, in conditions as varied as migraine, diabetic neuropathy, and fibromyalgia, antidepressants have an established role in the alleviation of both pain and associated depressive symptoms. Despite the fact that much of the literature cited above concerns depression and chronic pain throughout the life cycle, it is particularly applicable to the elderly, who bear a disproportionate burden of physical suffering and pain.

ANTECEDENTS OF DEPRESSION IN LATE LIFE

Psychosocial Risk Factors

Advancing age by itself does not appear to be a risk factor for depression. The age-related effects on depression appear to be attributable to deteriorating physical health and subsequent disability (Roberts et al., 1997) (Table 3). Not infrequently, deteriorating health leads to placement in a long-term-care facility. This transition brings additional burdens: separation from one's home, family, and social support network. One study identified symptoms of depression in 12% of residents in long-term-care facilities (Parmelee et al., 1989). An additional 30%

TABLE 3 Prevalence of Depression in Patients with Selected Medical Conditions Common in the Elderly

Medical illness	Prevalence (%)
Cancer	6–50
Congestive heart failure	36.5
Coronary artery disease	8–44
Diabetes	11
End-stage renal disease	5
Multiple sclerosis	54
Myocardial infarction	15–20
Parkinson's disease	10–32
Rheumatoid arthritis	12.5
Stroke	25–50

Source: Adapted from McDaniel, 2000.

of nursing home residents experienced less severe but clinically significant depressive symptoms.

Throughout the life span, depression is two times more common in women. Because women outlive men, they are more likely to assume the role of caregiver (Fig. 3). In fact two-thirds of all caregivers are women (AMA Council of Scientific Affairs, 1993). Caregivers frequently feel unsupported, have health problems, and experience a high rate of depression (Eastwood et al., 1996). The prevalence of depression in women caregivers of demented elderly people reaches 45–47% (Livingston et al., 1996). In addition to the added risk of female gender, older individuals who have less education, are unmarried, whose health is deteriorating, and who are experiencing financial difficulties, negative life events, social isolation, as well as inadequate social support have an increased risk of depression (Kaplan et al., 1987). Psychosocial antecedents of depression include life events, chronic stress, and daily hassles. Older people do not experience stressful life events any more frequently than younger persons (Hughes et al., 1993). However, the types of events and of life's burdens vary with age. The elderly experience a disproportionate burden of stress from such transitions or events as retirement, the sudden onset of a physical illness, or the death of a spouse. The prevalence of clinical depression following spousal bereavement, for example, is as high as 50% (Reynolds et al., 1999; Zisook et al., 1994). Across the life cycle, impaired social support networks have been implicated in the etiology of depression (Landerman et al., 1989). In one study, women of all ages but not older men were protected against the impact of adverse life events by adequate social support (George et al., 1989). Men generally have fewer friends and are thought to have fewer available social supports (Blazer, 1999).

Sleep and Changes in Circadian Rhythm

Intractable chronic insomnia that lasts more than 12 consecutive months is associated with a 40-fold greater risk of developing a new episode of major depression (Ford and Kamerow, 1989). In comparison to young adults, older individuals take a longer time to fall asleep, awaken more frequently, and have more difficulty returning to sleep after awakening (Prinz et al., 1990; Vieth and Raskin, 1988). The use of hypnotic medications increases with age. Older women use more of these medications than older men (Morgan, 1987). Although the elderly comprise only 12% of the population of the United States, they receive 40% of all prescriptions for hypnotic drugs (Morgan, 1987). Some 14% of the elderly consume hypnotic drugs daily. The death rate among people who often use these drugs is 1.5 higher than among age-matched individuals who have never used them. Elevated autonomic arousal (Zepelin and McDonald, 1987) and greater susceptibility to external stimuli (Zepelin et al., 1984) may also predispose the older person to disturbed sleep. Finally sleep-related breathing disturbance, (snoring, obstructive sleep apnea), and periodic movements of sleep are more common in the elderly (Bliwise, 1994). Excessive daytime sleepiness in the elderly is commonly associated with sleep-related respiratory disturbances and depression (Pack et al., 1997).

Vascular Depression

There is now substantial evidence to suggest that cerebrovascular disease is a factor in the pathogenesis of late-life depression (Nebes et al., 2002). Individuals who develop depression for the first time in old age display a disproportionate number of subcortical hyperintensity lesions on T2-weighted magnetic resonance imaging (MRI) of the brain when compared to their age-matched counterparts without evidence of clinical depression (Krishnan et al., 1988; Coffey et al., 1989; Alexopoulos et al., 1997). The white matter microvascular lesions are commonly associated with cardiac risk factors such as hypertension, dyslipidemia, diabetes, and obesity. The presence of these lesions correlates clinically with cognitive dysfunction (Reifler et al., 1982; Emery and Oxman, 1992), deficits in executive function, (Alexopoulos et al., 2002), and a poor response to antidepressant medications (Coffey et al., 1989; Reifler et al., 1982). In fact, between 18 and 57% of the elderly with "vascular depression" may complain of memory loss. Longitudinal increases in the volume of white matter hyperintensities correlate with persistence of depression and a progressive decline in executive function (Nebes et al., 2002).

NATURAL HISTORY

The Longitudinal Course: Relapse and Recurrence

Depression is now recognized as a characteristically recurrent disorder. The rate of recurrence varies with the number of previous episodes and age. The patient who has experienced one episode has a 50% risk of having a second episode (Grady et al., 1997). Following a second episode, the risk rises to 75%. With a third episode, the risk of having a fourth episode rises to 90% (NIMH Consensus Development Conference Statement, 1985). Some studies demonstrate a worsening of the depressed patient's prognosis with advancing age. Although there is some controversy in this area, elderly depressed patients appear to be more prone to relapse, recurrence, and persistence of symptoms (Judd et al., 1998; Cole et al., 1999; Beekman et al., 2002). While a first episode at the age of 30 is associated with a 50% risk of recurrence, an episode at the age of 40 is associated with a 75% risk of recurrence. At the age of 50 years, the risk of having another episode is as high as 90% (Alexopoulos, 1989). In addition to the experience of a recurrence, persistent depression is more common in the elderly (Lebowitz et al., 1997). In a 6-year follow-up study of an elderly population, almost 60% of the cohort was depressed more than 60% of the time. Only 23% of the patients had true remissions, while 12% had remissions with recurrences; 32% had a chronic remitting course and 32% experienced chronic depression (Beekman et al., 2002). In a metanalysis of available studies, 50% of older patients displayed chronic depressive symptoms at follow-up (Cole et al., 1999). The clinical implication of this trend is that the elderly depressed frequently require lifelong antidepressant maintenance treatment (Lebowitz et al., 1997).

There is a growing consensus that cardiovascular disease contributes to the evolution of depressive symptoms. In the Cardiovascular Health Study (Steffens et al., 2002), 3236 patients were evaluated and followed for 7 years, providing an opportunity to examine the relationship between vascular pathology of the brain seen on neuroimaging and changes in depressive symptoms over time. The presence of small basal ganglial lesions and large cerebral cortical white matter lesions was associated with persistence of depression. Conversely, the presence of subcortical white matter lesions was associated with worsening of depression.

Characteristic Clinical Features of Depression in Late Life

The diagnosis of depression in late life is often elusive. This is true because neither the victim nor the health care professional may recognize the symptoms of depression in the context of multiple and complex physical problems (Lebowitz et al., 1997). The clinical presentation of late-life depression resembles that of depression experienced earlier in the life cycle, with some significant differences. *First*, a depressed mood is often less apparent than other classic depressive symptoms: anorexia, insomnia, anergia, loss of interest, and anhedonia. *Second*, insomnia is a more common complaint. Awakening in the middle of the night is more common than difficulty falling asleep. This may be related to a phase advance of circadian rhythms reported even among nondepressed older individuals (Bliwise, 1994). *Third*, the clinical cluster of anorexia and weight loss, a loss of interest, and psychotic features are more commonly observed in the depressed elderly (Blazer, 1994; Folks and Ford, 2002). Psychotic symptoms are present in 3.6% of elderly depressives in the community (Alexopoulos, 1996). Delusions of physical illness and feelings of guilt are the commonest psychotic symptoms encountered in the depressed elderly. *Fourth*, the depressed elderly more often experience cognitive deficits. Between 18 and 57% may present with cognitive impairment, which in many cases responds to antidepressant treatment. *Finally*, executive dysfunction is more commonly observed in late-onset depression (Lockwood et al., 2002). When compared to a group of younger depressed individuals, the elderly cohort demonstrates psychomotor slowing and performs poorly on tasks requiring set shifting, problem solving, and initiation of novel responses. This has recently been described (Alexopoulos et al., 2002) as the "depression–executive dysfunction (DED) syndrome" and is also characterized by reduced fluency, impaired visual learning, psychomotor retardation, and loss of interest. However, the classic neurovegetative depressive symptoms are generally mild.

Cost of Depression

There is now exhaustive evidence that patients with depression in a primary care setting utilize more general medical services than patients without the diagnosis of depression. The direct cost of depression treatment represents only a small portion of the cost burden. The computerized medical record system of a large-staff model health maintenance organization (HMO) was used to identify a cohort of 6257 patients with the diagnosis of depression (Simon et al., 1995). The authors compared the cost accrued by this group to a sample of 6257 primary care patients without depression managed in the same system of care. The patients with the diagnosis of depression accrued higher annual health care costs for every examined category of care (Fig. 7). Patients with diabetes and concurrent depression make more ambulatory care visits and incur significantly higher (fivefold) total health care costs than their nondepressed counterparts (Egede et al., 2002).

The studies cited above (Simon et al., 1995; Egede et al., 2002) are representative of the general population and cut across the life cycle. However, considering that older persons have a disproportionate burden of physical illness, the cost of concurrent depression in the elderly is also disproportionately high.

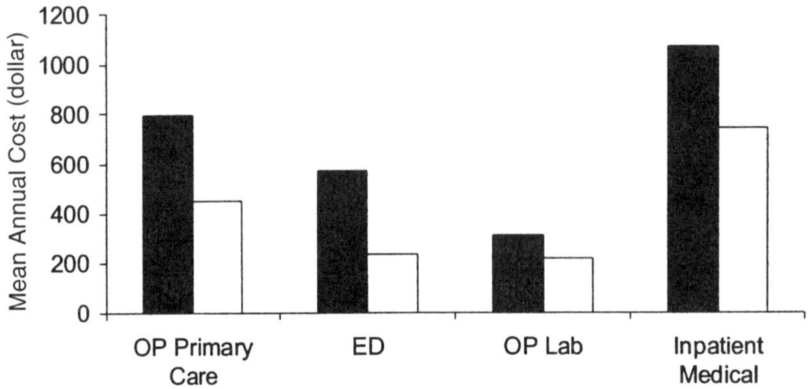

FIGURE 7 The influence of depression on the cost of medical care (n = 12,514). (From Simon et al., 1995.)

Unutzer et al. examined the costs of medical care in a cohort of 2558 elderly patients in a large-staff model HMO during a period of 4 years. The authors used the Center for Epidemiological Studies Depression (CES-D) scale as a measure of depressive symptoms (Unutzer et al., 1997). The patients with depressive symptoms made greater use of services in all categories of medical care: inpatient admissions, outpatient visits, laboratory tests, emergency department visits, number of prescriptions, number of ancillary visits, and number of optometry visits. Their total health care costs were 50% higher than the costs of those without depressive symptoms. The cost increase could not be explained by the differential use of specialty mental health services, which accounted for only 1% of general medical services. Yet another group (Callahan et al., 1994) examined the cost of medical care for 1711 older patients in an inner-city primary care clinic for 9 months. Patients with CES-D scores of 16 or greater made 38% more outpatient visits and incurred 61% greater outpatient charges. Elderly community residents with depressive symptoms tend to overutilize general medical services but not specialty mental health services (Ganguli et al., 1995). Older patients may be more sensitive to the stigma of mental illness, may request services less, may have less access to services, and may refuse a referral to a mental health specialist more often than younger patients (Unutzer et al., 1997). Unfortunately, primary care providers may be less likely to recognize and treat depression (Banazak, 1996).

Undertreatment of Depression in the Elderly

The recognition of depression in the elderly is hindered by the common co-occurrence of physical illness in this population. The average older person may suffer from as many as six concurrent different ICD-9 medical disorders. As a result, the depressed elderly are far more likely to present in the general medical setting rather than a mental health setting (Koenig et al., 1997). The overlap of physical and depressive symptoms commonly obscures the diagnosis of depression. Nonpsychiatric physicians may attribute recognized depressive symptoms such as fatigue and anorexia to the medical disorder and miss the opportunity for intervention with antidepressants. It is estimated that only one-half of those with major depression receive treatment for depression even after their nonpsychiatrist physicians are alerted to the diagnosis (Rapp et al., 1991). Fewer than 20% of depressed elders in the community and primary care populations are detected or adequately treated (Cole and Yaffe, 1996). And even when these patients are recognized and treated, the therapeutic interventions are too often inadequate. More than half of depressed patients who received treatment remained depressed after 1 year (Katon et al., 1995). Factors leading to treatment failure include inadequate instructions to patients concerning the disorder and the antidepressants, subtherapeutic doses of antidepressants, and inadequate length to treatment (Hirschfield et al., 1997). In a primary care setting, more than one-third of patients failed to refill their initial prescription (Lin et al., 2000), and nearly half stopped their antidepressants within 3 months (Lin et al., 1995). The consequences of underrecognition and inadequate treatment include excess morbidity from physical illness, premature mortality, and suicide (Lebowitz et al., 1997).

Increased Mortality Associated with Depression

Depression is associated with excess mortality (Rovner et al., 1991; Fredman et al., 1999; Zubenko et al., 1997). Zubenko et al. followed a cohort of 809 elderly patients for 5.75 years to evaluate the impact of common late-life mental disorders on life expectancy. The standard mortality ratio for the patients with mood disorders was 1.5 Saz et al. followed 1080 elderly patients for 4.5 years (Saz et al., 2002). The presence of depression was associated with a threefold increase in mortality. As anticipated, the presence of psychotic symptoms increased the risk of death almost fourfold. Surprisingly even dysthymia was associated with increased mortality (Fig. 8). These findings are consistent with numerous other studies (Rovner et al., 1991), which report an association between depression in the elderly and excess mortality.

Suicide

The suicide rate increases disproportionately with advancing age, with much of the increase accounted for by the high rate among white males. The old comprised 12.7% of the population of the United States in 1999 but committed 18.8% of the suicides. The young comprised 13.9% of the population and committed 13.4% of the suicides (Hoyert et al., 1999). The old old (over age 85)

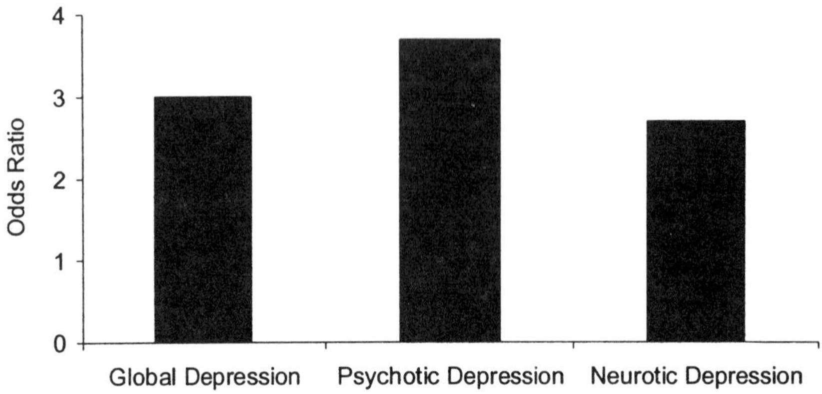

FIGURE 8 The influence of psychiatric illness on mortality rates in the elderly (Zaragoza, Spain, 1999). (From Saz et al., 1999.)

had the highest suicide rate of all age groups: 19.2 suicide deaths per 100,000 population. White men have a dramatically higher suicide rate than white women, black men, and black women (Fig. 9). White men over age 85 had a suicide rate of 65 per 100,000. This was six times greater than the overall national average (Cronwell, 1994). The elderly tend to make fewer suicide attempts and are more often successful. They tend to use more lethal means, such as firearms (Fig. 10). Many older adults who have committed suicide visited a primary care physician very close to the time of the suicide: 20% visited their family doctor on the day of suicide, 40% within 1 week, and 70% within 1 month of the suicide (Miller, 1976; Conwell et al., 2000). Conwell et al. compared a group of 42 suicides aged 60 and older who visited a primary care provider within 30 days of death and 196 age-matched patients from a primary care group practice. As expected, the presence of depressive illness was a common antecedent to suicide. Additionally, the completed suicides had substantially greater burdens of physical illness and corresponding functional limitations than the control subjects (Conwell et al., 2000).

CONCLUSIONS

Unless adequately recognized and treated, as the population ages, late-life depression is likely to achieve catastrophic importance, tarnishing the "golden years" for many older adults. Recognition can be improved in several ways: by acknowledging that depression in later life manifests itself differently from

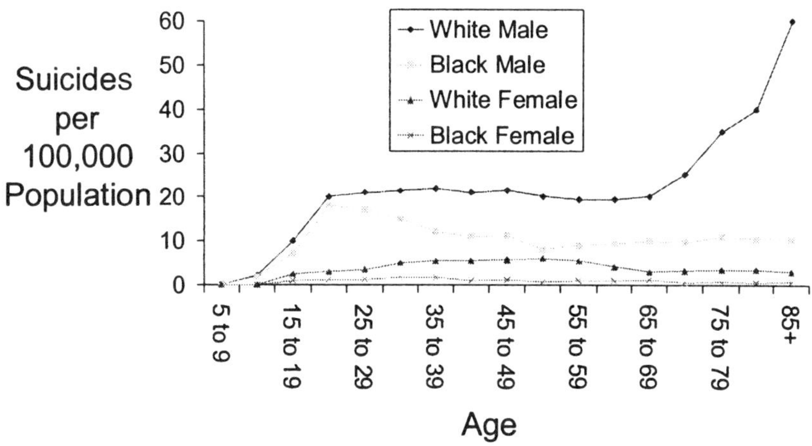

FIGURE 9 U.S. suicide rate, 1999. (From Centers for Disease Control and Prevention, 2002.)

depression in younger adults, by increasing patient awareness of the importance of depressive states, and by helping primary care clinicians to make the distinction between depression and the normal process of aging or the pathological symptoms associated with medical illnesses. Furthermore, the threshold for treatment must be lowered. Physicians have tended to withhold the use of anti-

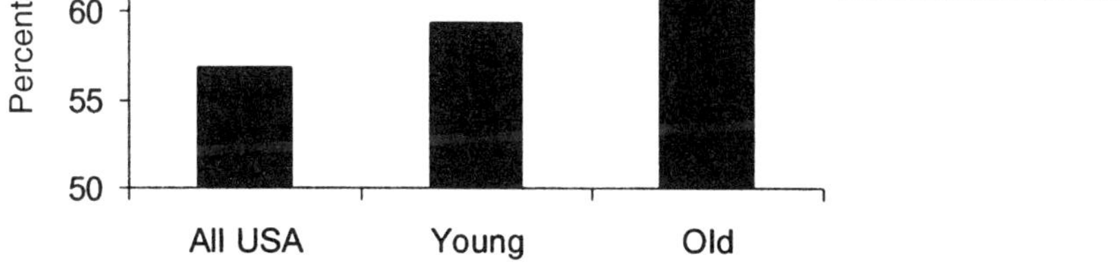

FIGURE 10 Percentage of U.S. suicides committed with firearms. (From Hoyert et al., 1999.)

depressants to all but the most profoundly depressed individuals. It is now apparent that subsyndromal, dysthymic, and minor depression (DSM-IV) are highly prevalent among the elderly and are accompanied by substantial disability, physical morbidity, and excess mortality (Lyness, 1999). Until recently, there has been limited evidence to recommend pharmacotherapy for either minor depression or dysthymia. However , there is increasing evidence that appropriate treatment can produce improvement in patients with minor depression (Williams et al., 2000; and see Chap. 9 in this book).

ACKNOWLEDGMENT

The author would like to thank Dr. Christopher Colenda, Chairman, Department of Psychiatry, Michigan State University, for his invaluable review of the manuscript, suggestions, and critical comments.

REFERENCES

Alexopoulos GS. Affective disorders. In: Sadavoy J, Lazarus LW, Jarvik JF, Grossberg GT, eds. Comprehensive Review of Geriatric Psychiatry—II. 2nd ed. Washington, DC: American Psychiatric Press, 1996a.

Alexopoulos GS. Geriatric Depression in Primary Care. Int J Geriatr Psychiatry 1996: 11:397–400.

Alexopoulos GS, Abrams RC. Depression in Alzheimer's disease. Psychiatr Clin North Am 1991; 14(2):327–340.

Alexopoulos GS, Kiosses DN, Klimstra S, Kalayam B, Bruce ML. Clinical presentation of the depression—"executive dysfunction syndrome" of late life. Am J Geriatr Psychiatry 2002; 10:98–106.

Alexopoulos GS, Meyers BS, Young RC, Campbell S, Silbersweig D, Charlson M. "Vascular depression" hypothesis. Arch Gen Psychiatry 1997; 54:915–922.

Alexopoulos GS, Young RC, Abrams RC, Myers B, Shamoian CA. Chronicity and relapse in geriatric depression. Biol Psychiatry 1989; 26:551–564.

AMA Council on Scientific Affairs. Physicians and family caregivers: a model for partnership. JAMA 1993; 269:1282–1284.

Astrom M, Adolfson R, Asplund K. Major depression in stroke patients: A three-year longitudinal study. Stroke 1993; 24:976–982.

Banazak DA. Late-life depression in primary care. J Gen Intern Med 1996; 11:163–167.

Barrett JE, Barrett JA, Oxman TE, Gerber PD. The prevalence of psychiatric disorders in a primary care practice. Arch Gen Psychiatry 1988; 45:1100–1106.

Beekman ATF, Geerlings SW, Deeg DJH, Smit JH, Schoevers RS, de Beurs E, Braam AW, Penninx BWJH, van Tilburg W. The natural history of late-life depression: a 6-year prospective study in the community. Arch Gen Psychiatry 2002; 59:605–611.

Blazer D. Geriatric Psychiatry. In: Hales RE, Yudofsky SC, Talbott JA, eds. The American Psychiatric Press Textbook of Psychiatry, 2nd ed. Washington, DC: American Psychiatric Press, 1994, pp 1405–1421.

Blazer D. Depression and the older man. Med Clin North Am 1999; 83:1305–1316.

Blazer DG II. Epidemiology of late-life depression. In: Schneider LS, Reynolds CF III, Lebowitz BD, et al, eds. Diagnosis and Treatment of Depression in Late Life: Results of the NIH Consensus Development Conference. Washington, DC: American Psychiatric Press, 1994, pp 9–19.

Blazer D, Williams CD. The epidemiology of dysphoria and depression in an elderly population. Am J Psychiatry 1980; 137:439–444.

Bliwise DL. Normal aging. In: Kryger MH, Roth T, Dement WC, eds. Principles and Practice of Sleep Medicine, 2nd ed. Philadelphia: Saunders, 1994, pp 26–39.

Blumenthal JS, Williams RS, Wallace AG, et al. Physiologic and psychologic variables predict compliance to prescribed exercise therapy in patients recovering from myocardial infarction. Psychosom Med 1982; 44:519–527.

Bouckoms AJ. Chronic pain: neuropsychopharmacology and adjunctive psychiatric treatment. In: Rundell JR, Wise MG, eds. Textbook of Consultation Liaison Psychiatry. Washington, DC: American Psychiatric Press, 1996, pp 1006–1037.

Breibart W. Suicide risk and pain in cancer and AIDS patients. In: Chapman CR, Foley KM, eds. Current and Emerging Issues in Cancer Pain: Research and Practice. New York: Raven Press, 1993, pp 49–66.

Breslau N, Schultz LR, Stewart WF, Lipton RB, Lucia VC, Welch KMA. Headache and major depression: is the association specific to migraine? Neurology 2000; 54:308–313.

Butters MA. Changes in cognitive functioning following treatment of late-life depression. Am J Psychiatry 2000; 157(12):1949–1954.

Centers for Disease Control and Prevention. April 26, 2002.

Coffey CE, Figiel FS, Djang WT, Saunders WB, Weiner RD. White matter hyperintensity on MRI clinical and neuroanatomic correlates in the depressed elderly. J Neuropsychiatry Clin Neurosci 1989; 1:135–144.

Cole MG, Bellavance F, Mansour A. Prognosis of depression in elderly community and primary care populations: a systematic review and meta-analysis. Am J Psychiatry 1999; 156:1182–1189.

Cole MG, Yaffe MJ. Pathway to psychiatric care of the elderly with depression. Int J Geriatr Psychiatry 1996; 11:157–161.

Colenda CC, Schneider LS, Katz IR, Alexopoulos GS, Reynolds CF. Late-life depression. In: Levenson JL, ed. Depression. Philadelphia: American College of Physicians, 2000, pp 169–200.

Conwell Y, Lyness JM, Duberstein P, Cox C, Seidlitz L, DiGiorgio A, Caine ED. Completed suicide among older patients in primary care practices: a controlled study. J Am Geriatr Soc 2000; 48:23–31.

Conwell Y. Suicide in elderly patients. In: Schneider LS, Reynolds CF III, Lebowitz BD, Friedhoff AJ, eds. Diagnosis and Management of Depression in Late Life. Washington, DC: American Psychiatric Press, 1994, pp 397–418.

Cummings JL. Depression and Parkinson's disease: a review. Am J Psychiatry 1992; 149:443–454.

Cydulka RK, Meldon SW, Emerman CL, Moffa DA, et al. Utility of clinical characteristics in identifying depression in geriatric ED patients. Am J Emerg Med 1999; 17: 522–525.

Devanand DP, Sano M, Tang MX, et al. Depressed mood and the incidence of Alzheimer's disease in the elderly living in the community. Arch Gen Psychiatry 1996; 53:175–182.

Eastwood R, Herrmann H, Singh B, Bloch S, Schofield H. Australia: survey of caregiving. Lancet 1996; 347(8998):402.

Egede LE, Zheng D, Simpson K. Comorbid depression is associated with increased health care use and expenditures in individuals with diabetes. Diabetes Care 2002; 25:464–470.

Emery VO, Oxman TE. Update on the dementia spectrum of depression. Am J Psychiatry 1992; 149:305–317.

Fabacher DA, Raccio-Robak N, McErlean MA, Milano PM, Verdile VP. Validation of a brief screening tool to detect depression in elderly ED patients. Am J Emerg Med 2002; 20:99–102.

Federoff JP, Spencer WC, Rabins PV, et al. Are depressive symptoms nonspecific in patients with acute stroke? Am J Psychiatry 1991; 148:1172–1176.

Folks DG, Ford CV. Clinical features of depression and Dysthymia. In: Copeland JRM, Abou-Saleh MT, Blazer DG, eds. Principles and Practice of Geriatric Psychiatry, 2nd ed. New York: Wiley, 2002, pp 407–412.

Ford DE, Kamerow DB. Epidemiological study of sleep disturbances and psychiatric disorders: an opportunity for prevention? JAMA 1989; 262:1479–1484.

Fishbain DA, Goldberg M, Meagher BR, et al. Male and female chronic pain patients categorized by DSM-III psychiatric criteria. Pain 1986; 26:181–197.

Fisher R, Simamyi M, Danielczyk W. Depression in dementia of the Alzheimer type and multi-infarct dementia. Am J Psychiatry 1990; 147:1484–1487.

Frasure-Smith N, Lesperance F, Talajic M. Depression following myocardial infarction: impact on six-month survival. JAMA 1993; 270:1819–1825.

Fredman L, Magaziner J, Hebel JR, et al. Depressive symptoms and 6-year mortality among elderly community-dwelling women. Epidemiology 1999; 10:54–59.

Fulop G, Strain JJ, Vita J, et al. Impact of psychiatric comorbidity on length of hospital stay for medical/surgical patients: a preliminary report. Am J Psychiatry 1987; 144:878–882.

Gallagher RM, Moore P, Chernoff I. The reliability of depression diagnosis in chronic low back pain: a pilot study. Gen Hosp Psychiatry 1995; 17:399–413.

Ganguli M, Gilby J Seaberg E, et al. Depressive symptoms and associated factors in a rural elderly population: the MoVIES project. Am J Geriatr Psychiatry 1995; 3:144–160.

German PS, Shapiro S, Skinner EA. Mental health of the elderly: use of health and mental health services. J Am Geriatr Soc 1985; 33:246–252.

George LK, Blazer DG, Hughes DC, et al. Social support and the outcome of major depression. Br J Psychiatry 1989; 154:478–485.

Glassman AH, Shapiro PA. Depression and the course of coronary artery disease. Am J Psychiatry 1998; 155:4–11.

Grady TA, Sederer LI, Rothschild AJ. Depression. In: Sederer LI, Rothschild AJ, eds. Acute Care Psychiatry: Diagnosis and Treatment. Baltimore: Williams & Wilkins, 1997, pp 83–121.

Hasin D, Link B. Age and recognition of depression: implication for a cohort effect in major depression. Psychol Med 1988; 18:683–688.

Hirschfield RMA, Keller MB, Panico S, et al. The National Depressive and manic-depressive association consensus statement on the undertreatment of depression. JAMA 1997; 277:333–340.

Hoyert DL, Arias E, Smith BL, Murphy SL, Kochaneck KD. Deaths: Final Data for 1999. National Vital Statistics Report, 49(8). DHHS Publication No. (PHS) 2001-1120. Hyattsville, MD: National Center for Health Statistics, 1999.

Hughes DC, DeMallie D, Blazer DG. Does age make a difference in the effects of physical health and social support on the outcome of a major depressive episode? Am J Psychiatry 1993; 150:72.

Judd LL, Akiskal HS, Maser JD, Zeller PJ, Endicott J, Coryell W, Paulus MP, Kunovac JL, Leon AC, Mueller TI, Rice JA, Keller MB. A prospective 12-year study of subsyndromal and syndromal depressive symptoms in unipolar major depressive disorders. Arch Gen Psychiatry 1998; 55:694–700.

Katon W, Egan K, Miller D. Chronic pain: lifetime psychiatric diagnoses, and family history. Am J Psychiatry 1985; 142:1156–1160.

Katon W, Schulberg H. Epidemiology of depression in primary care. Gen Hosp Psychiatry 1992; 14:237–247.

Katon W, von Korff M, Lin E, et al. Collaborative management to achieve treatment guidelines: impact on depression in primary care. JAMA 1995; 273:1026–1031.

Klerman GL, Lavori PW, Rice J, et al. Birth-cohort trends and rates of major depressive disorders among relatives of patients with affective disorder. Arch Gen Psychiatry 1985; 42:689–695.

Knauper B, Wittchen H. Diagnosing major depression in the elderly: evidence for response bias in Standardized diagnostic interviews. J Psychiatr Res 1994; 28:147–164.

Koenig HG, Blazer DG. Epidemiology of geriatric affective disorders. Clin Geriatr Med 1992; 8(2):235–251.

Koenig HG, George LK, Meador KG. Use of antidepressants by nonpsychiatrists in the treatment of medically ill hospitalized depressed elderly patients. Am J Psychiatry 1997a; 154:1369–1375.

Koenig HG, George LK, Peterson BL, Pieper CF. Depression in medically ill hospitalized older adults: prevalence, characteristics, and course of symptoms according to six diagnostic schemes. Am J Psychiatry 1997b; 154:1376–1383.

Koenig HG, Goli V, Shelp F, Kudler HS, Cohen HJ, Blazer DG. Major depression in hospitalized medically ill men. Int J Geriatr Psychiatry 1992; 7:25–34.

Krishnan KRR, Hays JC, Tupler LA, George LK, Blazer DG. Clinical and phenomenological comparisons of late-onset and early onset depression. Am J Psychiatry 1995; 152:785–788.

Krishnan KRR, Goli V, Ellinwood EH, France RD, Blazer DZ, Nemeroff CB. Leucoencephalopathy in patients diagnosed as major depression. Biol Psychiatry 1988; 23:519–522.

Landerman R, George L, Campbell R, et al. Alternative models of the stress buffering hypothesis. Am J Commun Psychol 1989; 17:625–642.

Lebowitz BD, Pearson JL, Schneider LS, Reynolds CF, Alexopoulos GS, Livingston M, Conwell Y, Katz IR, Meyers BS, Morrison MF, Mossey J, Niederehe G, Parmelee P. Diagnosis and treatment of depression in late life: consensus statement update. JAMA 1997; 278:1186–1190.

Lin EH, Katon WJ, Simon GE, et al. Low-intensity treatment of depression in primary care: is it problematic? Gen Hosp Psychiatry 2000; 22:78–83.
Lin E. The role of the primary care physician in patients' adherence to antidepressant therapy. Med Care 1995; 33:67–74.
Livingston G, Manela M, Katona C. Depression and other psychiatric morbidity in carers of elderly people living at home. Br Med J 1996; 312(7024):153–156.
Lockwood KA, Alexopoulos GS, Van Gorp WG. Executive dysfunction in geriatric depression. Am J Psychiatry 2002; 159:1119–1126.
Lyness JM. The importance of subsyndromal depression in older primary care patients: prevalence and associated functional disability. J Am Geriatr Soc 1999; 47:647–652.
Massie MJ, Holland JC. Depression in the cancer patient. J Clin Psychiatry 1990; 51(S7): 12–17.
Meldon SW, Emerman CL, Schubert DS. Recognition of depression in geriatric ED patients by emergency physicians. Ann Emerg Med 1997; 30:442–447.
McDaniel JS. Depression, medical illness, and health care. In: Levenson JL, ed. Depression. Philadelphia: American College of Physicians, 2000, pp 1–21.
McDaniel JS, Musselman DL, Porter MR, et al. Depression in patients with cancer: diagnosis, biology, and treatment. Arch Gen Psychiatry 1995; 52:89–99.
McGuire MH, Rabins. Mood disorders. In: Coffey CE, Cummings JL, eds.Textbook of Geriatric Neuropsychiatry. Washington DC: American Psychiatric Press, 1994, pp 246–260.
Miller M. Geriatric suicide: the Arizona study. Gerontologist 1976; 18:488–495.
Morgan K. Sleep and Aging: A Research-Based Guide to Sleep in Later Life. Baltimore: Johns Hopkins University Press, 1987.
Morris PL, Robinson RG, Andrzejewski P, et al. Association of depression with 10 year post-stroke mortality. Am J Psychiatry 1993; 150:124–129.
Murray CJL, Lopez AD. The Global Burden of Disease. Geneva: World Health Organization, 1996.
Musselman DL, Evans DL, Nemeroff CB. The relationship of depression to cardiovascular disease: epidemiology, biology, and treatment. Arch Gen Psychiatry 1998; 55:580–592.
Myers JK, Weissman MM, Tischler GL, Holzer CE, Leaf PJ, Orvaschel H, Anthony JC, Boyd JH, Burke JD, Kramer M, Stoltzman R. Six-month prevalence of psychiatric disorders in three communities. Arch Gen Psychiatry 1984; 41:959–967.
Nebes RD, Reynolds CF, Boada F, Meltzer CC, Fukui MB, Saxton J, Halligan EM, DeKosky ST. Longitudinal increase in the volume of white matter hyperintensities in late-onset depression. Int J Geriatr Psychiatry 2002; 17:526–530.
NIMH Consensus Development Conference Statement. Mood disorders: pharmacologic prevention of recurrences. Am J Psychiatry 1985; 142:469–476.
Noyes R, Kathol RG. Depression and cancer. Psychiatr Dev 1986; 2:77–100.
Pack AI, Dinges DF, Gehrman PR, et al. Sleepiness in the elderly, role of sleep apnea. A case control report approach. Sleep Res 1997; 26:453.
Parmelee PA, Katz IR, Lawton MP. Depression among institutionalized aged: assessment and prevalence estimation. J Gerontol 1989; 44:M22–M29.
Penninx BWJH, Beekman ATF, Honig A, Deeg DJH, Schoevers RA, van Eijk JTM, van Tilburg W. Depression and cardiac mortality: results from a community-based longitudinal study. Arch Gen Psychiatry 2001; 58:221–227.

Prinz P, Vitiello M, Raskind M. Geriatrics: sleep disorders and aging. N Eng J Med 1990; 323:520–526.
Rabins PV. Barriers to diagnosis and treatment of depression in elderly patients. Am J Geriatr Psychiatry 1996; 4(suppl 1):S79–S83.
Rapp SR, Parisi SA, Wallace CE. Comorbid psychiatric disorders in elderly medical patients. J Am Geriatr Soc 1991; 39:124–131.
Reifler BV, Larson E, Hanley R. Coexistence of cognitive impairment and depression in geriatric patients. Am J Psychiatry 1982; 139:623–626.
Reifler BV, Larson E, Teri L, Poulsen M. Dementia of the Alzheimer's type and depression. J Am Geriatr Soc 1986; 34:855–859.
Reynolds CF, Miller MD, Pasternak RE, et al. Treatment of bereavement-related major depressive episodes in late life: a controlled study of acute and continuation treatment with nortriptyline and psychotherapy. Am J Psychiatry 1999; 156:202–208.
Roberts RE, Kaplan GA, Shema SJ, Strawbridge WJ. Does growing old increase the risk for depression? Am J Psychiatry 1997; 154:1384–1390.
Robinson RG, Starr LB, Kubos KL, et al. A two-year longitudinal study of poststroke mood disorders: findings during the initial evaluation. 1983; 14:736–744.
Robinson RG, Bolduc P, Price TR. A two-year longitudinal study of poststroke depression: diagnosis and outcome at one and two-year follow-up. Stroke 1987; 18: 837–843.
Rovner BW, German PS, Brant IJ, et al. Depression and mortality in nursing homes. JAMA 1991; 265:993–996.
Rovner BW, Kafonek S, Filipp L, Lucas MJ, Folstein MF. Prevalence of mental illness in a community nursing home. Am J Psychiatry 1986; 143:1446–1449.
Sano M, Stern Y, Williams JBW, Cote L, Rosenstein R, Mayeux R. Coexisting dementia and depression in Parkinson's disease. Arch Neurol 1989; 46:1284–1286.
Saravay SM, Lavin M. Psychiatric comorbidity and length of stay in the general hospital: a critical review of outcome studies. Psychosomatics 1994; 35:233–252.
Saz P, Launer LJ, Dia JL, De-La-Camara C, Marcos G, Lobo A. Mortality of Depression in the Elderly. Int J Geriatr Psychiatry 1999; 14(12):1031–1038.
Schneider J. 100 and counting. US News & World Report, June 3, 2002 p 86.
Select Committee on Aging, US House of Representatives. Exploding the Myths: Caregiving in America. Washington, DC: US Government Printing Office, 1987, p 60.
Shah A, Herbert R, Lewis S, et al. Screening for depression among acutely ill geriatric inpatients with a short geriatric depression scale. Age Aging 1997; 26:217–221.
Simon GE, VonKorff M, Barlow W. Health care costs of primary care patients with recognized depression. Arch Gen Psychiatry 1995; 52:850–856.
Smith DWE. Centenarians: human longevity outliers. Gerontologist 1997; 37:200–207.
Snowdon J. The prevalence of depression in old age (editorial). Int J Geriatr Psychiatry 1990; 5:141–144.
Steffens DC, Krishnan KR, Crump C, Burke GL. Cerebrovascular disease and evolution of depressive symptoms in the cardiovascular heatlh study. Stroke 2002; 33:1636–1644.
Steffens DC, Skoog I, Norton MC, et al. Prevalence of depression and its treatment in an elderly population: the Cache County study. Arch Gen Psychiatry 2000; 57: 601–607.

Surridge DHC, Williams-Erdahl DL, Lawson JS, et al. Psychiatric aspects of diabetes mellitus. Br J Psychiatry 1984; 145:269–276.

Tariot PN, Podgorski CA, Blazina L, Leibovici A. Mental disorders in the nursing home: another perspective. Am J Psychiatry 1993; 150:1063–1069.

Weissman MM, Bruce ML, Leaf PJ et al. Affective disorders In: Robins LN, Regier DA, eds. Psychiatric Disorders in America. New York, Free Press, 1991.

Weissman MM, Leaf PJ, Tischler GL et al. Affective disorders in five United States communities. Psychol Med 1988; 18(3):141–153.

Weissman MM, Leaf PJ, Holzer CE III et al: The epidemiology of depression: An update on sex differences in rates. J Affective Disord 1984; 7:179–188.

Wilcox SM, Himmelstein DU, Woolhandler S. Inappropriate drug prescribing for the community-dwelling elderly. JAMA 1994; 272:292–296.

Williams JW, Barrett J, Oxman T, Frank E, Katon W, Sullivan M, Cornell J, Sengupta A. Treatment of dysthymia and minor depression in primary care: a randomized controlled trial in older adults. JAMA 2000; 284:1519–1526.

Winokur G. The concept of secondary depression and its relationship to comorbidity. Psychiatr Clin North Am 1990; 123:567–583.

Wragg RE, Jeste DV. Overview of Depression and psychosis in Alzheimer's Disease. Am J Psychiatry 1989; 146:577–587.

Unutzer J, Patrick DL, Simon G, Grembowski D, Walker E, Rutter C, Katon W. Depressive symptoms and the cost of health services in HMO patients aged 65 and older. JAMA 1997; 277:1618–1623.

U.S. Census Bureau. *National Projections Program, Population Division*. Washington, DC: U.S. Census Bureau, 1996.

Veith R, Raskind M. The neurobiology of aging: does it predispose to depression? Neurobiol Aging 1988; 9:101–117.

Wragg RE, Jest DV. Overview of depression and psychosis in Alzheimer's disease. Am J Psychiatry 1989; 146(5):577–587.

Young R. Update on Parkinson's disease. J Am Acad Fam Physicians 1990; 59(8):2155–2170.

Zepelin H, McDonald CS. Age differences in autonomic variables during sleep. J Gerontol 1987; 42:142–146.

Zepelin H, McDonald CS, Zammit GK. Effects of age on auditory awakening thresholds. J Gerontol 1984; 39:294–300.

Zesiewicz TA, Gold M, Chari G, Hauser RA. Current issues in depression in Parkinson's disease. Am J Geriatr Psychiatry 1999; 7:110–118.

Zisook S, Shuchter SR, Sledge PA, et al. The spectrum of depressive phenomena after spousal bereavement. J Clin Psychiatry 1994; 55:29–36.

Zonderman AB, Costa PT. The absence of increased levels of depression in older adults: evidence from a national representative study. Scientific Abstracts of the Annual Meeting of the American Psychological Association, 1991.

Zubenko GS, Mulsant BH, Sweet RA, Pasternak RE, Tu XM. Mortality of elderly patients with psychiatric disorders. Am J Psychiatry 1997; 154:1360–1368.

2

Barriers to the Safe and Effective Treatment of Late-Life Depression

Helen H. Kyomen
McLean Hospital, Belmont, and Harvard Medical School, Boston, Massachusetts, U.S.A.

Gary L. Gottlieb
Harvard Medical School and Brigham and Women's Hospital, Boston, Massachusetts, U.S.A.

INTRODUCTION

Depressive illnesses, including major depression and subsyndromal depressive conditions, are common in the elderly. Major depression has been reported to occur in 1–3% of the general elderly population (1–8), and an additional 8–16% have clinically significant, subsyndromal depressive symptoms (5,6,9). In medically ill elderly and nursing home residents, the prevalance of significant subsyndromal depressive symptoms may be as high as 44% (10). One study following elderly patients longitudinally estimated the 9-month incidence rate of depressive symptoms to be 11–12% (11). Another study reported that the incidence of first-onset depression in the general elderly (age ≥ 65 years) population was 12 per 1000 person-years in men and 30 per 1000 person-years in women aged 70–85 (12).

Despite the substantial prevalence and incidence of depressive conditions in the elderly, no more than half with diagnosable depressive symptoms are reliably identified (13–15). Diagnosis is often complicated by comorbid medical illness, cognitive impairment, and adverse life events. Only about 35–40% of the elderly with identified depressive signs and symptoms receive appropriate treatment for these problems (16–17). These figures suggest that as many as 70–80% of elderly with a depressive illness or significant depressive symptoms are not receiving indicated intervention. In addition, among elderly persons treated for depression, compliance with treatment is frequently incomplete (18).

Taken together, these circumstances—common occurrence of depression among elderly persons, obscured identification of these depressive signs and symptoms, insufficient provision of indicated interventions for these depressive conditions, and inadequate compliance with treatment among treated patients—suggest that there are important operative barriers to care among elderly persons with depression. The identification of these barriers to care may be a useful early step in their attenuation.

This chapter discusses barriers to care for depression in the elderly. The salient barriers to care are multiform and related to patient, provider, organizational/financial, interventional, and societal issues. Suggestions for an action and research agenda to improve the care of elderly with depression closes the discussion.

PATIENT-RELATED BARRIERS TO CARE

Patient-related barriers to care range from emotional and physiological changes occurring in the elderly patient due to the depressive condition, through problems of exacerbation of co-occurring medical illnesses, to difficulties based in the psychosocial network, economic status, and ethnocultural background of the patient.

Depressive illness in elderly patients, just as in younger adults, can range from mild symptoms suggesting a subsyndromal state to a full-scale major depression with psychotic features. Available data indicate that older adults use considerably fewer than expected mental health services relative to the prevalence of depressive disorders (17,19). Many patients may have a gradual, insidious onset of the depressive illness that progressively impairs their ability to retain insight into their condition. In contrast to depression experienced by many younger adults, many elderly persons with depression do not endorse affective symptoms of sadness or dysphoria and may experience the illness differently from younger adults (20, 21). Thus, the elderly patient may not be able to detect the depressive illness–related changes that are occurring and may not recognize the need to seek evaluation for a consequential illness.

Those elderly who do recognize that affective symptoms are having a significant impact on their lives may not acknowledge that these symptoms may need to be assessed and treated by mental health professionals. If somatic concerns predominate, the affective symptoms may be experienced as stemming from physical illness, needing assessment by the family doctor. Indeed, this approach may be favored by many elderly patients, especially where there are concurrent medical conditions (22,23). Alternatively and very commonly, the depressive condition may be considered as something that patients can take care of on their own or that will go away with time (23).

Even when the depressive condition is recognized and the need for mental health evaluation is acknowledged, impaired motivation, confidence, and self-esteem and feelings of guilt heightened by the depressive illness may deter the patient from seeking help. The patient may feel hopeless and believe that no assistance is available, or, if sought, that the aid will be ineffective. The patient, due to thought disturbances from the depressive illness or lack of knowledge about the available health benefits, may feel that the financial resources or health insurance to pay for physician visits, medications, or other treatments are inadequate (24,25). The tasks of identifying appropriate sources of care and then going to get this assistance can feel overwhelming to an elderly person experiencing disabling depressive symptoms. Obtaining transportation to a treatment site may be perceived as eminently problematic, especially for elderly living in regions where mental health care services are limited (26).

Many elderly persons believe that there is a stigma associated with depression or other mental illnesses and that there is a negative connotation associated with having depression or needing to seek and receive ongoing treatment for it (27). These stigmatization issues, often linked with ageism, can become accentuated in the depressed state, to the extent that self-esteem plummets and feelings of guilt about having a mental illness or being "too old to be worth helping" supervene, further dissuading the patient from seeking treatment.

Isolation and inadequate social supports, common among the elderly, present additional obstacles to care (28). Isolated older adults are at risk of deteriorating emotionally and physically from a clinical depression. They may have such severe anhedonia and even anorexia that they do not buy food or ask others to help them with food shopping, resulting in inadequate food or fluid intake, which can lead to dehydration, metabolic derangement, and nutritional deficits (29). In turn, these conditions may result in confusion, weakness, and frailty, leading to diminished motivation and reduced ability to seek help.

Even if the patient manages to seek treatment, he or she may de-emphasize depressive symptoms because other problems, in particular somatic symptoms, are more easily discussed (30). Elderly patients often have limited knowledge of psychiatric techniques and treatments (31). In view of the questionable specificity of psychiatric treatment for depression in elderly patients (32), patient desire can significantly influence the provider's treatment plan and affect outcome adversely (33). When queried, few older adults with depressive symptoms discuss their complaints with their primary care providers, and the majority of these individuals refuse psychiatric referral when it is offered (34). Similarly, demand for rapid relief or treatment of perceived somatic or behavioral symptoms may obscure complete evaluation and compromise appropriate diagnostic assessment.

Even if an appropriate treatment plan to address the depressive condition is defined, there may be limited adherence to the recommended treatments. This lack of compliance may be due to a limited understanding of the need for acute and ongoing treatment or of medication directions (35,36), or it may be related to the patient's reluctance to follow through with recommendations due to depressive illness–related symptoms such as decreased motivation or nihilistic thinking. Suicidal ideation may develop (37), and suicide may increasingly be seen as a reasonable or even inevitable choice, prevailing over any thoughts of recovery through treatment. For a substantial fraction of elderly depressed patients, this is a mortal risk if the means for a successful suicide attempt are available and the risk of discovery is low (38). The rates of active suicide rise and are greatest for elderly Caucasian men as compared to Caucasian women and black men and women. "Passive suicide," commonly seen in geriatric settings, occurs when individuals stop eating and taking fluids or needed medications. To our knowledge, there are no controlled studies of this phenomenon.

Increasingly, language and communication barriers due to failing sensorial and cognitive abilities and, for ethnic minority elderly, the inability to convey information adequately due to language and cultural differences are important impediments to care for elderly persons with depressive symptoms. To our knowledge, no data estimating the extent and severity of these communication and cultural barriers currently exist. Anecdotally, this is widely recognized as an important concern.

In summary, patient-related barriers to care for elderly persons with depressive symptoms include complexity of multiple psychiatric and medical problems, patient-provider communication issues, stigmatization and other attitudinal issues, compliance difficulties, and ethnocultural differences.

PROVIDER-RELATED BARRIERS TO CARE

Providers in this context are health care professionals who are in direct treatment roles, providing care to elderly patients.

Provider-related barriers to care stem from a number of issues, including nonrecognition or misdiagnosis of a depressive condition in an elderly patient, initiation of suboptimal or even inappropriate evaluation and treatment, and lack of patient referral for additional expert geropsychiatric evaluation and management.

The subtlety of some depressive symptoms in many elderly patients and the similarity of these symptoms to effects of primary medical disorders, which are highly prevalent in this population, may limit the ability of even the most adept clinician to diagnose and treat depressive disorders effectively. Indeed, depressive conditions in the elderly are often unrecognized by health care professionals. (17,39,40) This may occur because the older patient may assert anxiety or various somatic concerns such as pain, fatigue, or insomnia without explicitly endorsing a depressed mood. Various factors—including inherent differences in how elderly experience depressive illness compared to younger patients; the coexistence of additional medical illness, the symptoms of which may be accentuated due to the patient's depression; or the patient's reluctance to acknowledge symptoms of a mental illness which can be perceived as stigmatizing—may contribute to this presentation (20,21,30).

There is further diagnostic complication if the patient also is experiencing psychotic features, delirium, or dementia, which commonly occur in elderly patients (42–45). Depression in the presence of delusions, delirium, and/or dementia can be especially difficult to establish. Depressive signs and symptoms can mimic features of delirium or dementia; for instance, cognitive disturbances, apathy, anhedonia, and sleep problems can accompany depression, delirium, and dementia. In these contexts, a diagnosis of a possible depressive illness may not receive priority consideration. Frequently, there is limited history from both the patient and collateral historians. Elders with depression or depressive symptoms may underreport the severity of their symptoms (46). Respondents may not agree on key history issues (47,48). Screening instruments used to identify depression may yield high false-positive and false-negative results (49). Unless the clinician has substantial experience with elderly patients enduring depression with and without psychotic features, delirium, and/or dementia, these problems may go unrecognized and be managed inadequately.

Between one-half and two-thirds of all psychiatric care delivered to older adults is provided by primary care providers in the general health care sector (50–52). Primary care providers are a diverse group, comprising largely general practitioners, family practitioners, internists, and gynecologists. The majority of these providers have limited training in the special needs of older adults with depression. Yet most elderly patients with depression are evaluated and treated in primary care settings, and elderly patients are less likely than younger patients to see a mental health specialist. (19,53,54)

Some clinicians may unintentionally subject the presenting signs and symptoms of depression to stigmatization (55) and ageist-based misinterpretations, so that the patient is seen to be tired, eating less, or sleeping poorly due to a "normal aging" process. The frequent result is failure to evaluate for depression.

The time constraints and economic incentives inherent in the setting of primary care practice limit the time available to perform extensive diagnostic assessments and to distinguish disorders of mood from concomitant medical morbidity. Systematic screening for mental disorders generally, and depressive symptoms in particular, in primary care practices confirm a substantial prevalence of untreated psychiatric symptoms and disorders in these settings (56–59). Several studies indicate that primary care providers identify and then appropriately treat and/or refer only a small proportion of the older patients with depression in their practices (34,56,60). One recent study reported that primary care providers are more than 50% less likely to record a diagnosis of depression in elderly patients as compared to younger adult patients (61). Older patients in academic medical center primary care and Medicare Health Maintenance Organization (HMO) settings have been found to have low rates of treatment for depression, ranging from 4–7% of all persons studied and to 12–25% of patients with probable depression [Centers for Epidemiologic Studies Depression Scale (CES-D) score ≥21] (11,56).

Nearly 80% of elderly patients with psychiatric diagnoses receive treatment only with psychotropic drugs for their psychiatric diagnoses (51). Most of this treatment is provided by primary care practitioners. Nearly 85% of all older adults see a primary care physician at least once per year, and most make multiple visits (51). About 10% of medical visits by older adults are associated with prescription of a psychotropic medication (62,63). Primary care providers are also responsible for the overwhelming majority of psychiatric care and psychotropic prescription in institutional settings. Approximately 50–60% of nursing home patients are prescribed some kind of psychotropic medication in any given year (64–65). The rates of depression among the elderly are higher for nursing home patients than for noninstitutionalized, non-medically ill elderly (66). It has been estimated that more than 9 out of 10 nursing home residents who would benefit from treatment for psychiatric disorders, including depressive symptoms and major depression, receive no treatment whatsoever (10,67). This estimate may be conservative, as other data indicates that a substantial proportion of nursing home residents who receive psychiatric treatment are not treated for the correct disorder or are not treated with the appropriate intervention (10,51,68).

But not all of the assessment difficulties associated with depressive conditions in elderly persons relate to underrecognition. In some elderly patients, depressive conditions may be overdiagnosed, perhaps due to misinterpretation of the symptoms of other medical or psychiatric problems as caused by an underlying depression, and patients may be prescribed inappropriate treatment. One study suggests that, in an acute hospital settings, approximately 40% of specialty referrals for depression involved problems other than depression, including delirium, dementia, and anxiety (69). This can be of importance if the presumption of depression delays other medical, neurological, or psychiatric assessments.

If a depressive illness is considered and diagnosed, the severity of the illness may be misjudged, so that appropriate referrals to experts in geropsychiatry are not considered. As a result, adequate evaluation for suicide risk, mood-congruent delusions, or other psychiatric illness such as bipolar disorder may not occur, leading to treatment noninitiation or suboptimal/inappropriate interventions.

Treatments for depression in the elderly include pharmacological agents; psychotherapy, including individual, couples, family, and group therapies; psychosocial treatments, including behavioral and milieu interventions; electroconvulsive therapy (ECT); and, in some centers, transmagnetic stimulation (TMS). Some providers may not consider this range of possible treatments. The plan of treatment for an elderly patient is frequently much more complicated than that for a younger patient due to medical and social comorbidities requiring expert multidisciplinary care.

In summary, provider-related barriers to care affecting elderly patients with depression extend from depression-identification problems with older patients to provider difficulties in the selection and application of appropriate treatments.

ORGANIZATIONAL AND FINANCIAL BARRIERS TO CARE

Barriers to care related to organizational and financial factors include organization-specific mission and philosophy issues, availability of a sufficiently wide range of different modalities of psychiatric care to depressed elderly, financial incentives/disincentives, and transportation issues.

The diverse group of professionals and paraprofessionals who provide mental health services to older adults work in a fragmented system. They have limited commonality in training, philosophy, therapeutic approach, and objectives of care. These providers deliver care to elders with depressive symptoms under conditions of extraordinary uncertainty. Even in severe geriatric depression, definitions of illness remain controversial and triage and clinical decision making are not well standardized.

The mental health specialty sector providing care to older adults is composed of a large and growing group of diversely trained professionals and paraprofessionals from several major disciplines: nursing, social work, counseling, psychology, and psychiatry. Unquantified amounts of nonspecialty services are provided to elders with depressive symptoms by social workers and caseworkers in social agencies and by clergy in religious settings. Training in diagnosis and management among these providers is highly variable. Considering the complexity and sublety of geriatric depression, it is highly likely that case identification among these providers is incomplete, and appropriate referral almost surely is limited to settings that are relatively well connected to the mental health specialty sector or where innovative training programs have been initiated.

The availability of specialty training for the care of older adults in each of these disciplines is limited although growing in recent years. Virtually all of the disciplines have developed minimum criteria for specialty psychiatric training and for subspecialty training in geriatrics (70). Nursing, social work, psychology, and psychiatry have all undertaken extensive efforts to increase subspecialty geriatric training (71–75) and to provide incentives for trainees to pursue careers focused on the care of elderly patients (74,75). However, only a small fraction of the growing supply of mental health providers receive substantial exposure to and supervision in the care of older adults during their formal training experience (70).

Even with improvement in standardization of training, there remains considerable variability in the skills and objectives of providers from each of the disciplines. Each of the provider disciplines involved in mental health care for older adults has a unique ethos. Standards for training have been linked traditionally to the philosophy and the identified tasks that have been associated with each provider group. Additionally, the dominance of private practice by mental health providers in an environment of limited economic resources has led to vigorous competition among disciplines (52). The equivocal nature of criteria for treatment of depression in elderly patients has permitted providers from different disciplines to treat patients in accordance with their training, but in ways that do not necessarily reflect current knowledge-based practice.

Mental health specialty care is provided in a large variety of settings, few of which are designed specifically for the care of older adults. Private practice continues to dominate psychiatric service delivery (76), although this is steadily changing with the continued growth of managed care plans. Private practitioners maintain that geriatric depression and other late-life psychiatric disorders do not fit with their chosen style of practice. They also question the appropriateness of traditional psychiatric treatments to problems associated with aging. For example, some psychiatrists in private practice attribute their avoidance of geriatric patients to the complex nature of the care of elderly patients, who commonly have co-occuring medical problems. They claim that the resources required by this population are matched poorly with the structure of solo and group private psychiatric practice. (77,78) Similarly, community mental health centers (CMHCs), designed primarily to serve younger, chronically mentally ill patients often have limited programs for and expertise in the care of older adults with depression, particularly in the presence of medical comorbidity (79). CMHCs are commonly inadequately integrated with the social service agencies and the network of primary care providers in the community from which referrals are likely to originate (63). Several innovative programs have improved access to care for older adults with mental disorders. These programs have been successful largely because of their ability to recruit specialty-trained geriatric clinicians and because of innovative programs linking them to social agencies that provide services for older adults (80–83).

In recent years, mental health specialty providers in general and private psychiatric hospital settings have become more actively involved in providing geriatric mental health services. However, the nature of traditional general hospital and private psychiatric inpatient facilities, steeped in milieu therapies for behavioral control and functional improvement for younger populations, limits access to appropriate care for older adults who have concomitant medical disorders requiring acute attention. The advent of medical psychiatric units and geropsychiatric inpatient units (50,84–86) has provided a new resource for the treatment of frail, elderly depressed patients in acute-care settings.

Clinical uncertainty is said to emanate from three key factors: [1] the ability of the clinician to classify the existence of illness; [2] the ability of the clinician to understand the probability of a successful outcome given a specific treatment; and [3] the correspondence of the clinician's desires and benefits with those of the patient (87). Providers of mental health services to older adults have substantial variability in training, treatment philosophy, economic incentives, and perceived available treatment options. In a well-organized delivery system, this diversity could provide a richness of service delivery alternatives to meet the complex needs of older adults. However, given the fragmentation of the current service delivery system and the substantial barriers to access, this diversity has the effect of increasing the level of uncertainty that individual providers face in clinical decision making. The somewhat paradoxical result is that the appropriate matching of services to needs is less likely to occur for elderly depressed patients.

Some health services organizations may choose to de-emphasize care of the older mentally ill patient because of a perception that provision of such services will project a negative public image. For example, some clinics may wish to project a health and wellness image and accordingly emphasize treatment putatively focused on maintaining health among those who are relatively young, healthy, and with "intact" minds. Providing care to the elderly with mental illness may not accord well with this image.

In most health services organizations, there is vigorous competition for limited financial resources, and in this context, provision of care for mental illness may not be considered to be adequately profitable. Certainly, compared to many inpatient surgical procedures, the revenue generated in outpatient psychiatric care to elderly patients may not be substantial. This revenue-generation focus can have a profound effect on the way some health services organizations view and provide care to elderly patients with depressive symptoms.

Even in organizations (or organizational components) with a strong commitment to providing health care to the aged with mental illness, there can be important, sometimes unrecognized, barriers to care. There may be limited availability of psychiatric and/or mental health expertise, limited access to some care modalities (such as ECT), and a constrained pharmacy formulary so that options for pharmacological care are significantly reduced. The latter situation can be especially problematic if a patient needs a nonformulary drug to continue ongoing maintenance treatment or because of adverse reactions to drugs on formulary.

The growth of managed care in the general health care sector is likely to affect access to appropriate psychiatric care for older adults. As health maintenance organizations (HMOs) have gained increased market penetration throughout the country and while federal regulations have provided incentives for the inclusion of Medicare populations, older adult participation in HMOs have grown steadily (70,88). Of 40 million Americans enrolled in Medicare currently (96% of eligibles), more than 5.3 million (13.3%) elect to participate in the Medicare + Choice plans authorized under the 1997 Balanced Budget Act (88). The Medicare + Choice plans resemble a traditional HMO plan in that members are permitted to obtain services only from providers who participate in the plan or on referral from the plan, with monthly payment by Medicare of a fixed capitation amount to the insurer or HMO the Medicare beneficiary chooses. Medicare-eligible persons choosing Part B coverage currently pay a premium of about $50 per month (fiscal year 2002 = $54) for this coverage, and many choose to supplement this coverage with "Medigap insurance" purchased from private insurers. Inpatient Medicare benefits under Part B supplemental coverage are subject to 20% copayment, with some services also subject to a $100 annual deductible. Prior to the enactment of the Health Insurance Portability and Accountability Act (HIPAA) of 1996 (Public Law 104-191, 1996) (89), mental health services were treated in a discriminatory manner by Medicare, with a 50% copayment required instead of the 20% to which other medical services were subject (88). The HIPAA legislation, an effort by Congress to establish parity for mental health benefits, changed copayment requirements from the previously discriminatory 50% beneficiary–50% Medicare formula for inpatient mental health services to the 80–20% formula applied for all other medical services. However, for outpatient mental health care, the 50% beneficiary–50% Medicare arrangement continues.

Medicare Part A (inpatient services) are provided all Medicare beneficiaries at no premium cost. Part A covers inpatient hospital services, skilled nursing facility (SNF) benefits following a 3-day hospital visit, home health visits following a hospital or SNF stay, and certain other services. A copayment of $196 per day is required of Medicare beneficiaries for hospital stay days 61–90; this increases to $396 per day for days 91–150, and then to 100% of all costs after day 150. SNF care costs nothing during the first 20 days, after which a $99 per day copayment is required until day 100, after which the beneficiary pays all costs (88).

Nothing in these Medicare Part A provisions affects patients with depression or depressive symptoms any differently from the way that general hospital patients with other medical problems are affected. But because of the chronicity of depressive symptoms, these financial constraints impact much more heavily on Medicare beneficiaries with depression or other chronic medical problems than on Medicare enrollees whose medical problems are more episodic and less persistent over time. In this sense, these Medicare coverage rules differentially affect elderly persons with depression and other chronic problems.

Yet in practical terms, these Medicare Part A requirements for beneficiary participation in the payment for acute inpatient and SNF care probably do not have a significant deterrent effect on care seeking. In these situations, the need for care is so strong that, for the beneficiary, viable alternatives are not available. For Medicare Part B, the situation is quite different. Here, the 50% copayment and the need to pay for prescription drugs, either out of pocket or through one of the Medigap insurance coverages (for which the insurance premium costs are paid out of pocket), may have a substantial deterrent effect among elderly Medicare beneficiaries with depression.

It is widely understood that out-of-pocket expenditures by Medicare beneficiaries for depression treatment and other mental health services are substantial. But data giving credible estimates of the magnitude of out-of-pocket expenditures specific to depression care and to other mental health services are not available. Because we believe that these direct beneficiary payments for depression treatment can be an important barrier to care, perhaps one of the most important such barriers, we review here the available data on out-of-pocket expenditures by Medicare beneficiaries for health services generally. By applying an appropriate factor estimating the likely proportion of these general out-of-pocket expenditures that are made in payment for depression care, the reader can obtain a reasonable estimate of this important factor.

One recent estimate of beneficiary-paid, out-of-pocket expenditures for general health services is that 19.0% of income was spent for health services by elderly Medicare beneficiaries in 1995 (90). For low-income Medicare beneficiaries with incomes below the federally defined poverty level (but still without Medicaid coverage), about half of available income was spent out-of-pocket for health care services in 1997 (91). The beneficiaries with incomes between 100 and 125% of the poverty level (and still not enrolled in Medicaid) spent an estimated 30% of their income on out-of-pocket health care costs if they were in a traditional fee-for-service program and about 23% if they were in a Medicare HMO (91). Costs of prescription drugs have increased dramatically in recent years. One recent estimate is that drug spending by the insured elderly rose more than 18% annually between 1997 and 2000 (91). The number of different medications prescribed for elderly persons with multiple medical problems, especially chronic or recurrent problems such as depression, has increased dramatically in recent years (93,94). Older patients use an average of three prescription and nonprescription drugs at any given time (95). The typical elderly nursing home resident is on five to eight prescription drugs, not including pro re nata (PRN) medications (96). Available data clearly show that Medicare enrollees without drug insurance (usually obtained as part of Medigap supplemental insurance coverage) consistently use fewer prescriptions and spend more out-of-pocket on medications than comparable Medicare beneficiaries with drug coverage (97,98). In addition, drug benefit caps have been found to reduce the use of needed medications by the frailest, community-dwelling elderly with multiple mental and physical illnesses, possibly leading to more hospitalization and institutionalization (99).

In sum, these data suggest that current requirements under the Medicare program for beneficiary copayment and, especially, for payment of prescription drugs represent substantial barriers to care for the elderly with chronic problems with depressive symptoms. Treatment for depression commonly although certainly not universally involves prescription medication treatment. Available data indicate clearly that substantial compromise in medication treatment of depression and other medical problems may be attributable to out-of-pocket payment requirements imposed by current Medicare regulations.

For elderly persons in managed care plans, an additional mechanism intended to control health care expenditures is the mental health "carve-out" (100). This mechanism provides for a separate preapproval and service limitation system, administered by a third-party contractor, for treatment of depression, substance abuse, and other mental health services. These carve-out contractors are most commonly large, for-profit companies or group practices specializing in managed mental health care. Psychiatric carve-outs may focus on utilization control, without prioritizing patient care and outcomes, and this may disproportionately impact certain covered subgroups that are primarily elderly (101). To our knowledge, no data quantifying whether these carve-out programs significantly affect the quality of care provided Medicare/Medicaid beneficiaries with depressive symptoms are yet available. However, these programs have been put into operation to attempt to control putative over utilization, so that it seems likely that their net effect is to reduce the volume of services provided elders with problems with depression. A review of carve out programs available to Medicare beneficiaries demonstrates a consistent lack of required training in the care of the elderly, lack of specific protocols for older adult care and a paucity of special services for institutionalized older persons. Additionally, the discontinuation of psychiatric and medical care in this population is perilous (70).

Transportation issues can be problematic for elderly persons seeking to access mental health services. Available data, while limited in scope, clearly indicate that utilization and accessibility vary closely together among elderly persons needing health services (102). Some health organizations invest in community outreach activities, providing transportation between patients' homes and the health care facilities at which services are delivered. However, these programs can be costly and are not common. Obviously, to the extent that unavailability of appropriate transportation inhibits the delivery of needed health services, this can be an important barrier to care for elderly persons with depression.

In summary, organizational and financial barriers to care include fragmentation of care issues, insurance copayment and deductible provisions that obstruct access to services, especially pharmaceutical services, and transportation issues.

TREATMENT/INTERVENTION–RELATED BARRIERS TO CARE

By intervention-related barriers, we mean issues embedded in the pathophysiology of the illness and related to somatic and psychotherapeutic treatments for depression.

There is a growing but still relatively underdeveloped understanding of the pathophysiology of depression in elderly (103,104). The dynamics leading to depressive illness are complex in any circumstance, and especially so in elderly patients, who may also be affected by various aging-related changes as well as a wide spectrum of medical problems. Mechanisms of action of various interventions used in the treatment of depression—including psychotropic medications, ECT, and various psychotherapeutic treatments—are still incompletely understood. Knowledge about the tolerability and effectiveness of the antidepressant medications among elderly patients varies widely by the type and dose of treatment (105–110).

There are very active research initiatives examining the risk factors, pathophysiology, diagnostic specificity, and progression over time of major depression and subsyndromal depressive conditions in the elderly. However, despite the vigor with which this research is being pursued, current knowledge remains relatively limited. Compared to other medical conditions that affect the elderly significantly, such as hypertension or myocardial infarction, current levels of scientific understanding of depression in the elderly are at nascent levels.

Diagnostic assignments are affected by the limited scientific knowledge about the etiology, risk factors, and longitudinal pathophysiology of late-life depression. This has resulted in the routine use among depressed elderly patients of nosologic diagnostic categories mostly devised for a younger population. A consequence of this practice has been a widespread willingness to consider that the treatment indications and prognostic circumstances associated with these nosologic categories apply equally well to elderly as to the younger patients who were clinical trial subjects upon which they were based. As well, and perhaps ominously, various pharmacological and nonpharmacological intervention strategies originally developed for younger patients have been extended for use with elderly patients, sometimes without the benefit of adequate safety, tolerability, and efficacy research. Over a dozen antidepressants are currently marketed. Many of these are widely used among elderly depressed patients, even though efficacy research specific to elderly patients has been carried out relatively infrequently and has yielded conflicting results (105,110).

There are data available that suggest that the unconstrained use among older patients of treatments for depression that were developed within nonelderly panels may result in suboptimal results. Data on adverse drug reactions (ADRs) indicate that these events are a leading cause of morbidity and mortality, with the highest incidence occurring in patients aged 60 and older. ADR incidence data specific to antidepressant medications and their concurrent use with other classes of medications are not yet available. Because the ADR risk is substantial among elderly patients, especially among elderly patients with multiple medical problems who frequently are treated with medications of several different types, we review the available data on ADR risk here, despite the circumstance that ADR data that are available currently are not depression care- or antidepressant-specific, and much of these data are not elderly-specific. The ADR risk among elderly patients is a notable barrier to effective and safe depression care, and we believe that it is important to review briefly the available data here despite the current unavailability of elderly-specific data.

A recent meta-analysis concludes that ADRs are among the leading causes of death, ranking fourth to sixth, depending on study inclusion rules (ahead of diabetes and pneumonia), and that about three-fourths of ADRs are dose-dependent (111). The risk of suffering an ADR increases exponentially with increasing numbers of prescribed drugs, and, as noted above, elderly patients frequently are on several prescription/nonprescription medications concurrently. It is estimated that more than half (51%) of deaths due to ADRs occur among persons aged 60 years or older (95). Preventability of ADRs has been assessed in several studies, including one focused solely on elderly people (112). In this study, it was estimated that about two-thirds of medication-related ADRs were considered to be preventable.

The drug class associated with most ADRs among elderly patients is analgesics, especially nonsteroidal anti-inflammatory drugs. Psychotropic medications, include antidepressants, are among the five or six other drug categories that are commonly involved in ADRs in elderly patients, along with cardiovascular drugs, antidiabetic medications, anticoagulants, and antibiotics. While data on the association of ADR incidence with polypharmacy and dosing levels in elderly patients are not available, some observers conjecture that these factors may be important contributors to the high rate of ADRs observed in elderly psychiatric patients (95,112).

Some authorities recommend that physicians give older patients lower initial doses than are prescribed for younger patients. The reasons for this recommendation include the following: [1] older patients have reduced rates of drug metabolism and elimination compared with younger adults; [2] chronic or multiple disease processes, which are common in older patients, may alter drug response; and [3] drug-drug interactions are a particular concern among older patients because of the high likelihood that they are taking more than one medication. Most practicing physicians rely on the *Physicians' Desk Reference* (PDR) for medication dosing information (113). Yet, the PDR does not provide recommendations for reduced initial doses for older patients for many medications. These include the widely prescribed antidepressants bupropion, citalopram, doxepin, mirtazapine, sertraline, trazodone, and venlafaxine (95).

Polypharmacy in the elderly possibly could be reduced in prevalence if there were regular reviews of therapy already prescribed. This would enable the identification of medicines no longer required, those without clear indication, those prescribed for adverse effects that could be avoided by therapy changes, and those that duplicate similar medicines. All of these actions would reduce the frequency of polypharmacy and thereby reduce the likelihood of life-threatening ADRs.

In addition to pharmaceutical treatments for geriatric depression, various nonpharmacological interventions are also widely used. Psychotherapeutic interventions include interpersonal psychotherapy, behavioral therapy, cognitive behavioral therapy, and psychodynamic therapy. Counseling/social interventions of various types have been used to treat depression in elderly patients (114). Scientific knowledge about the outcomes of such treatments in the elderly is very limited. In a recently published meta-analysis evaluating pharmacological and psychological treatments for older depressed patients, only five nonpharmaceutical studies met the meta-analytic inclusion criteria, even though these criteria included the somewhat indulgent limitation of age >55 years (105). In this meta-analysis, 55 pharmaceutical-based studies meeting inclusion criteria were identified. Results of the meta-analysis were that the nonpharmaceutical therapies were superior to placebo in terms of average percentage reduction in measured symptom severity and did not differ significantly from tricyclic antidepressants or selective serotonin reuptake inhibitors on this summary outcome measure. However, the authors caution that no firm conclusions about comparative efficacy between nonpharmaceutical treatments and either placebo or medication treatments could be drawn because the direct comparison data were insufficient for this purpose (105).

Efficacy research on other nonpharmacological interventions in elderly cohorts is equally sparse. For example, efficacy research on ECT in the elderly is very limited (115,116). The limited data that are available suggest that ECT therapy results in favorable outcomes in elderly with depression, who are less able to tolerate the prolonged response times common with pharmaceutical therapies (115). Transmagnetic stimulation (TMS) in adults is of limited and mostly experimental use at this time, but is showing potential as an alternative to ECT; in time, it may prove to be a viable treatment alternative for depressed elderly (117,118). Currently, data on the efficacy and safety of TMS among depressed elderly are lacking.

The association of depression in elderly patients with hypertension and other cardiovascular and related physical illness risk factors could result in a weakening of some barriers to care. Although there are numerous reports of linkages of depression with elevated mortality risk for patients with cardiovascular and other illnesses (119–121), as yet no credible scientific data have been published that indicate that effective depression treatment can result in mortality reduction. If it is found that treatment of a depressive illness can result in reduced mortality risk in patients with cardiovascular and other illnesses, this could lead to dramatic improvements in the evaluation and management of depressive illness in the elderly.

If the risk factors for depression in elderly could be established more clearly, targeted prevention strategies might be more effectively instituted to decrease the incidence and eventually the prevalence of late-life depression. Were the etiology and pathophysiology of depression in the elderly understood more clearly, more specific antidepressant therapies with greater effectiveness and fewer side effects might be developed. This holds for whether the assessment is subsyndromal or clinical depression, for these diagnostic domains can be imprecise, and it is frequently not clear which treatments or combination of treatments are likely to be most appropriate for elderly patients in these categories. Because the elderly patient may have a number of co-occurring psychiatric or medical conditions and likely has been prescribed more than one or even several prescription medications, with accompanying increased risk for illness-drug and drug-drug interactions, the development of effective and safe antidepressant treatments is a very high priority goal. The availability of antidepressant medications with improved tolerability and without sacrificing efficacy for use with the elderly depressed will likely ameliorate patients' attitudes toward treatment, and improve compliance with acute and relapse prevention treatment, resulting in improved long-term treatment effectiveness.

In summary, intervention-related barriers to safe and effective care for depression in the elderly include limitations in current understanding of pathophysiological and ethological issues of depression in this age group, limited efficacy data, significant risks associated with polypharmacy, and vulnerability to adverse drug reactions and treatment intolerance.

SOCIETAL BARRIERS TO CARE

Sociodemographic characteristics have been shown to influence patient demand and the use of mental health services in general populations (122–125). Sex, age, race, education, marital status, residence location, and attitudes toward mental health services exert independent effects on the likelihood of pursuing mental health care (126–128). Socioeconomic status may determine access both to primary care and to mental health specialty providers who are specially trained to provide services for older adults. Similarly, geographic location may be an important factor in determining access to appropriate care for depression in elderly persons (26).

The stigma associated with psychiatric disorder and the pursuit of mental health services by older adults has its roots in a culture and tradition that have discouraged the recognition and the importance of depression and other psychiatric syndromes. The controversial nature of psychiatric treatments makes them especially vulnerable to public scrutiny and potential regulation. Social and legal pressures from local communities controlling the use of psychotropic medications and electroconvulsive therapy may limit the availability of safe and effective treatments for geriatric depression (129,130).

Societal denial of the importance of psychiatric disorders and discrimination against individuals with mental disorders continues to exert an influence over public policy governing payment for health services. Although recent reforms in the Medicare program have decreased the discriminatory regulation of mental health services in comparison to services for other medical problems, these discriminatory policies continue in force in numerous ways within the Medicaid programs of the several states. For example, federal participation in Medicaid has been disallowed for young adults residing in nursing homes where more than 50% of the residents have primary psychiatric diagnoses (70). Similarly, limitations in Medicaid reimbursement levels provide disincentives for some hospitals and many private providers to deliver psychiatric care to older adults.

Data on ethnicity differences in rates of identification and treatment of depressive symptoms in elderly patients are limited. One study, using data from the 1997–1998 National Ambulatory Medical Care Surveys, determined that primary care physicians were 37% less likely to record a diagnosis of depression during visits by African Americans compared to Caucasians and 35% less likely to do so during visits by Medicaid patients compared to patients with private insurance coverage (61). In making these comparisons, the investigators controlled for symptom presentation. It is possible, although unlikely given the magnitude of these differences, that the African-American and Medicaid patients were 37 and 35%, respectively, less likely to present with significant depressive symptoms and that the diagnostic assignments thus were validly made. Another interpretation is that these differential rates reflect discriminatory societal attitudes. It is unknown if these differential diagnostic rates for African-Americans and Medicaid recipients obtain in geriatric populations. Perhaps future research of this kind can help to determine whether these rate differentials are due to actual differences in depression prevalence or are attributable to discriminatory attitudes.

In summary, societal barriers to care include discriminatory health policy factors that treat mental health services in ways that are substantively different from other medical services and inferior to them.

IMPROVING ACCESS TO CARE: AN ACTION AND RESEARCH AGENDA

Prevention

Identifying risk factors for depressive illness in later life through longitudinal epidemiological studies would be invaluable for instituting preventive strategies. For example, multidisciplinary collaborative trials to reduce risk factors for cerebrovascular disease may help to prevent a form of late-onset depression with cerebrovascular etiology (131). Providing informative bulletins through different media to familiarize the public with depressive signs and symptoms in the elderly and the identifying depression with well-known figures or celebrities may help to destigmatize depression, raise the population's consciousness regarding depression, and encourage patients with depressive symptoms to seek help. Routine screening of at-risk individuals for depression and suicide, followed by appropriate evaluation and management over time, may improve patient access to care and moderate the incidence, prevalence, and progression of late-life depression (132,133).

Translational Research

Translational research suggests a bridging of knowledge gained through basic and clinical scientific work to application in the clinical realm. Inherent in applying these concepts to the elderly is the focus on change as a person becomes older. Important are [1] identifying and harnessing molecular mechanisms regarding the etiology and pathophysiology of depression over time and as a person ages; [2] unveiling longitudinal genotypic and phenotypic markers for depressive illness that are practicable, sensitive, and specific and can be identified cost-effectively; [3] developing longitudinal dimensional and categorical models of depressive illness; [4] shaping diagnostic criteria applicable to depression in the elderly; and [5] emphasizing pathways out of depression and into health in later life. These can impact the diagnostic and interventional capabilities of medical and scientific realms.

Interventional Studies

Changes in pharmacokinetics and pharmacodynamics in aging individuals, and uncertainties around medical comorbidities, polypharmacy, and adverse effects in the elderly make it imperative to conduct drug intervention trials with elderly subjects. The approval of the U.S. Food and Drug Administration (FDA) for antidepressant drug use in older patients may be made contingent on clinical trials in the elderly. In addition to the safety, efficacy, and tolerability of the interventions, additional measures to assess impact on compliance, functional ability, cognitive capabilities, well-being, and comorbid physical illnesses such as cardiovascular disease or diabetes mellitus may be especially relevant in the elderly.

Investigations of nonpharmacological interventions are just as important and include ECT, TMS, psychotherapeutic, psychosocial, behavioral and milieu interventions as well as case management. Alternative interventions such as exercise and nutritional supplements, as well as ethnic minority/cultural group and gender issues, also warrant scientific appraisal. Ethnocultural factors influence presentations of mental disorders, description of psychiatric symptoms, and diagnoses and treatments received. Ethnic and gender differences in pharmacokinetics and pharmacodynamics contributing to differential drug responsiveness deserve investigation as well. Efficacy of pharmacological versus nonpharmacological interventions in the elderly, alone or in combination, also needs further exploration.

Because geriatric depression is a chronic and/or recurrent illness, it is necessary to study the course of the illness longitudinally, over extended time periods of at least 18 to 24 months. Most of the existing outcomes research in geriatric depression has been limited to studies a few weeks or months in length.

Health Services Research

Managed care and long-term care have greatly influenced the delivery of health care to the elderly. Although interventional studies may help to uncover efficacious treatments, health services research may be better suited to determine if, in "real world" situations, the treatments are effective. Health services research should consider whether treatments are truly effective, with the financial and other constraints placed on treatments due to managed care and other considerations. Interventional clinical trials typically utilize stringent inclusion and exclusion criteria, so that the population studied may not be representative of the many patients who are frail; have multiple comorbid illnesses such as delirium, dementia, cardiovascular disease, or diabetes; and are taking multiple medications. Population-based studies could also establish study samples more representative of the general ill elderly population and may be able to identify morbidity risks associated with depression in such an ill population. Also needed are data that identify the morbidity risks associated with the use of antidepressant medication in combination with other commonly used treatments for medical problems in frail elderly. The roles of specialty mental health services, development and implementation of practice guidelines, and evaluation of outcomes are important to explore. Systematic research designed to assess the impact among elderly of depression on functioning, mortality, and quality of life is needed.

Training

Training in geriatric mental health needs to be improved at all levels, including patients, clinicians of various backgrounds, public workers who may come in contact with elderly living alone, the public at large, and policy makers. Patients who know more about depression and how it interacts with medical conditions may be more willing to seek and continue with treatment for depression and volunteer for studies on depression. Training collaborations among existing mental health services and centers with expertise on geriatric psychiatry and gerontology may help to improve and extend services for the elderly. Patients and service organizations may be more active in letting their needs be known to government officials to influence mental health policy and insurance groups to achieve greater mental health parity, improve insurance coverage for prescription drugs with the lifting of arbitrary drug benefit caps, pay for clinical trials, and contribute data for research.

REFERENCES

1. Narrow WE, Rae DS, Robins LN, Regier DA. Revised prevalence estimates of mental disorders in the United States—using a clinical significance criterion to reconcile two surveys' estimates. Arch Gen Psychiatry 2002; 59:115–123.
2. Beekman ATF, Copeland JRM, Prince MJ. Review of community prevalence of depression in later life. Br J Psychiatry 1999; 174:307–311.
3. Cole MG, Bellavance F, Mansour A. Prognosis of depression in elderly community and primary care populations: A systematic review and meta-analysis. Am J Psychiatry 1999; 156:1182–1189.
4. Cole MG, Yaffe MJ. Pathway to psychiatric care of the elderly with depression. Int J Geriatr Psychiatry 1996; 11:157–161.
5. NIH Consensus Development Conference. Diagnosis and treatment of depression of late life. JAMA 1992; 268:1018–1029.
6. Blazer D. Depression in the elderly. N Engl J Med 1989; 320:164–166.
7. Bland RC, Newman SC, Orn H. Prevalence of psychiatric disorders in the elderly in Edmonton. Acta Psychiatr Scand (Suppl) 1988; 338:57–63.
8. Regier DA, Myers JK, Kramer M, Robins LN, Blazer DG, Hough RL, Eaton WW, Locke BZ. The NIMH Epidemiologic Catchment Area Program: historical context, major objectives, and study population characteristics. Arch Gen Psychiatry 1984; 41:934–941.
9. Unutzer J, Patrick DL, Simon G, Grembowski D, Walker E, Rutter C, Katon W. Depressive symptoms and the cost of health services in HMO patients aged 65 years and older. JAMA 1997; 277:1618–1623.
10. Teresi J, Abrams R, Holmes D, Ramirez M, Elmicke J. Prevalence of depression and depression recognition in nursing homes. Soc Psychiatry Psychiatr Epidemiol 2001; 36:613–620.
11. Callahan CM, Hui SL, Nienaber NA, Musick BS, Tierney WM. Longitudinal study of depression and health services use among elderly primary care patients. J Am Geriatr Soc 1994; 42:833–838.
12. Palsson SP, Ostling S, Skoog I. The incidence of first-onset depression in a population followed from the age of 70 to 85. Psychol Med 2001; 31:1159–1168.

13. Mulsant BH, Ganguli M. Epidemiology and diagnosis of depression in late life. J Clin Psychiatry 1999; 60(suppl 20):9–15.
14. Gottlieb GL. Barriers to care for older adults with depression. In: Schneider LS, Reynolds CF III, Lebowitz BD, et al, eds. Diagnosis and Treatment of Depression in Late Life. Washington, DC: American Psychiatric Press, 1994, pp 377–396.
15. Gorman PS, Shapiro S, Skinner EA, Von Korff M, Klein LE, Turner RW, Teitelbaum ML, Burke J, Burns BJ. Detection and management of mental health problems for older patients by primary care providers. JAMA 1987; 257:489–493.
16. Lenze EJ, Miller MD, Dew MA, Martire LM, Mulsant BH, Begley AE, Schulz R, Frank E, Reynolds CF III. Subjective health measures and acute treatment outcomes in geriatric depression. Int J Geriatr Psychiatry 2001; 16:1149–1155.
17. Crawford MJ, Prince M, Menezes P, Mann AH. The recognition and treatment of depression in older people in primary care. Int J Geriatr Psychiatry 1998; 13: 172–176.
18. Shah PN, Maly RC, Frank JC, Hirsch SH, Reuben DB. Managing geriatric syndromes—what geriatric assessment teams recommend, what primary care physicians implement, what patients adhere to. J Am Geriatr Soc 1997; 45:413–419.
19. Goldstrom ID, Burns BJ, Kessler LG, Feuerberg MA, Larson DB, MIller NE, Cromer WJ. Mental health services use by elderly adults in a primary care setting. J Gerontol 1987; 42:147–153.
20. Gallo JJ, Rabins PV. Depression without sadness: alternative presentations of depression in late life. Am Fam Physician 1999; 60:820–826.
21. Gottfries CG. Is there a difference between elderly and younger patients with regard to the symptomatology and aetiology of depression? Int Clin Psychopharmacol 1998; 13(suppl 5):S13–S18.
22. Katona C, Livingston G, Manela M, Leek C, Mullan E, Orrell M, D'Ath P, Zeitlin D. The symptomatology of depression in the elderly. Int Clin Psychopharmacol 1997; 12(suppl 7):S19–23.
23. Sherrill JT, Frank E, Geary M, Stack JA, Reynolds CF. Psychoeducational workshops for elderly patients with recurrent major depression and their families. Psychiatr Serv 1997; 48:76–81.
24. Raccio-Robak N, McErlean MS, Fabacher DA, Milano PM, Verdile VP. Socioeconomic and health status differences between depressed and nondepressed ED elders. Am J Emerg Med 2002; 20:71–73.
25. Mickus M, Colenda CC, Hogan AJ. Knowledge of mental health benefits and preferences for type of mental health providers among the general public. Psychiatr Serv 2002; 51:199–202.
26. Fortney J, Rost K, Zhang M, Warren J. The impact of geographic accessibility on the intensity and quality of depression treatment. Med Care 1999; 37:884–893.
27. Sirey JA, Bruce ML, Alexopoulos GS, Perlick DA, Raue P, Friedman SJ, Meyers BS. Perceived stigma as a predictor of treatment discontinuation in young and older outpatients with depression. Am J Psychiatry 2001; 158:479–481.
28. Mistry R, Rosansky J, McGuire J, McDermott C, Jarvik L, UPBEAT Collaborative Group. Social isolation predicts re-hospitalization in a group of older American veterans enrolled in the UPBEAT Program. Int J Geriatr Psychiatry 2001; 16: 950–959.

29. Elie M, Cole MG, Primeau FJ, Fellavance F. Delirium risk factors in elderly hospitalized patients. J Gen Intern Med 1998; 13:204–212.
30. O'Connor DW, Rosewarne R, Bruce A. Depression in primary care 1: elderly patients' disclosure of depressive symptoms to their doctors. Int Psychogeriatr 2001; 13:359–365.
31. Orne MT. Psychotherapy: toward an appropriate basis for reimbursal. In: Taintor Z, Widern P, Barrett SA, eds. Cost Considerations in Mental Health Treatment: Settings, Modalities and Providers. Series EN, No 2 (DHHS Publ No ADM-84-1295). Washington, DC: US Government Printing Office, 1984, pp 55–60.
32. Karasu TB. The specificity versus nonspecificity dilemma: toward identifying therapeutic change agents. Am J Psychiatry 1986; 143:687–695.
33. Smith ML, Glass GV, Miller TI. The benefits of psychotherapy. Baltimore: Johns Hopkins University Press, 1980.
34. Waxman HM, Carner EA. Physicians' recognition, diagnosis and treatment of mental disorders in elderly medical patients. Gerontologist 1984; 24:23–30.
35. Lauber C, Nordt C, Falcato L, Rossler W. Lay recommendations on how to treat mental disorders. Soc Psychiatry Psychiatr Epidemiol 2001; 36:553–556.
36. Salzman C. Medication compliance in the elderly. J Clin Psychiatry 1995; 56 (suppl 1):18–22.
37. Alexopoulos GS, Bruce ML, Hull J, Sirey JA, Kakuma T. Clinical determinants of suicidal ideation and behavior in geriatric depression. Arch Gen Psychiatry 1999; 56:1048–1053.
38. Szanto K, Gildengers A, Mulsant BH, Brown G, Alexopoulos GS, Reynolds CF III. Identification of suicidal ideation and prevention of suicidal behaviour in the elderly. Drugs Aging 2002; 19:11–24.
39. Pouget R, Yersin B, Wietlisbach V, Burnand B, Bula CJ. Depressed mood in a cohort of elderly medical inpatients: prevalence, clinical correlates and recognition rate. Aging Clin Exp Res 2000; 12:301–307.
40. Bair DB. Frequently missed diagnosis in geriatric depression. Psychiatr Clin North Am 1998; 21:941–971.
41. Garrard J, Rolnick SJ, Nitz NM, Luepke L, Jackson J, Fischer LR, Leibson C, Bland PC, Heinrich R, Waller LA. Clinical detection of depression among community-based elderly people with self-reported symptoms of depression. J Gerontol (Series A) 1998; 53:92–101.
42. Sandberg O, Gustafson Y, Brannstrom B, Bucht G. Clinical profile of delirium in older patients. J Am Geriatr Soc 1999; 47:1300–1306.
43. Serretti A, Lattuada E, Cusin C. Gasperini M, Smeraldi E. Clinical and demographic features of psychotic and nonpsychotic depression. Comp Psychiatry 1999; 40:358–362.
44. Lacro JP, Jeste DV. Geriatric psychosis. Psychiatr Q 1997; 68:247–260.
45. Farrell KR, Ganzini L. Misdiagnosing delirium as depression in medically ill elderly patients. Arch Intern Med 1995; 155:2459–2564.
46. Lyness JM, Cox C, Curry J. Cornwell Y, King DA, Caine ED. Older age and the underreporting of depressive symptoms. J Am Geriatr Soc 1995; 43:216–221.
47. Heun R, Muller H. Interinformant reliability of family history information on psychiatric disorders in relatives. Eur Arch Psychiatry Clin Neurosci 1998; 248:104–109.

48. Long K, Sudha S, Mutran EJ. Elder-proxy agreement concerning the functional status and medical history of the older person: the impact of caregiver burden and depressive symptomatology. J Am Geriatr Soc 1998; 46:1103–1111.
49. Papassotinopoulos A, Heun R. Screening for depression in the elderly: a study on misclassification by screening instruments and improvement of scale performance. Prog Neuropsychopharmacol Biol Psychiatry 1999; 23:431–446.
50. Ettner SL, Hermann RC. Provider specialty choice among Medicare beneficiaries treated for psychiatric disorders. Health Care Finance Rev 1997; 18:43–59.
51. Burns BJ, Taube CA. Mental health services in general medical care and in nursing homes, In: Fogel BS, Furino A, Gottlieb GL, eds. Mental Health Policy for Older Americans: Protecting Minds at Risk. Washington, DC: American Psychiatric Press, 1990, pp 53–83.
52. Gottlieb GL. Market segmentation. In: Fogel BS, Furino A, Gottlieb GL, eds. Mental Health Policy for Older Americans: Protecting Minds at Risk. Washington DC: American Psychiatric Press, 1990, pp 135–155.
53. Pingitore D, Snowden L, Sansone RA, Klinkman M. Persons with depressive symptoms and the treatments they receive: a comparison of primary care physicians and psychiatrists. Int J Psychiatry Med 2001; 31:41–60.
54. Olfson M, Shea S, Feder A, Fuentes M, Nomura Y, Gameroff M, Weissman MM. Prevalence of anxiety, depression, and substance use disorders in an urban general medicine practice. Arch Fam Med 2000; 9:876–883.
55. Raue PJ, Meyers BS. An overview of mental health services for the elderly. New Dir Ment Health Serv 1997; 76:3–12.
56. Unutzer J, Simon G, Belin TR, Datt M, Katon W, Patrick D. Care for depression in HMO patients aged 65 and older. J Am Geriatr Soc 2000; 48:1011–1013.
57. Von Korff M, Shapiro S, Burke JD, Teitelbaum M, Skinner EA, German P, Turner RW, Klein L, Burns B. Anxiety and depression in a primary care clinic. Arch Gen Psychiatry 1987; 44:152–156.
58. Wilkinson G. Overview of Mental Health Practices in Primary Care Settings, with Recommendations for Future Research, Series DN, No 7 (DHHS Publ No ADM-86-1467). Washington, DC: US Government Printing Office, 1986.
59. Zung WWK. Recognition and treatment of depression in a family medicine practice. J Clin Psychiatry 1983; 44:3–6.
60. German PS, Shapiro S, Skinner EA, Von Korff M, Klein LE, Turner RW, Teitelbaum ML, Burke J, Burns BJ. Detection and management of mental health problems of older patients by primary care providers. JAMA 1987; 257:489–493.
61. Harman JS, Schulberg HC, Mulsant BH, Reynolds CF III. The effect of patient and visit characteristics on diagnosis of depression in primary care. J Fam Pract 2001; 50:1068.
62. Schneider LS. Pharmacological considerations in the treatment of late life depression. Am J Geriatr Psychiatry 1996; 4(suppl 1):S51–S65.
63. Lebowitz BD, Niederehe G. Concepts and issues in mental health and aging. In: Birren JE, Sloane RB, Cohen GD, eds. Handbook of Mental Health and Aging, 2nd ed. San Diego, CA: Academic Press, 1992, pp 3–26.
64. Grossberg GT, Grossberg JA. Epidemiology of psychotherapeutic drug use in older adults. Clin Geriatr Med 1998; 14:1–5.

65. Beardsley RS, Larson DB, Burns BJ, Thompson JW, Kamerow DB. Prescribing of psychotropics in nursing home patients. J Am Geriatr Soc 1989; 37:327–330.
66. Nelson JC. Diagnosing and treating depression in the elderly. J Clin Psychiatry 2001; 62(suppl 24):18–22.
67. Burns BJ, Kamerow DB. Psychotropic drug prescriptions for nursing home residents. J Fam Pract 1988; 26:155–160.
68. Mort JR, Aparasu RR. Prescribing of psychotropics in the elderly—why is it so often inappropriate? CNS Drugs 2002; 16:99–109.
69. Boland RJ, Diaz S, Lamdan RM, Ramchandani D, McCartney JR. Overdiagnosis of depression in the general hospital. Gen Hosp Psychiatry 1996; 18:28–35.
70. Gottlieb GL. Managed Behavioral Healthcare Standards, Guidelines, and Competencies for Older Adults with Mental Illness. Rockville, MD: Center for Mental Health Services, SAMSHA, 1998.
71. Fichtner CG, Hardy D, Patel M, Stout CE, Simpatico TA, Dove H, Cook LP, Grossman LS, Giffort DW. A self-assessment program for multidisciplinary mental health teams. Psychiatr Serv 2001; 52:1352–1357.
72. Howe JL, Hyer K, Mellor DJ, Lindeman D, Luptak M. Educational approaches for preparing social work students for interdisciplinary teamwork on geriatric health care teams. Soc Work Health Care 2001; 32:19–42.
73. Belza B. Baker MW. Maintaining health in well older adults: initiative for schools of nursing and The John A. Hartford Foundation for the 21st century. J Gerontolog Nurs 2000; 26:8–17.
74. Cohen GD. The future of mental health and aging. In: Birren JE, Sloane RB, Cohen GD, eds. Handbook of Mental Health and Aging, 2nd ed. San Diego, CA: Academic Press, 1992, pp 894–914.
75. Mezey MD, Lynaugh JE. The teaching nursing home program: outcomes of care. Nurs Clin North Am 1989; 24:769–780.
76. Zarin DA, Pincus HA, Peterson BD, West JC, Suarez AP, Marcus SC, McIntyre JS. Characterizing psychiatry with findings from the 1996 National Survey of Psychiatric Practice. Am J Psychiatry 1998; 155:397–404.
77. Mitchell JB, Cromwell J, Schurman R, et al. Psychiatric office practice study: Final Report submitted to the National Institute of Mean Health. Needham, MA: Health Economics Research, 1989.
78. Mitchell JB, Schurman J. Practice patterns and earnings of private psychiatrists: report submitted to National Institute of Mental Health. Needham, MA: Health Economics Research, 1986.
79. Shear MK, Greeno C, Kang J, Ludewig D, Frank E, Swartz HA, Hanekamp M. Diagnosis of nonpsychotic patients in community clinics. Am J Psychiatry 2000; 157:581–587.
80. Moak G, Borson S. Mental health services in long-term care—still an unmet need. Am J Geriatr Psychiatry 2000; 8:96–100.
81. Rosenheck R. Primary care satellite clinics and improved access to general and mental health services. Health Serv Res 2000; 35:777–790.
82. Lebowitz BD, Light E, Bailey F. Mental health center services for the elderly: the impact of coordination with area agencies on aging. Gerontologist 1987; 27:699–702.
83. Light E, Lebowitz BD, Bailey F. CMHCs and elderly services: an analysis of

direct and indirect services and service delivery sites. Community Ment Health J 1986; 22:294–302.
84. Kominski G, Andersen R, Bastani R, Gould R, Hackman C, Huang D, Jarvik L, Maxwell A, Moye J, Olsen E, Rohrbaugh R, Rosansky J, Taylor S, Van Stone W. UPBEAT: the impact of a psychogeriatric intervention in VA medical centers. Unified Psychogeriatric Biopsychosocial Evaluation and Treatment. Med Care 2001; 39:500–512.
85. Weintraub D, Mazour I. Clinical and demographic changes over ten years on a psychogeriatric inpatient unit. Ann Clin Psychiatry 2000; 12:227–231.
86. Fogel BS, Kroessler D. Treating late-life depression on a medical-psychiatric unit. Hosp Community Psychiatry 1987; 38:829–831.
87. Wennberg JE, Barnes BA, Zubkoff M. Professional uncertainty and the problem of supplier-induced demand. Soc Sci Med 1982; 16:811–824.
88. Fronstin P, Weinstein M. Medicare in the 21st century. Benefits Q 2001; 17:14–23.
89. Public Law No. 104-191, 110 Stat. 2023 (1996), 42 U.S.C. 1320(d)-3. The Health Insurance Portability and Accountability Act of 1996.
90. Crystal S, Johnson RW, Harman J, Sambamoorthi U, Kumar R. Out-of-pocket health care costs among older Americans. J Gerontol B Psychol Sci Soc Sci 2000; 55:S51–S62.
91. Gross DJ, Alecxih L, Gibson MJ, Corea J, Caplan C, Brangan N. Out-of-pocket health spending by poor and near-poor elderly Medicare beneficiaries. Health Serv Res 1999; 34:241–254.
92. Thomas CP, Ritter G, Wallack SS. Growth in prescription drug spending among insured elders. Health Affairs 2001; 20:265–277.
93. Poisal JA, Chulis GS. Medicare beneficiaries and drug coverage. Health Affairs 2000; 19:248–256.
94. Steinberg EP, Gutierrez B, Momani A, Boscarino JA, Neuman P, Deverka P. Beyond survey data: a claims-based analysis of drug use and spending by the elderly. Health Affairs 2000; 19:198–211.
95. Cohen JS. Avoiding adverse reactions: effective lower-dose drug therapies for older patients. Geriatrics 2000; 55:54–56, 59–60, 63–64.
96. Monette J, Gurwitz JH, Avorn J. Epidemiology of adverse drug events in the nursing home setting. Drugs Aging 1995; 7:203–211.
97. Lillard LA, Rogowski J, Kington R. Insurance coverage for prescription drugs: effects on use and expenditures in the Medicare population. Medical Care 1999; 37:926–936.
98. Stuart B, Grana J. Ability to pay and the decision to medicate. Med Care 1998; 36:202–211.
99. Forress EE, Soumerai SB, McLaughlin TJ, Ross-Degnan D. Utilization of essential medications by vulnerable older people after a drug benefit cap: importance of mental disorders, chronic pain, and practice setting. J Am Geriatr Soc 2001; 49:793–797.
100. Frank RG, Huskamp HA, McGuire TG, Newhouse JP. Some economics of mental health "carve-outs."Arch Gen Psychiatry 1996; 53:933–937.
101. Kihlstrom LC. Managed care and medication compliance: implications for chronic depression. J Behav Health Serv Res 1998; 25:367–376.

102. Field KS, Briggs DJ. Socio-economic and locational determinants of accessibility and utilization of primary health care. Health Social Care Community 2001; 9: 294–308.
103. Gareri P, Falconi U, De Fazio P, De Sarro G. Conventional and new antidepressant drugs in the elderly. Prog Neurobiol 2000; 61:353–396.
104. Robinson RG, Chemerinski E, Jorge R. Pathophysiology of secondary depressions in the elderly. J Geriatr Psychiatry Neurol 1999; 12:128–136.
105. Gerson S, Belin TR, Kaufman A, Mintz J, Jarvik L. Pharmacological and psychological treatments for depressed older patients: a meta-analysis and overview of recent findings. Harv Rev Psychiatry 1999; 7:1–28.
106. Kyle CJ, Petersen HE, Overo KF. Comparison of the tolerability and efficacy of citalopram and amitriptyline in elderly depressed patients treated in general practice. Depress Anxiety 1998; 8:147–153.
107. Montgomery SA. Efficacy and safety of the selective serotonin reuptake inhibitors in treating depression in elderly patients. Int Clin Psychopharmacol 1998; 13(suppl 5):S49–S54.
108. Volz HP, Gleiter CH. Monoamine oxidase inhibitors. A perspective on their use in the elderly. Drugs Aging 1998; 13:341–355.
109. Amrein R, Stabl M, Henauer S, Affolter E, Jonkanski I. Efficacy and tolerability of moclobemide in comparison with placebo, tricyclic antidepressants, and selective serontin reuptake inhibitors in elderly depressed patients: a clinical overview. Can J Psychiatry 1997; 42:1043–1050.
110. Schneider LS, Olin JT. Efficacy of acute treatment for geriatric depression. Int Psychogeriatr 1995; 7(suppl):7–25, 1995.
111. Lazarou J, Pomeranz BH, Corey PN. Incidence of adverse drug reactions in hospitalized patients: a meta-analysis of prospective studies. JAMA 1998; 279:1200–1205.
112. Cunningham G, Dodd TRP, Grant DJ, McMurdo MET, Richards RME. Drug-related problems in elderly patients admitted to Tayside hospitals, method for prevention and subsequent reassessment. Age Aging 1997; 26:375–382.
113. Physicians' Desk Reference, 56th ed. Montvale NJ: Medical Economics Co, 2002.
114. Freudenstein U, Jagger C, Arthur A, Donner-Banzhoff N. Treatments for late life depression in primary care—a systematic review. Fam Pract 2001; 18:321–327.
115. Kelly KG, Zisselman M. Update on electroconvulsive therapy (ECT) in older adults. J Am Geriatr Soc 2000; 48:560–566.
116. Tew JD, Mulsant BH, Haskett RF, Prudic J, Thase ME, Crowe RR, Dolata D, Begley AE, Reynolds CF III, Sackeim HA. Acute efficacy of ECT in the treatment of major depression in the old-old. Am J Psychiatry 1999; 156:1865–1870.
117. Hasey G. Transcranial magnetic stimulation in the treatment of mood disorder: a review and comparison with electroconvulsive therapy. Can J Psychiaty 2001; 46: 720–727.
118. McNamara B, Ray JL, Arthurs J, Boniface S. Transcranial magnetic stimulation for depression and other psychiatric disorders. Psychol Med 2001; 31:1141–1146.
119. Blazer DG, Hybels CF, Pieper CF. The association of depression and mortality in elderly persons: a case for multiple, independent pathways. J Gerontol A Biol Sci Med Sci 2001; 56:M505–M509.

120. Ariyo AA, Haan M, Tangen CM, Rutledge JC, Cushman M, Dobs A, Furberg CD. Depressive symptoms and risks of coronary heart disease and mortality in elderly Americans. Circulation 2000; 102:1773–1779.
121. Schulz R, Beach SR, Ives DG, Martire LM, Ariyo AA, Kop WJ. Association between depression and mortality in older adults: the Cardiovascular Health Study. Arch Intern Med 2000; 160:1731–1732.
122. Husaini BA, Sherkat DE, Levine R, Bragg R, Holzer C, Anderson K, Cain V, Moten C. Race, gender, and health care service utilization and costs among Medicare elderly with psychiatric diagnoses. J Aging Health 2002; 14:79–95.
123. Kales HC, Blow FC, Bingham CR, Roberts JS, Copeland LA, Mellow AM. Race, psychiatric diagnosis, and mental health care utilization in older patients. Am J Geriatr Psychiatry 2000; 8:301–309.
124. Baker FM. Further reflections on race, psychiatric diagnosis, and mental health care utilization in older persons. Am J Geriatr Psychiatry 2000; 8:297–300.
125. Swartz MS, Wagner HR, Swanson JW, Burns BJ, George LK, Padgett DK. Administrative update: utilization of services: I. Comparing use of public and private mental health services: the enduring barriers of race and age. Community Mental Health J 1998; 34:133–144.
126. Wells KB, Manning WG, Duan N, Newhouse JP, Ware JE Jr. Sociodemographic factors and the use of outpatient mental health services. Med Care 1986; 24: 75–85.
127. Gallo JJ, Cooperpatrick L, Lesikar S. Depressive symptoms of whites and African Americans aged 60 years and older. J Gerontol (Series B) 1998; 53:277–286.
128. Leaf PJ, Livingston MM, Tischler GL, Weissman MM, Holzer CE III, Myers JK. Contact with health professionals for the treatment of psychiatric and emotional problems. Med Care 1985; 23:1322–1337.
129. Curlik S, Frazier D, Katz I. Psychiatric aspects of long-term care. In: Sadavoy J, Lazarus LW, Jarvik LF, eds. Comprehensive Review of Geriatric Psychiatry. Washington, DC: American Psychiatric Press 1991, pp 547–564.
130. Gottlieb GL. Diversity, uncertainty and variations in practice: the behaviors and clinical decision-making of mental health care providers In: Taube CA, Mechanic D, Homann AA, eds. The Future of Mental Health Services Research. DHHS Publ No ADM-89-1600. Washington, DC: US Government Printing Office, 1989, pp 225–251.
131. Alexopoulos GS, Meyers BS, Young RC, Campbell S, Silbersweig D, Charleson M. "Vascular depression" hypothesis. Arch Gen Psychiatry 1997; 54:915–922.
132. Gottlieb GL. Financial issues. In: Sadovay J, Lazarus LW, Jarvik LF, eds. Comprehensive Review of Geriatric Psychiatry. Washington, DC: American Psychiatric Press, 1991, pp 667–686.
133. Gottlieb GL. Cost implications of depression in older adults. Int J Geriatr Psychiatry 1988; 3:191–200.

3

Diagnosing Depression in Later Life

Janet Lawrence and Donald Davidoff
McLean Hospital, Belmont, and Harvard Medical School, Boston, Massachusetts, U.S.A.

Yosef Berlow
McLean Hospital, Belmont, Massachusetts, U.S.A.

INTRODUCTION: DEPRESSION THROUGH THE STAGES OF ADULTHOOD

As people age, they become even more heterogeneous as a group than when younger. Each individual's differing life experiences, social connections, and medical issues are superimposed on already unique personality traits and abilities. Similarly, the clinical presentations of depression can become more heterogeneous in later life. Our most widely used diagnostic system, the *Diagnostic and Statistical Manual of Mental Disorders* (DSM-IV-TR™) (American Psychiatric Association, 2000), is based on categorization of clusters of co-occurring symptoms derived from empirical data obtained predominantly in younger populations. In some cases, therefore, it fails to capture the more subtle and varied manifestations of depression in the elderly, resulting in failure of clinicians to diagnose and treat this condition.

Although the DSM-IV-TR acknowledges the greater prominence of cognitive symptoms in late life, there is strikingly more emphasis on the differences in presentation of depression in children and adolescents than in the elderly, in spite of the fact that a hallmark of depression, the "depressed" mood, is denied by many elderly depressed adults. Furthermore, changes in sleep, appetite, and energy can be hard to distinguish from those due to age or nonpsychiatric illnesses. In addition, thoughts about death are not unusual in this age group, and suicidal behavior is relatively much more frequent. The diagnosis of major depression requires five or more of the nine symptoms listed in Table 1, occurring during the same 2-week period and causing clinically significant distress or impairment in social, occupational, or other important areas of functioning. The presence of either depressed mood or anhedonia is required.

The insistence on the presence of at least five depressive symptoms may not be sufficiently sensitive to detect elderly patients with a clinically significant mood disorder characterized by a lesser number of clearly identifiable symptoms (Blazer, 1989). The less frequent reporting of depressed mood by elderly patients with other signs and symptoms suggestive of depression has been explained in a variety of ways. Elders, especially men, feel uncomfortable acknowledging psychological symptoms. They may deny feelings of depression, if asked, or focus on somatic complaints as a more appropriate "ticket" to justify medical care. In turn, the somatic symptoms of depression (e.g., fatigue) may be difficult for the patient to distinguish from those of coexisting physical illness. The phenomenon of "somatosensory amplification" (Barsky, 1992), in which psychological distress increases the perception of somatic symptoms, is also thought to increase patients' focus on somatic complaints. Somatic presentations of depression have generally also been considered to be more likely in some cultures than others (Koenig et al., 1993). However, Simon et al. (1999), in studies of primary care patients, suggested that the prevalence of somatic presentation was more strongly influenced by its definition and the type of

TABLE 1 DSM-IV Criteria for Major Depressive Episode

Symptom	DSM-IV diagnostic criteria for major depressive episode
Depressed mood	Depressed mood most of the day, on most days
Anhedonia	Markedly decreased interest or pleasure in most activities
Weight change	Substantial unintentional weight loss or gain
Sleep disturbance	Insomnia or hypersomnia most days
Psychomotor change	Psychomotor retardation or agitation most days
Lack of energy	Fatigue or loss of energy most days
Excessive guilt	Feelings of excessive guilt or worthlessness most days
Poor concentration	Diminished ability to think or concentrate most days
Suicidal ideation	Recurrent thought of death or suicide

Source: Adapted from Whooley and Simon, 2000.

health care available, occurring most frequently when patients lack a close relationship with their physician, regardless of the cultural setting. In any case, the frequency with which somatic complaints predominate in elderly depressives suggests that an atypical presentation of depression should be considered among the differential diagnostic assessment of patients presenting only with physical symptoms that cannot be explained on the basis of a nonpsychiatric illness. Even a vehement disavowal of depressed mood or a syndrome of depression in such patients must be interpreted in the light of all available information (Lyness et al., 1995). In addition to the emphasis on somatic concerns, additional differences have been noted between the psychological expression of depression in the elderly as compared to younger adults. Feelings of decreased self-esteem and worthlessness are more frequently reported in the elderly, and ruminative thinking (in which the individual dwells on particular themes or ideas) may be prominent. Guilt and feelings of failure, by contrast, are more common in younger patients (Burkhart, 2000). Hopelessness about the future and thoughts about death may be more normative in the elderly and are not sufficient to indicate depression in the absence of other symptoms (Burns et al., 1999).

Cognitive impairment, more frequent among elderly than among younger adults, presents a further difficulty in assessment of depressive symptoms. When memory or insight is reduced, an individual is rendered less fully able to report the presence of symptoms. Especial care must be taken with such individuals to observe clues such as behavioral disturbances (e.g., weeping, pacing, handwringing, avoidance of social interaction) and depressive thought content, which may be expressed in a fragmented way due to language impairment. These may be combined with more typical depressive symptoms such as anorexia, sleep disturbance, and anhedonia. When moderate to severe dementia is present, family members are often more aware than the patient of abnormal shifts in affect and mood. They are therefore essential informants during evaluation and monitoring (Ballard et al., 1996).

An important recent development in diagnosing depression among demented patients is the development by Olin and colleagues (2002) of diagnostic criteria for depression in Alzheimer's disease. These include the stipulation that at least three of the following symptoms be present during the same 2-week period: depressed mood, anhedonia, social withdrawal, tearfulness (in less verbal patients), or decreased positive affect or pleasure in response to social contracts or usual activities (Olin et al., 2002).

The presence of comorbid medical illnesses, common among the elderly, is another factor confounding the diagnosis of depression in later life (Lyness et al., 1996). As discussed more fully in Chapter 6, medical illnesses bear a complex and interactive relationship to depression. While certain illnesses such as Parkinson's disease can produce depressive symptoms, others such as coronary artery disease can produce symptoms that overlap those of depression.

Several approaches have been suggested for assessing the symptoms of medical illness that relate to the diagnosis of depression (Lyness et al., 1996), including counting only those symptoms thought to be etiologically related to depression (closer to DSM-IV-TR); counting all symptoms, regardless of etiology; or counting only affective and cognitive symptoms. The more inclusive approach is supported by some research (Koenig et al., 1995).

INSTRUMENTS FOR THE IDENTIFICATION OF DEPRESSION

Despite the obstacles to diagnosis just described, it is vitally important not to overlook cases of depression in the elderly, which, even in the most impaired individuals, may be responsive to treatment. Much effort has been devoted, therefore, to the development of screening strategies for case detection and rating scales to track the severity of the illness and its response to treatment (Blazer, 1989).

Some of these scales are used both in older and younger patients, some are designed for self-report, and others utilize interviews by trained or untrained observers to gather information from the patient or a family member or other caregiver. The advantages, disadvantages, and potential utility of each instrument will be described briefly. Information is provided about the sensitivity and specificity of some of these scales in older people; however, comparisons are made less reliable by the derivation of these numbers from different populations. Few studies have directly compared scales in the same population; of these, a number designate as the "gold standard" scales (e.g., the Hamilton Depression Rating Scale) that were not developed for the detection of depression in older adults.

Hamilton Depression Rating Scale (HAMD)

The HAMD (1960, 1967) is familiar to many psychiatric clinicians and is the most commonly used and best validated scale in the general adult population. Other, newer scales are often compared to this for validity; however, its emphasis on somatic symptoms has the potential to result in overdiagnosis of depression when applied to older adults, especially those with medical illnesses. It also requires a clinician trained in its administration, which limits its utility in nonpsychiatric settings. Using a cutoff score of 16, this scale has been reported to have a sensitivity of 87.5% and a specificity of 99.1% in a community-dwelling geriatric population (Mottram et al., 2000).

Beck Depression Inventory (BDI)

The BDI (1961) is a brief (20-minute), 21-item self-report scale that is widely used, but not specifically developed, for the geriatric population. As with other self-report scales, it suffers from the limitations imposed by patients' denial or lack of awareness of depressive symptoms. Although other cutoff scores have been used, a common choice is 17, which has been shown to differentiate patients with moderate depression from those without depressive symptoms with a sensitivity of 87% and a specificity of 85% (Beck et al., 1961; Burns et al., 1999).

Zung Self-Rating Depression Scale (SDS)

The SDS (1965) is a brief self-administered instrument with 20 statements, each representing a different depressive symptom. For 10 of these statements, a positive response indicates the presence of depressive symptoms. A negative response to any of the other 10 statements indicates the presence of depressive symptoms. Responses are rated from 1 to 4, covering the range from "a little of the time" to "most of the time." A scoring key is provided. Low scores indicate a low likelihood of depression. The final score is expressed as an index derived by converting the sum of the raw score values to a percentage of the maximum score of 80, with percentages greater than 50% suggesting depression (Zung, 1983). Using this cutoff score among geriatric patients, the sensitivity and specificity of the SDS have been reported to be 76% and 82%, respectively (Okimoto et al., 1982).

Montgomery Asberg Depression Rating Scale (MADRS)

The MADRS (1979) was designed especially to be sensitive to change in depression and is thus commonly used in antidepressant treatment trials. The scale requires a trained interviewer and measures apparent and reported sadness; inner tension; changes in sleep, appetite, and concentration; lassitude; inability to feel; and pessimistic and suicidal thoughts. Like the HAMD, it was not designed specifically to address geriatric depression. In a geriatric population, the sensitivity and specificity have been reported to be 72% and 98.9% using 21 as a cutoff score (Mottram et al., 2000).

Geriatric Depression Scale (GDS)

The original 30-item GDS (Yesavage, 1983) was developed by gathering 100 yes/no questions related to depression in the elderly and analyzing which 30 correlated best with the total score. The 15-item scale (GDS-S) (Sheikh, 1986) correlates with the 30-item scale and can be used as a briefer screening instrument, with a cutoff score of between 5 and 7 suggesting depression. With a cutoff score of 5/15, sensitivity of the GDS-S is reported to be 92% and specificity 81% (Lyness et al., 1997).

The GDS is a self-report scale and therefore does not require a trained interviewer. It is quite commonly used in clinical practice. The value of the scale is, however, limited by the quality of information provided by the patient. Studies in patients with dementia have suggested that it is not accurate in assessing demented individuals, especially those with a Mini Mental State Examination (MMSE) score less than 15 (McGivney et al., 1994).

Center for Epidemiological Studies–Depression Scale (CES-D)

The CES-D (Radloff and Teri, 1986) is a brief (5-minute), 20-item, self-administered screen that has been used in large studies of the general population and has been found to be useful as well in assessing elderly adults. It compares favorably to the use of the GDS in terms of sensitivity and specificity, which have been reported as 92% and 87% using a cutoff score of 21/60 (Lyness et al., 1997).

Cornell Scale for Depression in Dementia

The Cornell Scale (Alexopoulos et al., 1988) is a 19-item instrument that allows the clinician to collect information by observation and interview with the patient and from an informant. By incorporating multiple sources of information, this scale overcomes some of the difficulties of an instrument based solely on self-report, which, as noted previously, is often unreliable in dementia. The scale is correlated to the HAMD and thus suffers from some of the same limitations in terms of the symptomatology covered. A cutoff score of 7 has been reported to yield a sensitivity of 90% and specificity of 75% (Vida et al., 1994).

Brief Assessment Schedule Depression Cards (BASDEC)

The BASDEC assessment tool (Adshead et al., 1992) is designed for use in hospitalized geriatric patients, where privacy might be an issue. The patient is handed a deck of 19 cards with statements about depressive symptoms and is asked to place each of the cards into one of two piles, "True" or "False." The positive predictive value of this test was similar to that of the GDS, with sensitivity of 71% and specificity of 74% noted in this population.

Minimum Data Set Depression Rating Scale

This scale (Burrows et al., 2000) was developed by gathering results from the routine evaluation of nursing home patients using the Minimal Data Set of the Residential Assessment Instrument, which includes material about mood symptoms. These results were correlated with the Hamilton and Cornell scales to identify seven mood items, which could be used for screening this population and which compared favorably as an instrument with the 15-item GDS. With a cutoff score of 3, sensitivity was reported as 91% and specificity as 69% (Burrows et al., 2000).

LABORATORY TESTING

To date, no practical biological markers of depression aid in the diagnosis of depression. With older patients, however, laboratory testing is quite useful in identifying potentially treatable medical causes of depressive symptoms. This is true especially in patients presenting with an initial depressive episode in later life. Useful tests include complete blood count and chemistry panel, thyroid function tests, B_{12}, RBC folate, and urinalysis. When clinically indicated, laboratory testing may also be appropriate for the confirmation of other possible, but more unusual, causes of depression such as infectious diseases (VDRL, Lyme antibody titer), inflammatory or connective tissue diseases (ESR, ANA), endocrine disturbances (LH, FSH, testosterone, serum cortisol), drugs of abuse, or heavy metal poisoning (toxicology).

NEUROIMAGING

Computed tomography (CT) or structural magnetic resonance imaging (MRI) techniques have not yet proven helpful in establishing the diagnosis of depression, although localized left hemisphere infarcts (Robinson et al., 1984) and decreases in prefrontal volume (Kumar et al., 1998) have been associated with the presence of depression. More typically, MRI is useful in identifying the presence of nonpsychiatric pathological states that may produce depression-like symptoms. Subdural hematomas, cerebrovascular disease, normal pressure hydrocephalus, mass lesions, or certain infectious conditions may be detected in this way (van Crevel et al., 1999). MRI findings, too, can be considered along with other factors relevant to forecasting a patient's prognosis. The presence of extensive subcortical hyperintensities on MRI, for example, suggests a less robust response to treatment (Lloyd et al., 2001; Simpson et al., 1998).

Functional imaging of depressed patients' brains appears a promising area of current research. Depression in the elderly has been associated with reductions in whole brain glucose metabolic rate on PET scanning (Kumar, 1993; Meltzer et al., 1998). Increases in frontal myo-inositol/creatine and choline/creatine ratios on proton magnetic resonance spectroscopy have also been noted (Kumar et al., 2002). EEG can also provide an inexpensive, noninvasive screen of general brain activity that may have the potential to be a useful secondary screening investigation in depressed patients with suspected cognitive impairment or other CNS pathology (Kaszniak et al., 1979; Markland, 1990; Radermecker, 1977; Robinson et al., 1994).

SCREENING FOR LATE-LIFE DEPRESSION IN PRIMARY CARE

While screening instruments and rating scales for depression have been developed and implemented in many environments, screening in primary care is of particular importance. The PCP is usually the first line of treatment for the elderly (Gallo et al., 1995); unfortunately, as reviewed in greater detail elsewhere in this book, there are a number of barriers to detection (Blank et al., 2001; Williams-Russo, 1996). The presentation of depression is often confounded by concurrent medical problems, cognitive difficulties, and multiple medications. In addition, primary care physicians may not be sufficiently trained to recognize mood disturbances or may underestimate the value and importance of treatment in the elderly. They may feel that depression is of lesser importance than medical problems, or that it is a normal response to the losses associated with aging. In addition, the increasing time pressures and the rapid patient turnover in primary care make it more difficult to perform an in-depth interview and recognize changes in the patient's mood over time.

Screening tests would appear to be ideal as tools to increase case detection in primary care (Oxman, 1997) and are known to perform better than clinical impression alone (Mulrow et al., 1995). A review by Schade (1998), however, notes that the benefit of depression screening is hard to measure and remains controversial. Schade's data suggest that briefer tests, which have minimal costs in terms of time and personnel, perform as well as more complicated versions. Most screening tests, however, are based upon syndromal definitions of depression, which are more useful in hospital based research. In primary care settings, by contrast, up to 50% of patients with depressive symptoms and functional impairment are not adequately classified by current psychiatric categories (Barrett et al., 1988). The high prevalence in primary care populations of subsyndromal depressive states (described in detail in Chapter 4 of this book) is of particular importance. It is thus necessary to educate primary care providers in the use and limitations of currently available screening devices and to pursue research into alternative strategies (Gallo and Coyne, 2000).

In recent years, efforts have been made to screen for depression in the elderly in community settings, such as senior centers or libraries. National Depression Screening Day (NDSD), started in 1991, has become a large and successful program for screening and for educating the public about depression in general (Greenfield et al., 1997). In addition, NDSD has helped to destigmatize the illness and its treatment. The initial programs utilized the Zung Self-Rating Depression Scale (1965) and it was reported that a relatively large proportion of individuals screening positive sought subsequent care (Greenfield et al., 2000). More recently, the specially developed Harvard Department of Psychiatry National Depression Screening Day Scale (HANDS) has been used. Since 1998, an additional version of the screening program has been available for older individuals and has utilized the 15-item GDS. The results of the elderly outreach effort have not been reported to date; however, based upon the authors' experience with large-scale community-based memory screening (Lawrence et al., 2002), the success of such an endeavor may be limited by both the willingness of the older individual to seek treatment and its local availability.

LATE-ONSET DEPRESSION: A SUBSET OF DEPRESSION IN LATER LIFE

In the discussion of late-life depression, a distinction is often made between late-onset depression (that occurring for the first time in later life) and depression in late life that is a recurrence of an illness with earlier onset. Earlier onset illness is more commonly associated with a positive family history of depression and substance abuse, while later onset depression is more commonly associated with observable brain abnormalities, especially microvascular changes visible by neuroimaging techniques. Studies have investigated whether late-onset depression differs from late-life depression in terms of course and prognosis. While Reynolds et al. (1998) suggested that response to treatment was similar in both groups, other than the observation that earlier age of onset may predict a slower remission, other studies have gathered evidence that supports a different viewpoint (Alexopoulos et al., 1996; Caine et al., 1993). These studies have found that individuals with onset of depression after 60 may show a more intractable course of illness.

Some of the reported differences in outcome between late-onset and late-life depressions may be related to sample selection and whether a specific study included individuals who are more cognitively impaired or physically ill—characteristics associated with a poorer prognosis. It appears well established, however, that late-onset illness is associated with more structural brain abnormalities, such as enlarged ventricles and white matter hyperintensities (Krishnan and Gadde, 1996) and cognitive change. In a number of individuals, the cognitive changes develop into full-blown dementia of the vascular or Alzheimer type (Lebowitz et al., 1997). A worse outcome might intuitively be expected, therefore, in patients whose depression first began later in life.

DISTINGUISHING BETWEEN UNIPOLAR AND BIPOLAR DISORDERS

In order to provide appropriate treatment, unipolar depression must be distinguished from depression occurring in the context of a bipolar disorder. This can be rendered more difficult in the elderly population, where mania can present with increased irritability and confusion rather than with the euphoria, increased energy, hyperactivity, and mental content reflecting increased sexual interest, religiosity, and grandiosity more typical of younger adults (Shulman and Herrmann, 1999). Mania in the elderly can therefore be difficult to distinguish from an agitated unipolar depression.

As with unipolar depression, a distinction can also be made between early- and late-onset bipolar disorder. Schurhoff and colleagues (2000) found that earlier onset bipolar disorder was associated with more psychotic features, more mixed episodes, greater comorbidity with panic disorder and worse response to lithium prophylaxis than late-onset disorder. Late-onset bipolar disorder has also been associated in several studies with right hemisphere subcortical hyperintensities, which may represent vascular changes (Berthier et al., 1996; McDonald et al., 1991).

DEPRESSION AND DEMENTIA

One of the more vexing problems in accurately diagnosing depression in the elderly involves understanding the relationship between cognitive impairment and mood symptoms. Whether depression and dementia are related—and if so, the nature of the relationship— is a critical question. When depression is accompanied by cognitive symptoms that lead to a misdiagnosis of dementia, an elder may be subjected to the nihilistic attitude of "why bother doing anything?" and hence not receive treatment that might result in symptom remission and restoration of quality of life. Furthermore, when depression is a prodrome for dementia (Chen et al., 1999; Devanand et al., 1996; Raskind, 1998), recognition and assessment can in some cases lead to an early diagnosis and more effective treatment approach. When depression reflects an introspective awareness of loss of function due to underlying organic pathology, it may be important to address both the cognitive impairment and the associated depressive reaction (Berger et al., 1999; Dufouil et al, 1996; Geerlings et al., 2000).

Even in the absence of dementia per se, the presence of depression typically implies some degree of cognitive inefficiency. Diagnostic criteria for major depressive disorder include decline in concentration as well as apathy and abulia (DSM-IV-TR). A depressed individual who attends poorly to stimulus material, concentrates inadequately on the material to be processed, and lacks motivation will perform less than optimally on neuropsychological testing. Aging, too, contributes to cognitive inefficiency. The primary criteria for diagnosis of dementia in the elderly are cognitive in nature (DSM-IV-TR, NINCDS) and require that there be a disturbance of memory (Kindermann and Brown, 1997). Yet even before information can be stored in memory, it must be perceived, attended to, ordered, and understood. Furthermore, it must be communicated in some way after retrieval from memory storage (Bassuk et al., 1999). The apparent disturbance of memory seen in many older depressed patients may represent impairment of one of these associated cognitive functions rather than an inability to store or retrieve information. Precise characterization of a patient's cognitive difficulties by means of neuropsychological assessment can be diagnostically revealing.

"PSEUDODEMENTIA" AND THE DEMENTIA SYNDROME OF DEPRESSION

As early as the turn of the last century, Wernicke (1900) coined the term "pseudodementia" to refer to a group of prisoners, who during questioning, attempted to play the role of demented patients by providing immediate reflexive "I don't know" responses and giving tangential answers. Kiloh (1961) revived the term in describing a global cognitive decline that could be reversed by appropriate treatment of an underlying medical or psychiatric condition. Since that time the term "pseudodementia" has implied an acquired deterioration of cognitive function resembling that seen in organic dementia but whose origin and subsequent course are reversible (Caine, 1981; Caine, 1986; Cummings, 1989; Lamberty and Bieliauskas, 1993; Lishman, 1987; Sachdev et al., 1990; Wells, 1979). The etiologies of such cognitive decline vary (e.g., medication toxicity, hysteria, neuroendocrinological or other systemic illnesses), but there is agreement that the most common cause of pseudodementia is depression. In addition, there has been some thought that pseudodementia is not "pseudo" at all but rather is either a prodrome or the first expression of a true dementing process. As a result, the more specific term "dementia syndrome of depression" has been recommended and increasingly is used (Cummings, 1989).

While Wernicke (1900) clearly referred to pseudodementia as a form of malingering and Kiloh (1961) made it clear that the term is purely descriptive and carries no diagnostic meaning, it has commonly come to be used as a "pseudodiagnosis" (Lamberty and Bieliauskas, 1993). It is primarily applied to the elderly and implies both etiologic and prognostic implications beyond its originally descriptive purpose. Caine (1986), in attempting to characterize patients with pseudodementia, described deficits in cognition (e.g., arousal, attention concentration, visuoperceptual, executive function, memory and language), mood and affect, intellectual function, and personality function. Validity of the syndrome is supported by observations in some studies of improved cognitive functioning when such patients receive treatment directed at the mood disorder (Bassuk et al., 1998; Butters et al., 2000; La Rue et al., 1986; Rabins et al., 1984). Other studies, by contrast, have found an increased risk for subsequent organic dementia in patients who show cognitive symptoms consistent with a diagnosis of pseudodementia (Berger et al., 1999; Chen et al., 1999; Devanand et al., 1996; Geerlings et al., 2000). What then is to be made of the terms "pseudodementia" and "dementia syndrome of depression?" How are these terms of clinical value in assessment and prognosis? Much of the confusion in studies of cognition and depression in the elderly stems from the heterogeneity of depression as discussed earlier in this chapter. Are the cognitive dysfunctions seen in elderly depressed patients indicative of primary impairments or are they secondary to affective factors? If the former, do they predict further cognitive decline, and if the latter, are they merely transient in nature? In addition, the issue of whether such cognitive deficits are a function of depression or are related to inefficiencies resulting from normal aging must be addressed to fully explicate the relationship between depression and cognition in the geriatric population.

MAJOR DEPRESSION AND COGNITION IN YOUNGER ADULTS

Even younger depressed adults have been reported to perform poorly on cognitive tasks when compared with nondepressed individuals of the same age cohort. Following the DSM-IV-TR criteria for major depressive disorder, such poor performance has been attributed to impairments of attention, concentration, and memory (Burt et al., 1995; Cassens et al. 1990; Cavenar et al., 1979; Sweet, 1983). Veiel (1997), however, points out that most of these studies have serious methodological flaws and that there has been little attempt to delineate the nature and extent of cognitive deficits in young and middle-aged individuals with clearly diagnosed major depression.

Veiel (1997) performed a meta-analysis on 13 studies done since 1975 on individuals who were less than 60 years old, were diagnosed with major depression, and had no other known causes for cognitive impairment. He examined nine cognitive domains (i.e., simple attention, verbal fluency, scanning/tracking, visuospatial function, verbal learning/acquisition, verbal learning/retention, nonverbal learning/acquisition, nonverbal learning/retention, and mental flexibility). In addition, he studied reaction time, a variable not usually measured in standardized neuropsychological tests but known to be sensitive to speed of mental processing. His analysis found that depressed individuals were severely impaired, compared to nondepressed individuals, in measures of mental flexibility and reaction time. Performance in other domains was noted to be highly variable. These functions are, however, dependent on many noncognitive factors. Veiel (1997) concluded that the cognitive deficits of patients with depression most closely resemble those of patients with frontal lobe syndrome.

A more recent study by Grant, Thase, and Sweeney (2001) noted that almost all cognitive domains have been implicated in studies of patients with depression. They administered complete neuropsychological batteries to two groups of individuals: one with clearly defined DSM-IV-TR nonbipolar, nonchronic major depressive disorder without psychotic features, and the other consisting of healthy controls. They reached the same conclusions as Veiel (1997), finding significant and consistent differences on parameters measuring mental flexibility and reaction time. They further noted that reaction time correlated inversely with assessed severity of depression.

It would appear that nongeriatric patients with major depression present with cognitive deficits primarily involving executive functions and psychometrically resemble individuals with frontal lobe syndrome. Reaction time appears to be a sensitive indicator of both the severity of the depression (Grant et al., 2001) and, in general, of the degree of frontal involvement (Gronwall, 1989).

MAJOR DEPRESSION AND COGNITION IN OLDER ADULTS

Memory complaints among the elderly are ubiquitous. Complaints also increase in frequency with severity of depression (Lamberty and Bieliauskas, 1993). Yet performance on neuropsychological measures of memory demonstrates no consistent problems with memory function. Most studies suggest the contrary—that at worst there are only the subtlest of differences between healthy and depressed elders. Small differences have been noted in the acquisition of new information, although additional evidence suggests these differences primarily involve simple attention and/or depth of encoding (Craik and Lockhart, 1972; Weingartner et al., 1981). Repeated presentation of information eliminates even these differences (Weingartner et al., 1981). Likewise, rates of forgetting, recall, and retrieval all appear to be equivalent for depressed and healthy elderly individuals (Lamberty and Bieliauskas, 1993). Burt and colleagues (1995) did find that depression and memory impairment are significantly associated, but the magnitude of the association was quite small compared with the magnitude of the association between memory impairment and dementia.

Similarly, no obvious differences in terms of receptive and expressive language distinguish healthy from depressed elders. Emery and Breslau (1989) did note subtle deficits on measures of naming, repetition, reading, and verbal comprehension for elders with depression. They point out, however, that the magnitude of these differences was much smaller than the magnitude of the differences between depressed and demented elders. Verbal fluency has been shown to be impaired on controlled oral word association tasks (Hart et al., 1988), but this difficulty vanishes when the task is made less effortful through the use of categorical rather than phonemic cues. It would therefore appear that the apparent inefficiency of a depressed cognition derives from slowed mentation and decreased effort rather than from primary language problems. A recent study by Lockwood, Alexopoulos, and van Gorp (2002) attempted to characterize the neuropsychological presentation of elders with major depression. In examining four subject groups consisting of normal and depressed adults between 20 and 60 and normal and depressed elders (older than 61) on a variety of standardized neuropsychological measures, they found that the elders with major depression demonstrated significant impairments in executive functions when compared with either younger adults (with or without depression) or healthy elders. They noted particular deficits in initiation and inhibition, cognitive flexibility, complex mental manipulation, and processing speed. As with younger adults with depression, it appears that the cognitive profile of individuals with late-life depression resembles that seen in those with frontal lobe syndrome. Lockwood, Alexopoulos, and van Gorp (2002) further note that these executive inefficiencies are more pronounced in older depressed individuals than in younger ones. They hypothesize that age-related changes in metabolism and the volume of prefrontal and orbital frontal areas may provide an explanation for their findings.

COGNITION AND NORMAL AGING

The issue of cognitive functioning and normal aging must be addressed in order to provide a context for assessing elders' performance on neuropsychological tests. As individuals age, a series of anatomic, biochemical, physiologic, pharmacologic, and support system changes underlie the progressive involution of the nervous system and the development of cognitive inefficiencies. Both Davidoff (1994) and Albert (1994) have reviewed the nature of these changes, which imply impairment in the domains of memory and executive functions as well as in speed of processing. In other words, "crystallized" intelligence—which relies on the use of previously stored information manipulated in familiar ways—remains fairly constant even through the eighth decade of life. "Fluid" intelligence—which requires the manipulation of novel material in unfamiliar and complex ways—begins to show deterioration as early as the fifth decade of life (Davidoff, 1994; Dufouil et al., 1996; Veiel, 1997). Furthermore, this increasing inefficiency is exacerbated by generally slowed mental processing speed. The point at which such changes intrude in everyday life and the actual magnitude and rate of change varies on an individual basis and with particular cognitive domains. Hence, cognitive dysfunctions in healthy elders do not arise uniformly and are subject to a wide range of individual variations. While much progress has been made in establishing age-related normative comparisons for many standardized neuropsychological tests, caution must still be exercised in interpreting the nature and extent of cognitive deficits in a specific elderly individual.

SUBJECTIVE MEMORY COMPLAINTS

Elders with depression report more cognitive complaints than either healthy elders or demented individuals (Berger et al., 1999; Grut et al., 1993). Nonetheless, formal neuropsychological examination reveals that depressed individuals often underestimate their own memories, which on objective testing are often within the normal range (Grut et al., 1993). By contrast, an abnormal degree of abulia and apathy are often observed in depressed elders. It has been shown that the use of stimuli with high affective valence can improve selective attention, and hence, memory, for otherwise normal individuals who are functioning in a diminished state of consciousness (Davidoff et al., 1984; Paul, 1964). Furthermore, Rapaport (1942) has postulated that in such a diminished state, affect plays an organizing and directing role in the processing of information. Care must therefore be taken in both the selection of mental test materials and in the affective tone of actual presentation of such tests to the individual.

DEMENTIA WITH DEPRESSION

Dementia is often accompanied by depression, requiring in assessment a sensitivity to the manner in which each disorder impairs cognitive functioning. It is known, for example, that the prevalence of depression among elders with a primary degenerative dementia is markedly greater than in the general elderly population (Bassuk et al., 1998). Some studies find major depressive disorder in 10% to 30% of individuals with dementia (Cancellaro, 2001). This phenomenon of comorbidity occurs particularly in the earlier stages of dementia, when the individual still retains a reflective sense of self and can appreciate his or her own failing cognitive abilities (Migliorelli et al., 1995; Ott and Fogel, 1992). Furthermore, some studies suggest that elders manifesting cognitive dysfunction are, in fact, more vulnerable to the cognitive sequelae of depression and may demonstrate apparent exacerbation of impairment in particular cognitive domains (e.g., memory) (Veiel, 1997).

IN SEARCH OF CLARITY

The exact nature of the relationship between depression and dementia remains unresolved. Is an episode of depression that occurs years before the development of clinically significant dementia a prodrome, a risk factor, or an unrelated event? Can a major depressive episode be a consequence of the awareness of encroaching cognitive decline secondary to dementia even before clear clinical manifestations of organic brain disease are observable to others? As early as 1915, Kraepelin (1915), on the basis of longitudinal observation, expressed his belief that depression is a common prodrome of dementia in the elderly. In contrast, Roth (1955) found late-life depression to be unrelated to the eventual development of a dementing illness. A variety of studies continue to seek resolution of the issue of cause—consequence or happenstance (Bassuk et al., 1998;

Beekman et al., 2002; Chen et al., 1999; Geerlings et al., 2000; Kramer-Ginsberg et al., 1999; Lamberty and Bieliauskas, 1993; Lavretsky and Kumar, 2002; Raskind, 1998; Veiel, 1997; Yaffe et al., 1999).

Recent studies by several groups of investigators all demonstrate a moderately increased risk for later diagnosis of dementia in older patients with depressed mood and/or a diagnosis of major depressive disorder at baseline (Bassuk et al., 1998; Chen et al., 1999; Devanand et al., 1996). These findings apply, however, only to those individuals in whom cognitive impairment is already apparent at baseline. It appears that for such individuals (i.e., those with depressed mood and some degree of cognitive impairment), depression may indeed be a prodrome for dementia. A study by Butters and colleagues (2000) provided additional support for the idea that depression without cognitive impairment may be different from depression with cognitive deficits in an elderly population. In this study, depressed elderly patients' performance on neuropsychological testing was shown to improve significantly following antidepressant treatment when baseline cognitive impairment was present, but not when such impairment was absent at baseline. In addition, Lamberty and Bieliauskas (1993), Lauretsky and Kumar (2002), and Kramer-Ginsberg and colleagues (1999) all found increased risk for significant cognitive impairment and the subsequent development of dementia in depressed patients with white matter findings on neuroimaging.

Speck and colleagues (1995) demonstrated an association between the development of Alzheimer's disease and episodes of depression occurring (and resolving) 10 years before the onset of Alzheimer's. They found no such relationship for episodes of depression less than 10 years before the beginning of significant cognitive impairment. In contrast, Jorm and colleagues (1991), in examining the association between history of depression and Alzheimer's disease, came to the conclusion that there was increased risk of primary degenerative dementia for any episode of depression, including those within 10 years of onset of dementia. Raskind (1998) suggests a neuroendocrinological explanation for this observed relationship between depression and dementia. He notes that late-life depression is associated with increased activity of the hypothalamic–pituitary–adrenal axis. The hippocampal pyramid neurons, which are known to be implicated in Alzheimer's disease, may in turn be especially vulnerable to increased circulating cortisol concentrations, therefore increasing the risk for developing Alzheimer's disease. Interestingly, a number of other studies found no relationship between depression and subsequent cognitive decline (Bassuk et al., 1998; Dufouil et al., 1996; Henderson et al., 1997).

At the current time, no single framework, "theory," or explanation has proven to be of general value in understanding the precise nature of the relationship between cognitive impairment and depressed mood or between depression and dementia. Nonetheless, neuropsychological testing can help shed some light on this debate. There is general agreement that the nature of cognitive impairments in depressed elders tends to be of a subtle nature, such that MMSE performance, for example, may be unrevealing (Butters et al., 2000; Geerlings et al., 2000). More extensive neuropsychological testing, however, is of significant value in delineating the nature and magnitude of the executive function deficits observed in depressed patients. Normative studies now make it possible to distinguish depression-associated cognitive inefficiencies from normal functioning in elders. Similarly, the diagnosis of dementia can be clarified through the use of neuropsychological testing.

The evaluation of the relationship of cognitive and mood symptoms in any individual patient remains the province of an interdisciplinary team. A careful history of the nature and progression of the symptoms is of critical importance in diagnosing the patient. Rapid onset of cognitive difficulties is more suggestive of depression than of dementia, which commonly takes years to develop. Subjective memory complaints are more common in elders with family history of depression and/or dementia, substance abuse history, and history of head trauma. These all provide critical data important to accurate diagnosis and appropriate treatment.

Until such time as a definitive theory is developed, it is suggested that a more precise "pseudonosology" be adopted. To that end, it is suggested that the term "pseudodementia" be reserved for individuals with major depression who evidence no positive findings on neuropsychological testing. This harks back to Wernicke's (1900) original use of the term to define individuals whose primary mode of response to questions is "I don't know." The use of the term "dementia syndrome of depression" would be applied to those individuals with major depression and significant cognitive impairment on formal testing. There is at least some strong evidence that such patients are at risk for developing dementia and that timely treatment with cholinesterase inihibitors may prolong quality of life. Finally, the term "dementia with depression" would be applied to those individuals who, on neuropsychological examination, meet criteria for a diagnosis of possible/probable dementia and who also have a DSM-IV-TR diagnosis of major depression or, alternatively, meet the new criteria for depression in dementia cited previously. Given the lack of subtlety of simple mental status testing (e.g., MMSE), it appears that formal neuropsychological evaluation can play a critical role in the identification of those elders who are at greatest risk and most likely to benefit from early interventions.

SUMMARY

Depression in the elderly is heterogeneous and often presents differently from depression in younger adults. Older patients may present with fewer symptoms, or a different spectrum of symptoms, than are required when diagnosing major depressive disorder in younger adults. Emphasis on somatic and cognitive concerns rather than psychological distress can distract the clinician from accurately diagnosing depression. In addition, comorbid medical and cognitive factors, including dementia, can further complicate the diagnosis of depression in the elderly by introducing confounding symptoms, which may cause the depression itself to be overlooked, underdiagnosed, and untreated. Current nosologic systems, such as the DSM-IV-TR, do not adequately describe the range of presentations of depression in the elderly. Hence, terms such as "pseudodementia," "dementia syndrome of depression," "subsyndromal depression," and "nonmajor depressive disorder" have each been utilized in an attempt to adequately describe the range of clinical pictures encountered. Consensus on nosology would be helpful in facilitating appropriate interventions and the further study of depression in this population.

In the interim, efforts to train nonpsychiatric care providers—who provide the bulk of care to the depressed elderly—in the utilization of appropriate screening methods and instruments may increase the rate of detection of depression and increase the opportunities for successful treatment. Furthermore, an understanding the limitations of such screening instruments will encourage the care provider to make referrals in difficult or questionable cases. As our understanding of late-life depression increases, it is to be hoped that an increasing number of affected individuals will be correctly detected, diagnosed, and offered the potential benefits of appropriate treatment.

REFERENCES

Adshead F, Cody DD, Pitt B. BASDEC: a novel screening instrument for depression in elderly medical inpatients. BMJ 1992; 305:397.

Albert MS. Age-related changes in cognitive function. In: Albert ML, Knoefel JE, eds. Clinical Neurology of Aging. New York: Oxford University Press, 1994:314–328.

Alexopoulos GS, Abrams RC, Young RC, Shamoian CA. Cornell Scale for Depression in Dementia. Biol Psychiatry 1988; 23:271–284.

Alexopoulos GS, Meyers BS, Young RC, Kakuma T, Feder M, Einhorn A, Rosendahl E. Recovery in geriatric depression. Arch Gen Psychiatry 1996; 53:305–312.

American Psychiatric Association. Diagnostic and Statistical Manual of Mental Disorders. Washington, DC: American Psychiatric Press, 2000.

Ballard C, Bannister C, Oyebode F. Depression in dementia sufferers. International Journal of Geriatric Psychiatry 1996; 11:507–515.

Barrett JE, Barrett JA, Oxman TE, Gerber PD. The prevalence of psychiatric disorders in a primary care practice. Arch Gen Psychiatry 1988; 45:1100–1106.

Barsky AJ. Amplification, somatization, and the somatoform disorders. Psychosomatics 1992; 33:28–34.

Bassuk SS, Berkman, LF, Wypij D. Depressive symptomatology and incident cognitive decline in an elderly community sample. Arch Gen Psychiatry 1998; 55:1073–1081.

Bassuk SS, Glass TA, Berkman LF. Social disengagement and incident cognitive decline in community-dwelling elderly persons. Ann Intern Med 1999; 131:165–173.

Beck A, Ward C, Mendelson M, Mock J, Erbaugh J. An inventory for measuring depression. Arch Gen Psychiatry 1961; 4:53–63.

Beekman AT, Geerlings SW, Deeg DJ, Smit JH, Schoevers RS, De Beurs E, Braam AW, Penninx BW, Van Tilburg W. The natural history of late-life depression: a 6-year prospective study in the community. Arch Gen Psychiatry 2002; 59:605–611.

Berger AK, Fratiglioni L, Forsell Y, Winblad B, Backman L. The occurrence of depressive symptoms in the preclinical phase of AD: a population-based study. Neurology 1999; 53:1998–2002.

Berthier ML, Kulisevsky J, Gironell A, Fernandez Benitez JA. Poststroke bipolar affective disorder: clinical subtypes, concurrent movement disorders, and anatomical correlates. J Neuropsychiatry Clin Neurosci 1996; 8:160–167,

Blank K, Cohen C, Cohen G. Failure to adequately detect suicidal intent in elderly patients in the primary care setting. Clinical Geriatrics 2001; 9:26–36.

Blazer D. Depression in the elderly. N Engl J Med 1989; 320:164–166.

Burkhart KS. Diagnosis of depression in the elderly patient. Prim Care Pract 2000; 4: 149–162.

Burns A, Lawlor B, Craig S. Assessment scales in old age psychiatry. London: Martin Dunitz, 1999.

Burrows AB, Morris JN, Simon SE, Hirdes JP, Phillips C. Development of a minimum data set–based depression rating scale for use in nursing homes. Age Ageing 2000; 29:165–172.

Burt DB, Zembar MJ, Niederehe G. Depression and memory impairment: a meta-analysis of the association, its pattern, and specificity. Psychol Bull 1995; 117:285–305.

Butters MA, Becker JT, Nebes RD, Zmuda MD, Mulsant BH, Pollock BG, Reynolds CF 3rd. Changes in cognitive functioning following treatment of late-life depression. Am J Psychiatry 2000; 157:1949–1954.

Caine E, Lyness J, DA K. Reconsidering depression in the elderly. Am J Geriatr Psychiatry 1993; 1:4–20.

Caine ED. Pseudodementia. Current concepts and future directions. Arch Gen Psychiatry 1981; 38:1359–1364.

Caine ED. The neuropsychology of depression: the pseudodementia syndrome. In: Grant I, Adams K, eds. Neuropsychological Assessment of Neuropsychiatric Disorders. New York: Oxford University Press, 1986:221–243.

Cancellaro LA. Depression or dementia? South Med J 2001; 94:663.

Cassens G, Wolfe L, Zola M. The neuropsychology of depressions. J Neuropsychiatry Clin Neurosci 1990; 2:202–213.

Cavenar JO, Maltbie AA, Austin L. Depression simulating organic brain disease. Am J Psychiatry 1979; 136:521–523.

Chen P, Ganguli M, Mulsant BH, DeKosky ST. The temporal relationship between depressive symptoms and dementia: a community-based prospective study. Arch Gen Psychiatry 1999; 56:261–266.

Craik FM, Lockhart RS. Levels of processing: A framework for memory research. Journal of Verbal Learning and Verbal Behavior 1972; 11:671–684.

Cummings JL. Dementia and depression: an evolving enigma. J Neuropsychiatry Clin Neurosci 1989; 1:236–242.
Davidoff DA. The recognition and treatment of dementia. In: Ellison JM, Weinstein CS, Hodel-Malinofsky T, eds. The Psychotherapist's Guide to Neuropsychiatry: Diagnostic and Treatment Issues. Washington: American Psychiatric Press, 1994: 487–556.
Davidoff DA, Butters N, Gerstman LJ, Zurif E, Paul IH, Mattis S. Affective/motivational factors in the recall of prose passages by alcoholic Korsakoff patients. Alcohol 1984; 1:63–69.
Devanand DP, Sano M, Tang MX, Taylor S, Gurland BJ, Wilder D, Stern Y, Mayeux R. Depressed mood and the incidence of Alzheimer's disease in the elderly living in the community. Arch Gen Psychiatry 1996; 53:175–182.
Dufouil C, Fuhrer R, Dartigues JF, Alperovitch A. Longitudinal analysis of the association between depressive symptomatology and cognitive deterioration. Am J Epidemiol 1996; 144:634–641.
Emery OB, Breslau LD. Language deficits in depression: comparisons with SDAT and normal aging. J Gerontol 1989; 44:M85–M92.
Gallo JJ, Coyne JC. The challenge of depression in late life: bridging science and service in primary care. JAMA 2000; 284:1570–1572.
Gallo JJ, Marino S, Ford D, Anthony JC. Filters on the pathway to mental health care: II. sociodemographic factors. Psychol Med 1995; 25:1149–1160.
Geerlings MI, Schoevers RA, Beekman AT, Jonker C, Deeg DJ, Schmand B, Ader HJ, Bouter LM, Van Tilburg W. Depression and risk of cognitive decline and Alzheimer's disease. Results of two prospective community-based studies in the Netherlands. Br J Psychiatry 2000; 176:568–575.
Grant MM, Thase ME, Sweeney JA. Cognitive disturbance in outpatient depressed younger adults: evidence of modest impairment. Biol Psychiatry 2001; 50:35–43.
Greenfield SF, Reizes JM, Magruder KM, Muenz LR, Kopans B, Jacobs DG. Effectiveness of community-based screening for depression. Am J Psychiatry 1997; 154: 1391–1397.
Greenfield SF, Reizes JM, Muenz LR, Kopans B, Kozloff RC, Jacobs DG. Treatment for depression following the 1996 National Depression Screening Day. Am J Psychiatry 2000; 157:1867–1869.
Gronwall D. Cumulative and persisting effects of concussion on attention and cognition. In: Levin HS, Eisenberg HM, Benton AL, eds. Mild Head Injury. New York: Oxford University Press, 1989:153–162.
Grut M, Jorm AF, Fratiglioni L, Forsell Y, Viitanen M, Winblad B. Memory complaints of elderly people in a population survey: variation according to dementia stage and depression. J Am Geriatr Soc 1993; 41:1295–1300.
Hamilton M. A rating scale for depression. Journal of Neurology, Neurosurgery and Psychiatry 1960; 23:56–62.
Hamilton M. Development of a rating scale for primary depressive illness. Br J Soc Clin Psychol 1967; 6:278–296.
Hart RP, Kwentus JA, Taylor JR, Harmer RM. Productive naming and memory in depression and Alzheimer's type dementia. Arch Clin Neuropsychol 1988; 3:313–322.

Henderson AS, Korten AE, Jacomb PA, Mackinnon AJ, Jorm AF, Christensen H, Rodgers B. The course of depression in the elderly: a longitudinal community-based study in Australia. Psychol Med 1997; 27:119–129.

Jorm AF, Van Duijn CM, Chandra V, Fratiglioni L, Graves AB, Heyman A, Kokmen E, Kondo K, Mortimer JA, Rocca WA, et al. Psychiatric history and related exposures as risk factors for Alzheimer's disease: a collaborative re-analysis of case-control studies: EURODEM Risk Factors Research Group. Int J Epidemiol 1991; 20(suppl 2):S43–S47.

Kaszniak AW, Garron DC, Fox JH, Bergen D, Huckman M. Cerebral atrophy, EEG slowing age, education, and cognitive functioning in suspected dementia. Neurology 1979; 29:1273–1279.

Kiloh LG. Pseudo-dementia. Acta Psychiatrica Scandinavica 1961; 37:336–351.

Kindermann SS, Brown GG. Depression and memory in the elderly: a meta-analysis. J Clin Exp Neuropsychol 1997; 19:625–642.

Koenig HG, Cohen HJ, Blazer DG, Krishnan KR, Sibert TE. Profile of depressive symptoms in younger and older medical inpatients with major depression. J Am Geriatr Soc 1993; 41:1169–1176.

Koenig HG, Pappas P, Holsinger T, Bachar JR. Assessing diagnostic approaches to depression in medically ill older adults: how reliably can mental health professionals make judgments about the cause of symptoms? J Am Geriatr Soc 1995; 43:472–478.

Kraepelin E. Clinical Psychiatry: A Textbook for Students and Physicians. New York: Macmillan, 1915.

Kramer-Ginsberg E, Greenwald BS, Krishnan KR, Christiansen B, Hu J, Ashtari M, Patel M, Pollack S. Neuropsychological functioning and MRI signal hyperintensities in geriatric depression. Am J Psychiatry 1999; 156:438–444.

Krishnan K, Gadde K. The pathophysiologic basis for late-life depression—imaging studies of the aging brain. Am J Geriatr Psychiatry 1996; 4:S22–S33.

Kumar A. Functional brain imaging in late-life depression and dementia. J Clin Psychiatry 1993; 54(suppl):21–25.

Kumar A, Jin Z, Bilker W, Udupa J, Gottlieb G. Late-onset minor and major depression: early evidence for common neuroanatomical substrates detected by using MRI. Proc Natl Acad Sci USA 1998; 95:7654–7658.

Kumar A., Thomas A, Lavretsky H, Yue K, Huda A, Curran J, Venkatraman T, Estanol L, Mintz J, Mega M, Toga A. Frontal white matter biochemical abnormalities in late-life major depression detected with proton magnetic resonance spectroscopy. Am J Psychiatry 2002; 159:630–636.

La Rue A, Spar J, Hill CD. Cognitive impairment in late-life depression: clinical correlates and treatment implications. J Affect Disord 1986; 11:179–184.

Lamberty GJ, Bieliauskas. Distinguishing between depression and dementia in the elderly: a review of neuropsychological findings. Arch Clin Neuropsychol 1993; 8: 149–170.

Lavretsky H, Kumar A. Clinically significant non-major depression: old concepts, new insights. Am J Geriatr Psychiatry 2002; 10:239–255.

Lawrence J, Davidoff D, Katt-Lloyd D, Connell A, Berlow Y, Savoie J. Is large scale community memory screening feasible? [Submitted.]

Lebowitz BD, Pearson JL, Schneider LS, Reynolds CF 3rd, Alexopoulos GS, Bruce ML, Conwell Y, Katz IR, Meyers BS, Morrison MF, Mossey J, Niederehe G, Parmelee P. Diagnosis and treatment of depression in late life: consensus statement update. JAMA 1997; 278:1186–1190.

Lishman WA. Organ Psychiatry. Oxford: Blackwell Scientific Publications, 1987.

Lloyd AJ, Grace JB, Jaros E, Perry RH, Fairbairn AF, Swann AG, O'Brien JT, McKeith IG. Depression in late life, cognitive decline and white matter pathology in two clinico-pathologically investigated cases. Int J Geriatr Psychiatry 2001; 16:281–287.

Lockwood KA, Alexopoulos GS, Van Gorp WG. Executive dysfunction in geriatric depression. Am J Psychiatry 2002; 159:1119–1126.

Lyness JM, Bruce ML, Koenig HG, Parmelee PA, Schulz R, Lawton MP, Reynolds CF 3rd. Depression and medical illness in late life: report of a symposium. J Am Geriatr Soc 1996; 44:198–203.

Lyness JM, Cox C, Curry J, Conwell Y, King DA, Caine ED. Older age and the underreporting of depressive symptoms. J Am Geriatr Soc 1995; 43:216–221.

Lyness JM, Noel TK, Cox C, King DA, Conwell Y, Caine ED. Screening for depression in elderly primary care patients: a comparison of the Center for Epidemiologic Studies–Depression Scale and the Geriatric Depression Scale. Arch Intern Med 1997; 157:449–454.

Markand ON. Organic brain syndromes and dementias. In: Daly D, Pedley T, eds. Current Practice of Clinical Neurophysiology: Electroencephalography. New York: Raven Press, 1990:371–400.

McDonald WM, Krishnan KR, Doraiswamy PM, Blazer DG. Occurrence of subcortical hyperintensities in elderly subjects with mania. Psychiatry Res 1991; 40:211–220.

McGivney SA, Mulvihill M, Taylor B. Validating the GDS depression screen in the nursing home. J Am Geriatr Soc 1994; 42:490–492.

Meltzer CC, Smith G, DeKosky ST, Pollock BG, Mathis CA, Moore RY, Kupfer DJ, Reynolds CF 3rd. Serotonin in aging, late-life depression, and Alzheimer's disease: the emerging role of functional imaging. Neuropsychopharmacology 1998; 18:407–430.

Migliorelli R, Teson A, Sabe L, Petracchi M, Leiguarda R, Starkstein SE. Prevalence and correlates of dysthymia and major depression among patients with Alzheimer's disease. Am J Psychiatry 1995; 152:37–44.

Montgomery SA, Asberg M. A new depression scale designed to be sensitive to change. Br J Psychiatry 1979; 134:382–389.

Mottram P, Wilson K, Copeland J. Validation of the Hamilton Depression Rating Scale and Montgomery and Asberg Rating Scales in terms of AGECAT depression cases. Int J Geriatr Psychiatry 2000; 15:1113–1119.

Mulrow CD, Williams JW Jr., Gerety MB, Ramirez G, Montiel OM, Kerber C. Case-finding instruments for depression in primary care settings. Ann Intern Med 1995; 122:913–921.

Okimoto JT, Barnes RF, Veith RC, Raskind MA, Inui TS, Carter WB. Screening for depression in geriatric medical patients. Am J Psychiatry 1982; 139:799–802.

Olin JT, Katz IR, Meyers BS, Schneider LS, Lebowitz BD. Provisional diagnostic criteria for depression of Alzheimer disease: rationale and background. Am J Geriatr Psychiatry 2002; 10:129–141.

Olin JT, Schneider LS, Katz IR, Meyers BS, Alexopoulos GS, Breitner JC, Bruce ML, Caine ED, Cummings JL, Devanand DP, Krishnan KR, Lyketsos CG, Lyness JM, Rabins PV, Reynolds CF 3rd, Rovner BW, Steffens DC, Tariot PN, Lebowitz BD. Provisional diagnostic criteria for depression of Alzheimer disease. Am J Geriatr Psychiatry 2002; 10:125–128.

Ott BR, Fogel BS. Measurement of depression in dementia: self vs. clinical rating. Int J Geriatr Psychiatry 1992; 7:899–904.

Oxman TE. New paradigms for understanding the identification and treatment of depression in primary care. Gen Hosp Psychiatry 1997; 19:79–81.

Paul IH. The effects of drug-induced aliteration in state of consciousness as retention of drive-related verbal material. J Nerv Ment Dis 1964; 138:367–374.

Rabins PV, Merchant A, Nestadt G. Criteria for diagnosing reversible dementia caused by depression: validation by 2-year follow-up. Br J Psychiatry 1984; 144:488–492.

Radermecker FJ. Degenerative diseases of the nervous system. In: Remond A, ed. Handbook of Electroencephalography and Clinical Neurophysiology, vol 15A. Amsterdam: Elsevier, 1977:162–191.

Radloff L, Teri L. Use of the Center for Epidemiological Studies–Depression Scale in older adults. Clin Gerontol 1986; 5:119–137.

Rapaport D. Emotions and Memory. New York: International University Press, 1942.

Raskind MA. The clinical interface of depression and dementia. J Clin Psychiatry 1998; 59(suppl 10):9–12.

Reynolds CF 3rd, Dew MA, Frank E, Begley AE, Miller MD, Cornes C, Mazumdar S, Perel JM, Kupfer DJ. Effects of age at onset of first lifetime episode of recurrent major depression on treatment response and illness course in elderly patients. Am J Psychiatry 1998; 155:795–799.

Robinson DJ, Merskey H, Blume WT, Fry R, Williamson PC, Hachinski VC. Electroencephalography as an aid in the exclusion of Alzheimer's disease. Arch Neurol 1994; 51:280–284.

Robinson RG, Starr LB, Lipsey JR, Rao K, Price TR. A two-year longitudinal study of post-stroke mood disorders: dynamic changes in associated variables over the first six months of follow-up. Stroke 1984; 15:510–517.

Roth M. The natural history of mental disorder in old age. J Ment Sci 1955; 101:281–301.

Sachdev PS, Smith JS, Anus-Lepan H, Rodriguez P. Pseudodementia twelve years on. J Neurol Neurosurg Psychiatry 1990; 53:254–259.

Schade CP, Jones ER Jr., Wittlin BJ. A ten-year review of the validity and clinical utility of depression screening. Psychiatr Serv 1998; 49:55–61.

Schurhoff F, Bellivier F, Jouvent R, Mouren-Simeoni MC, Bouvard M, Allilaire JF, Leboyer M. Early and late onset bipolar disorders: two different forms of manic-depressive illness? J Affect Disord 2000; 58:215–221.

Sheikh J YJ. Geriatric Depression Scale: recent findings and development of a short version. In: Brink TL, ed. Clinical Gerontology: A Guide to Assessment and Intervention. New York: Howarth Press, 1986.

Shulman KI, Herrmann N. The nature and management of mania in old age. Psychiatr Clin North Am 1999; 22:649–665.

Simon GE, VonKorff M, Piccinelli M, Fullerton C, Ormel J. An international study of the relation between somatic symptoms and depression. N Engl J Med 1999; 341: 1329–1335.
Simpson S, Baldwin RC, Jackson A, Burns AS. Is subcortical disease associated with a poor response to antidepressants? Neurological, neuropsychological and neuroradiological findings in late-life depression. Psychol Med 1998; 28:1015–1026.
Speck CE, Kukull WA, Brenner DE, Bowen JD, McCormick WC, Teri L, Pfanschmidt ML, Thompson JD, Larson EB. History of depression as a risk factor for Alzheimer's disease. Epidemiology 1995; 6:366–369.
Sweet JJ. Confounding effects of depression on neuropsychological testing: five illustrative cases. Clin Neuropsychology 1983; 5:103–109.
van Crevel H, van Gool WA, Walstra GJ. Early diagnosis of dementia: which tests are indicated? What are their costs? J Neurol 1999; 246:73–78.
Veiel HO. A preliminary profile of neuropsychological deficits associated with major depression. J Clin Exp Neuropsychol 1997; 19:587–603.
Vida S, Des Rosiers P, Carrier L, Gauthier S. Depression in Alzheimer's disease: receiver operating characteristic analysis of the Cornell Scale for Depression in Dementia and the Hamilton Depression Scale. J Geriatr Psychiatry Neurol 1994; 7: 159–162.
Weingartner H, Cohen RM, Murphy DL, Martello J, Gerdt C. Cognitive processes in depression. Arch Gen Psychiatry 1981; 38:42–47.
Wells CE. Pseudodementia. Am J Psychiatry 1979; 136:895–900.
Wernicke C. Grundiss der Psychiatric I Klinischen Vorlesungen. Leipzeig, Germany: Thieme, 1900.
Whooley MA, Simon GE. Managing depression in medical outpatients. N Engl J Med 2000; 343:1942–1950.
Williams-Russo. Barriers to diagnosis of depression in primary care. Am J Geriatr Psychiatry 1996; 4:S84–S90.
Yaffe K, Blackwell T, Gore R, Sands L, Reus V, Browner WS. Depressive symptoms and cognitive decline in nondemented elderly women: a prospective study. Arch Gen Psychiatry 1999; 56:425–430.
Yesavage JA BT, Rose TL, Lum O, Huang V, Adey M, Leirer VO. Development and validation of a geriatric depression screening scale: a preliminary report. Journal of Psychiatric Research 1983; 17:37–49.
Zung W. A self-rating scale for depression. Arch Gen Psychiatry 1965; 12:63–70.
Zung W. Self-rating scales for psychopathology. In: Crook T, Ferris S, Bartus R, eds. Assessment in geriatric psychopharmacology. New Canaan, CT: Mark Powley Associates, 1983:145–151.

4

Geriatric Nonmajor Depressive Syndromes
Dysthymia, Subsyndromal Depression, and Other Nonmajor Depressive Disorders in the Elderly

Jennifer L. Woehr
McLean Hospital, Belmont, and Harvard Medical School, Boston, Massachusetts, U.S.A.

Martin Goldstein
Weill Medical College of Cornell University, New York, New York, U.S.A.

INTRODUCTION

Mild to moderate depressive symptoms in the elderly are sometimes regarded by clinicians or family members as a natural consequence of aging. Substantial evidence, however, indicates that such symptoms have important individual and public health consequences (Beekman et al., 2002). Dysthymic disorder, minor depression, and related conditions are thought to affect as many as 15% of community-dwelling elders (Blazer, 1994) and as many as 70% of those living in long-term care settings (Mulsant and Ganguli, 1999), contributing to widespread functional impairment and morbidity (Rollman and Reynolds, 1999).

Studies consistently report undertreatment of elderly patients with depressive symptomatology in both primary care and nursing home settings, suggesting that greater attention must be paid to recognizing nonmajor depressive disorders (Lavretsky and Kumar, 2002).

Although clinical attention and research on late-life mood disorders have focused on major depression, much depressive symptomatology in the elderly is not adequately accounted for by criteria belonging to major depression as outlined in DSM-III through DSM-IV-TR (Flint, 2002). It is increasingly evident that DSM-IV criteria for major depression and other depressive disorders fail to detect the less florid symptom profiles that may in fact be the most common expressions of depressed mood in later life. There are two major explanations for this, each requiring careful conceptualization. First, *DSM-IV criteria for major depression do not adequately capture the heterogeneity of expression of major depression in late life* (Caine et al., 1994). Second, and equally significant, the frequency and impact of less florid depressive syndromes in the elderly have only recently begun to achieve recognition. Just as major depression can have a variable expression in geriatric populations, nonmajor depression syndromes can be distinct from their counterpart disorders in younger populations (Geiselmann and Bauer, 2000). Consequently, the diagnosis, treatment, and related public health management of geriatric depressive syndromes require both (a) appreciation of the geriatric variants of major depression, and (b) delineation of clinically significant nonmajor depressive syndromes as expressed in the elderly (Beekman et al., 1997).

This chapter will discuss the range of depressive conditions encountered in older adults who do not meet criteria for major depressive disorder considered together under the heading of geriatric nonmajor depressive syndromes, or GNMDSs. These disorders comprise a continuum of vaguely defined and frequently overlapping categories. Discussion of GNMDSs is made more challenging by their variability in presentation, nonspecificity of symptoms, and inadequate etiological grounding. Furthermore, these categories include diagnostic criteria sets continually subject to revision due to evolving theoretical paradigms and etiological knowledge. Given the wide use and acknowledged clinical usefulness of diagnostic criteria sets such as those given in DSM-IV-TR, however, we will use DSM-IV-TR diagnostic terminology in this discussion when appropriate. For example, the term "dysthymic disorder" will refer specifically to the DSM-IV-TR category so defined, while the term "dysthymia" will be used to encompass closely related syndromes described in the psychiatric literature under that more general designation.

EVOLUTION OF THE CONCEPT OF NONMAJOR DEPRESSIVE DISORDERS

Historically, many attempts have been made to describe and classify clinically significant depressive syndromes that do not meet criteria for major depressive disorder. Terms such as "subsyndromal," "subthreshold," and even "subclinical" have been applied (Pincus et al., 1999). The history of conceptual development of nonmajor depression diagnostic categories is, in essence, the history of theorists, clinicians, and investigators grappling with the conceptual challenge of classifying subtle variations in clinical manifestation type, severity, and/or duration. A useful model for appreciating the challenges intrinsic to the task of generating an accurate and thorough account of geriatric nonmajor depressive phenomenology is provided by the evolution of the diagnostic construct of dysthymia. "Dysthymic disorder" was introduced as part of DSM-III in 1980 to encompass, as Akiskal (1990) described, "the heterogeneous realm of mixed characterologic and low-grade affective pathology." The introduction of dysthymic disorder was in part a by-product of the prospective follow-up of "neurotic depressives," which revealed recurrent unipolar or bipolar outcome in up to 40% of cases (Akiskal, 1990). "Dysthymic disorder" designated the large number of remaining "neurotic depressives" whose course was chronic and low-grade.

The introduction of the dysthymic disorder diagnosis was more than simply an expansion of our clinical vocabulary (Akiskal, 1990). It actually represented something of a paradigm shift from an earlier perspective that attributed protracted depressive symptomatology to character pathology. Recognition of dysthymic disorder meant the acknowledgement that some individuals displaying symptoms previously regarded as characterological would subsequently be considered to have a variant of a mood disorder. In part, this paradigm shift was driven by pharmacological research demonstrating the responsiveness of these less severe depressive symptoms to antidepressant treatment. Following in the wake of dysthymic disorder, other nonmajor depressive states have been described as an effort to help guide treatment and identify individuals whose symptoms might be responsive to pharmacological interventions.

AN OVERVIEW OF THE NONMAJOR DEPRESSIVE CATEGORIES

Clinical manifestations of GNMDS can fluctuate both interindividually and intraindividually, with the same patient meeting criteria for different diagnostic categories at different times during the course of illness. Table 1 lists a range of DSM-IV-TR diagnostic categories that include depressive symptoms below the severity threshold for major depressive disorder.

Dysthymic disorder is defined as a mild chronic depression of at least 2 years' duration, though often lasting much longer (Kocsis, 1998; Markowitz et al., 1992). DSM-IV-TR specifies early onset as before age 21 and late onset as 21 or over. Double depression indicates major depression superimposed on preexisting dysthymic disorder (McCullough et al., 2000; Keller et al., 1997; Keller and Shapiro, 1982). Concomitant personality disorders are common in

TABLE 1 DSM-IV-TR Diagnostic Categories with Nonmajor Depressive Symptoms

Major depression, single or recurrent episode, in partial remission
Depression NOS
• Minor depressive disorder
• Recurrent brief depressive disorder
Mood disorder due to a general medical condition, with depressive features
Dementia with depressed mood
Adjustment disorder with depressed mood
Substance-induced mood disorder with depressive features
Anxiety disorder with depressive features
Dysthymic disorder

young adults with dysthymia (Devanand et al., 1994). Klein et al. (1988) found that 39.5% of dysthymic disorder subjects whom he studied met diagnostic criteria for schizotypal or borderline personality disorder. Markowitz et al. (1992) reported axis II diagnoses in 85.3% of 43 subjects with dysthymic disorder, with an average of 1.7 axis II diagnoses per subject. Of note, most of the young adults with dysthymia in these studies suffered from double depression, and it is not clear if these findings hold in pure dysthymic disorder (Devanand et al., 1994).

Minor depressive disorder is a DSM-IV "potential category" with a set of diagnostic research criteria proposed for further studies (American Psychiatric Association, 1994). The essential feature of minor depression is one or more depressive episodes that resemble major depressive episodes in duration (2 weeks or longer) but manifest fewer symptoms and less impairment. Using this construct, minor depression can be conceptualized as part of a depressive spectrum defined by number, severity, and duration of symptoms. DSM-IV criteria notwithstanding, research literature on minor depression defines this condition with some variability (Lavretsky and Kumar, 2002). Rather than the narrower definition used in DSM-IV, "minor depression" has frequently denoted *all* clinically significant forms of depression that fail to meet criteria for major depression.

Little is known about the natural history of minor depression, in part because of its varying definitions. For example, approximately 20% of those diagnosed with minor depression have had a prior diagnosis of major depression (Judd et al., 1996), and some of these individuals might be more accurately understood as suffering from major depression in partial remission. The primary differences between minor depression and the more familiar category of dysthymic disorder relate to duration (minimum of 2 weeks versus 2 years), subjective experience of affective distress (*either* dysphoria *or* diminished interest versus dysphoria), and physiological exclusionary criteria (minor depression can have a physiological etiology, whereas dysthmic disorder cannot be diagnosed when a secondary physiological etiology exists). Of particular import is the fact that a patient with minor depression can meet diagnostic criteria without necessarily experiencing dysphoric mood. As a result, minor depression represents a type of "subsyndromal depression" in which somatic symptoms can be the most prominent features (Judd and Akiskal, 2002).

Due to inadequacies of current diagnostic terminology for nonmajor depression syndromes, clinicians and investigators frequently employ various other nonstandardized descriptors. Terms such as "subthreshold," "subsyndromal," and "subclinical" depression have been used to describe clinically significant symptoms of depression that linger over time.

The term *subthreshold major depression* describes patients who have fewer than five clinically significant depressive symptoms, therefore not meeting criteria for the diagnosis of major depression. An alternate term employed in longitudinal research on both adult and geriatric subjects is *subsyndromal depressive spectrum disorders* (Lavretsky and Kumar, 2002), a group of disease states operationally defined by the presence of any two or more concurrent symptoms of depression for most or all of the time, for at least 2 weeks, associated with evidence of social dysfunction, occurring in patients who do not meet criteria for diagnosis of minor depression, major depression, and/or dysthymic disorder (Judd et al., 1998).

Age at onset appears to contribute to differences in the clinical appearance of GNMDS between younger and older adults. Several investigators have focused on dysthymic disorder in particular in exploring these differences. In one study, 340 adult subjects with double depression entered a large multisite treatment study comparing treatment with sertraline or imipramine (Kocsis, 1998). The majority of subjects had onset of dysthymic disorder at an early age (i.e., before age 21); a substantial minority, however, reported onset of dysthymic disorder at later ages, including after age 50. Subjects with younger age at onset tended to be female, to have had a greater number of major depression episodes, to carry a greater number of comorbid personality disorders, and to report a greater number of family members with affective disorders (Kocsis, 1998). In contrast, there were no significant differences between early- and late-onset dysthymia for severity of depression, range of functional impairments, and treatment response. Age at clinical presentation, too, accounts for differences between older and younger dysthymics. Devanand and colleagues (1994) evaluated elderly outpatients with dysthymic disorder to determine whether they presented with the same clinical features as those reported in young adults with dysthymic disorder. Of 224 consecutive subjects, 51.3% (115) had major depression and 17.9% (40) met DSM-III criteria for dysthymic disorder. Table 2 summarizes key clinical features of the dysthymic disorder group.

These geriatric dysthymics showed features that differ from descriptions of younger dysthymics. While up to 90% of younger dysthymic patients report a major depressive episode at some point concurrent with their dysthymia, only 32.5% of this geriatric dysthymic group met criteria for major depression at *any* point in their lifetimes, suggesting a distinct difference in the natural history of geriatric compared to nongeriatric dysthymic disorder. Furthermore, younger adult dysthymics tend to have a female predominance, whereas the gender ratio for geriatric dysthymic subjects in the Devanand et al. (1994) study was approximately 1 : 1. In these subjects, major stressors, particularly medical disease, preceded dysthymia onset. Compared to younger dysthymics in other studies, comorbid substance abuse and anxiety disorders were infrequent in these older dysthymics. But most striking was the finding that only 10% of elderly dysthymic subjects had comorbid personality disorders; in younger cohorts, 50% or more have been found to have comorbid personality disorders (Devanand et al., 1994). Unfortunately, a shared feature between these older dysthymics and younger cohorts from other studies is a history of undertreatment (Devanand et al., 1994).

Two important caveats need to be kept in mind when interpreting the data from Devanand et al. (1994). First, these results indicate that dysthymic disorder is not uncommon among outpatients *presenting* to a geriatric depression clinic. However, since most elderly subjects with mild-to-moderate symptoms do not seek psychiatric care (Blazer, 1989), subjects in the Devanand et al. (1994) study may not be typical of community elderly with dysthymia (in contast, young adults with dysthymic disorder commonly present to outpatient psychiatric clinics). Also, although subjects in the Devanand et al. (1994) study met criteria for dysthymic disorder both cross-sectionally and historically, heavy reliance on subject self-report for age at dysthymia onset and occurrence of major depression, the possibility of inaccurate memory yielding report of a later age at onset, or underreporting of prior major depression, cannot be ruled out.

EPIDEMIOLOGY OF GNMDS

Multiple studies have investigated the epidemiology of nonmajor depressive syndromes among elders, though differences in sampling and syndromal definitions make meta-analysis difficult. Despite the obstacles to comparing these studies, one clear finding is that nonmajor depression syndromes are more common than major depressive disorder in geriatric populations. In fact, while the prevalence of major depression decreases with age, the prevalence of minor

TABLE 2 Clinical Characteristics of 40 Elderly Subjects with Dysthymic Disorder

Male	50%
Female	50%
Race	
Caucasian	85%
African American	12.5%
Hispanic	2.5%
Mean age	67.8 years
Marital status	
Never married	10.3%
Married	28.2%
Separated/divorced	35.9%
Widowed	25.6%
Mean education	14.7 years
Mean duration dysthymic disorder	12.5 years
Mean age at onset of dysthymia	55.2 years
Mean age at first-ever depressive episode	51.1 years
Employed	32.5%
Stressor history present	
Major stressors preceding dysthymia onset	
Separation/divorce	22.5%/75%
Bereavement	17.5%
Retirement	12.5%
Family problems	10%
Financial difficulties	7.5%
Major medical illness	5.0%
Multiple	20%
Major stressors in last 3 years	77.5%
Psychiatric diagnosis	
Dysthymic disorder	100%
Secondary subtype dysthymic disorder	2.5% (one subject)
Met major depression criteria earlier during dysthymic disorder	17.5%
Major depression in prior episode with remission before dysthymia onset	20%
Family history of depression	40%
Treatment history during dysthymic illness	
Medication only	27.5%
Psychotherapy only	15%
Medication and psychotherapy	25%
No treatment	32.5%

Table 2 *Continued*

Medical illnesses	
Concomitant major medical illness (any type)	52.5%
Hypertension	25%
Heart disease (any type)	25%
Prior myocardial infarction	5%
Nonpsychotropic medication with high potential to cause depression	2.5%
Comorbid psychiatric pathology	
Panic disorder	2.5%
Generalized anxiety disorder	10%
Personality disorder	10%
Past substance abuse	12.5%

Source: Adapted from Devanand et al., 1994.

depression and depressive symptoms seems to increase (Flint, 2002; Judd and Akiskal, 2002).

In the Epidemiologic Catchment Area study of five U.S. communities, data across all age groups reveal a point-prevalence of 10% for all depressive spectrum disorders, with major depression constituting 2.3% and minor depession 1.5% (Judd et al., 1997; Weissman et al., 1988). The overall prevalence rate of dysthymic disorder in the adult population was 3.1% (Judd et al., 1997). The highest prevalance was in the 45–64-year-old age group. In the geriatric population (over age 65), prevalence rates were 2% for men and 2.3% for women (Judd et al., 1997). These data would seem to suggest that the prevalence of dysthymia in the geriatric population is significant but somewhat lower than in the younger adult population. It should be noted, howver, that these findings were obtained with the Diagnostic Interview Schedule, an instrument with questionable sensitivity for detecting conditions of mild to moderate severity such as dysthymic disorder (Devanand et al., 1994; Eaton et al., 1985).

Even more prevalent than dysthymic disorder in the community elderly is the presence of other, milder depressive states. Blazer et al. (1987) found that 27% of community elderly report depressive symptoms, including mild dysphoria (19%), symptomatic depression (4%), and a mixed depressive and anxiety syndrome (1.2%). Jaffe et al. (1994) found that 17% of elders aged 65 and older met criteria for minor depression. Similarly, Judd and Akiskal (2002) reported that the combined prevalence of subsyndromal and minor depression in patients 64 and older was 10% to 24%, whereas levels of major depression in the same sample were estimated at only 5% to 10%. In a follow-up study of an Icelandic cohort born in 1931, Stefansson et al. (1991) found a high prevalence of dysthymia, 6.4%, among subjects in their late 50s.

The prevalences of nonmajor depression syndromes overall clearly vary across age groups. In Judd and Kunovac's 1998 analysis, the prevalences of subsyndromal and minor depression within the over-65 age group were 18.1% and 13.0%, respectively, markedly higher than the respective rates in nongeriatric populations. Interestingly, prevalence of nonmajor depressive syndromes appears to have a bimodal distribution across age groups in a cross-sectional assessment of the current population. Young adult nonmajor depression and nonmajor depression in the elderly are more prevalent than nonmajor depression in middle-aged adults (Judd and Kunovac, 1998). A dramatically increased prevalence of nonmajor depressive syndromes has been noted in persons over age 80 (Beekman et al., 1997; Ernst and Angst, 1995). Prevalence rates also are much higher among persons institutionalized in long-term care settings, with reported rates of 50% to 70% (Mulsant and Ganguli, 1999; Rosen et al., 2000).

ETIOLOGY OF PRIMARY GNMDS

Even though GNMDSs are most accurately conceptualized as comprising a spectrum of syndromes rather than specific diagnoses, some generalizations about etiology can be offered. Most reports on etiology have focused on adverse life events, individual attributes, and neurobiological factors. Each of these will be reviewed.

Adverse Life Events

Late life, subthreshold depressive syndromes are highly associated with environmental triggers, and evidence points to a preponderance of exogeneous rather than endogenous etiologies. Compared to younger peers, elders are far more likely to report experiencing a stressful life event at symptom onset (Devanand et al., 1994), and geriatric subjects with depressive symptoms report living through significantly more stressful life events than nondepressed peers (Pahkala et al., 1992). Furthermore, situational risk factors such as functional limitation, smaller contact networks, and less exchange of social support are even more strongly associated with minor than major depression among the elderly (Beekman et al., 1995).

One source of stress of particular importance among the elderly is medical illness and its associated functional limitations. Medical illness is strongly associated with both dysthymic disorder and minor depression, contributing to both the emergence and persistence of depressive symptoms (Lyness et al., 1997; Kocsis, 1998). Medical illness and consequent physical disabilities frequently rob individuals of the ability to pursue goals and engage in preferred activities (Rovner and Casten, 2002; Vali and Walkup, 1998). For example, among elders with physical disability and/or visual impairment, the loss of usual activities such as watching TV, reading, driving, walking, exercise, engaging in hobbies, and engaging in physical activities or routines are commonly reported (Rovner and Casten, 2002). Such changes constitute a major loss, leading to demoralization, low self-esteem, and diminished self-efficacy (Bandura, 1982; Rovner and Casten, 2002). Further, these changes often occur in close proximity to other major life events (such as retirement, interpersonal loss, and reduced income) that may also diminish individual autonomy and compound vulnerability to depressive syndromes.

All of the above constitute potential threats to emotional well-being, and the vast majority of patients with late-life dysthymia and subthreshold depression report one or more of these events occurring at the onset of affective symptomatology. Table 3 summarizes specific psychosocial stressors noted among dysthymic elders by Devanand and colleagues (1994).

Individual Attributes

Despite the frequency of adverse life events among older adults, the majority of elders do *not* experience chronic, reactive depressive symptomatology. Indeed, there is some evidence to suggest that many elders become more resilient with age, such that stressful life events may not confer the same emotional impact that younger individuals experience (Hughes et al., 1988; Zlotnick et al., 1996). Thus, although stressful life events do play a role in the onset of dysthymic disorder and other nonmajor depressive states, certain elders appear to be more vulnerable than others, with individual characteristics and coping styles modifying affective response. Studies assessing the relationship of depression to personality attributes suggest a complex and mutually reinforcing relationship, in which the emotional impact of adverse life events is mediated by individual differences and vulnerabilites. For example, the presence and severity of preexisting depressive symptoms in geriatric patients contribute to the subjective emotional impact of life events. Subthreshold depressives fall in between patients with major depression and patients with no depression on measures of reactivity (Devanand et al., 2002).

Mazure et al. (2002) examined stressful life events, personality characteristics, and their interactions among elders, with a number of notable findings. Elders most likely to be resilient included those with a high degree of autonomy, interpersonal independence, and recent positive achievements. In contrast, low desire for self-control, high needs for interpersonal approval and reassurance, and recent negative achievement events (such as financial loss) were associated with depressive symptomatology. Mazure and her colleagues discovered that the interaction between specific life events and personality characteristics was predictive of affective outcome. For example, although persons with high levels

TABLE 3 1-Year Prevalence of Adverse Life Events Among Dysthymic Elders

Adverse life event	Dysthymic subjects reporting (%)	Control group reporting (%)
Financial difficulties	30.4	27.5
Retirement	8.9	5.0
Loss of employment	10.1	5.0
New major physical illness	21.5	2.5
Other major physical illness	25.3	15.0
Physical illness of close family member	26.6	35.0
Accident or injury	5.1	10.0
Marital separation/divorce	0.0	2.5
Other marital difficulties	17.7	5.0
Major family conflict	30.4	22.5
Major conflict with friend/neighbors	12.0	7.5
Breakup of long-term relationship other than marriage	2.5	0.0
Separation from other close friend/relative	8.0	10.0
Death of spouse	1.3	0.0
Death of child	0.0	0.0
Death of parent	0.0	0.0
Death of sibling	3.8	2.5
Death of other relative or friend	29.1	30.0
Death of pet	3.8	7.5
Forced to leave/lose home	1.3	0.0
Voluntarily changed residence	3.8	0.0
Individual moved out of household	1.3	5.0
Individual moved into household	1.3	7.5
Difficulty getting adequate professional services	13.9	2.5
Victim of crime	8.9	5.0
Became caretaker for relative or friend	3.8	10.0

Source: Adapted from Devanand et al., 2002.

of autonomy are less likely to experience depressive symptoms overall, these individuals are at increased risk when stressful life events specifically diminish autonomy and opportunities for achievement. Similarly, persons with a high need for interpersonal approval and reassurance experienced the greatest affective vulnerability to events related to interpersonal conflict. In other words, stressful life events that affect personal vulnerabilities are most likely to contribute to depressive symptoms, and lifelong coping patterns subsequently become an important mediating variable in determining patient resiliency.

Neurobiological Factors

Although little is now known about the neurobiology of GNMDSs, genetic evidence suggests that nonmajor depression syndromes have similar pathogenic primary CNS mechanisms as other clinical states on the depressive disease spectrum. Family studies of depressive disorders designed to study the heritability of depression have found relationships among multiple depressive syndrome variants. Remick and colleagues (1996), in a representative study of this type, examined first-degee relatives of adult probands with minor depression, major depression, dysthymia, and double depression. When morbidity risks were calculated for the first-degree relatives, results showed comparable risks of depression. The authors concluded that recurrent depression, minor depression, and double depression were indistinguishable when considered from a genetic perspective.

SECONDARY GNMDS: MEDICAL AND NEUROLOGICAL CONSIDERATIONS

As with depression and mania, a "secondary" GNMDS can be conceptualized, representing a state of altered mood as a result of disturbances in physical functioning. Given the nonspecificity of mild-to-moderate depressive symptoms, the full range of systemic medical and neurological disease processes with capacity to affect CNS function can conceivably contribute to the genesis of secondary GNMDS. The geriatric population, with its greater burden of medical illness, is at risk for this form of GNMDS. Chapter 3 of this book addresses the medical differential diagnosis of geriatric depression in some detail. Here, the focus will be more on the relationship of GNMDS to cognitive impairment and to neurological illnesses associated with cognitive deficits.

The clinical interface of geriatric depressive syndomes with cognitive impairment is rich and complicated, likely representing multifactorial and layered pathogenic relationships (Raskind, 1998). Clinical assessment is complicated by the fact that dementia and depression are not only often comorbid but also are characterized by an overlapping constellation of symptoms.

Although most research in this area focuses on major depression, there are compelling theoretical and clinical reasons for considering the relevance of this research to the relationship between GNMDS and cognitve dysfunction as well. First, as discussed, geriatric major depression is itself a protean syndrome, with the capacity to present in a subthreshold, nonmajor depression–like, manner. Thus, it is important to consider the relationship of such subthreshold presentations of geriatric major depression with geriatric cognitive dysfunction. Second, just as a spectrum approach to depressive disease states appears especially applicable to geriatric depressive syndromes, there is increasing evidence to suggest that a similar spectrumlike approach should be applied to geriatric cognitive decline; hence, the development of diagnostic constructs such as *mild cogntive impairment* (MCI). MCI expands the territory upon which geriatric affective symptomalogy and geriatric cognitive dysfunction can interact.

Depending on temporal course and suspected causal relationships, the connection between GNMDS and cognitive impairment can be classified into one of several categories. GNMDS can precede, coincide with, or follow cognitive impairment and seemingly can cause, result from, or exist independently from GNMDS. These permutations will be considered in turn.

GNMDS Can Increase the Risk of Cognitive Impairment

GNMDS can constitute a risk factor, functioning via as yet inadequately identified pathways, for the later development of primary neurodegenerative geriatric cognitive dysfunction. Speck et al. (1995) employed a case-control design to evaluate the relationship between depression and onset of Alzheimer's disease (AD) in a large community-based sample of elderly. When data were analyzed by year of depression onset, an increased risk for development of AD was found in subjects who developed depression more than 10 years before the clinically detectable onset of cognitive and behavioral manifestations of AD (Raskind, 1998; Speck et al., 1995). Interestingly, in that study there was no increased AD risk for subjects experiencing a depression *within* 10 years of AD onset (Speck et al., 1995). A meta-analysis of other case-control studies, however, revealed that depression was a risk factor for subsequent development of AD throughout the patient's history (Raskind, 1998).

One can postulate many pathogenic causal explanations for how a depressive syndrome could function as a risk factor for development of a neurodegenerative dementia. For example, many investigators have theorized a neuro-endocrinological mechanism by which a geriatric depressive syndrome can contribute to cognitive dysfunction: geriatric depression can be associated with hypothalamic–pituitary–adrenal hyperactivity, resulting in exposure of the brain to excessive systemic glucocorticoid levels (Raskind, 1998). Animal models suggest that elevated corticosteroid concentrations can lower the threshold for age-associated hippocampal degeneration (Sapolsky et al., 1985). If this mechanism is relevant to humans, aggressive treatment of GNMDS might preventively reduce a risk factor for later cognitive impairment.

GNMDS Can Represent the Prodrome of Neurodegenerative Cognitive Disease

Depression can itself be an early symptom of several degenerative dementing processes. For example, a depressive syndrome occurring many years before the onset of cognitive impairment can be conceptualized as merely an early expression of the underlying neurodegenerative pathological process. Evidence supporting this includes the observation that despite initial remission via antidepressant therapy, almost half of elderly patients with dementia syndrome of depression (previously known as pseudodementia and discussed in detail in Chapter 3) subsequently develop irreversible degenerative dementias within 5 years. Those patients with depression unaccompanied by cognitive impairment develop dementia at rates more comparable to that of the general population.

GNMDS Can Contribute Directly to Cognitive Dysfunction

In some cases of GNMDS, cognitive symptoms may represent an epiphenomenon of the mood disturbance. Up to 55% of elders with depression develop cognitive impairment phenomenologically consistent with a dementia syndrome (Meyers, 1998). This syndrome—termed the *dementia syndrome of depression* or *depression-related cognitive impairment* (DRCI)—can occur in more subtle form in conjunction with GNMDS. Regrettably, neither clinical features nor currently available biological markers reliably differentiate elderly patients with a primary dementia from those with DRCI. Cognitive testing in DRCI reveals performance variability partly dependent on fluctuations of attention and effort during memory encoding. Careful bedside mental status or neuropsychological assessment is necessary to establish a genuine primary dementia in a patient with both affective symptomatology and cognitive deficits.

The co-occurring cognitive and mood symptoms of some GNMDS patients represent the appearance of mood symptoms as part of a neurodegenerative process. As discussed earlier, any disease process that affects CNS function can produce depressive symptoms. This is especially true of neurodegenerative processes that result in cognitive dysfunction (e.g., Alzheimer's disease, dementia with Lewy bodies, Parkinson's disease). The most prevalent of these will be discussed briefly.

Alzheimer's disease (AD) is the most common primary neurodegenerative dementia, accounting for approximately 65% of cases. Although mild memory dysfunction is likely to be the first evidence of Alzheimer's disease, AD can present in a variety of ways. Behavioral changes (e.g., decreased self-care), personality changes (e.g., increased irritability), and affective phenomenology, all potentially consistent with a GNMDS, can characterize initial presentation. And in fully expressed AD, a GNMDS can be a common clinical component. Not surprisingly, postmortem findings of degenerative changes in brainstem aminergic nuclei correlate with a history of depressive symptomatology complicating AD cognitive deficits.

Frontotemporal lobar dementias (FTLD) comprise a group of clinical syndromes resulting from degenerative processes that disproportionately affect circumscribed areas of frontal and/or frontotemporal cortex. Although FTLDs are much less common than AD, dementia with Lewy bodies, and vascular dementia, they are important to recognize because of their tendency to progress to severe disability. Their symptomatology, and especially the abulic presentation of frontal variant FTLD, can mimic a GNMDS. Not surprisingly, FTLD-associated behavioral disturbances can be erroneously attributed to primary psychiatric disease, often prompting initial patient presentation to a mental health clinician.

Dementia with Lewy bodies (DLB) is probably the second most common type of degenerative dementia after AD (Campbell et al., 2001). DLB is defined clinically by presence of dementia, gait/balance disorder, perceptual disturbances (e.g., hallucinations), delusions, heightened sensitivity to the adverse effects of traditional antipsychotics, and fluctuations in alertness. DLB has clinical features that overlap with AD and PD. DLB-related cognitive impairment can range from transient dysfunction to sustained dementia. DLB-associated depressive features can include neurovegetative derangement and dysthymia (Ballard et al., 2001).

Posterior cortical atrophy (PCA) is a selective lobar dementia characterized initially by disturbances of visual perception and integration (Benson et al., 1988). Involvement of the occipitoparietal region produces visuospatial and integrated attentional disturbances, with relative sparing of personality, insight, and memory until late in disease. Mild secondary depressive symptoms can be a component of this syndrome.

Parkinson's disease (PD), in nearly all affected patients, includes disturbances of mood and cognition at some point during the course of the illness (Brown and Marsden, 1984). PD-related depressive and cognitive symptoms can be considered a component of the spectrum of neuropsychiatric disturbances attendant to basal ganglia disorders. McHugh has described such basal ganglia disease-related disturbances as part of a "triadic syndrome" comprising depression, dementia, and dyskinesia (McHugh, 1989). It is likely that degeneration of brain-stem neuroadrenergic nuclei also contributes to PD-related depressive symptomatology.

DIAGNOSING GNMDS

Phenomenologically, nonmajor depressive disorders such as dysthymic disorder and minor depression are often described as similar to major depression but characterized by lesser number, severity, and/or duration of symptoms (American Psychiatric Association, 1994; Kessler et al., 1997; Remick et al., 1996). It is increasingly evident, however, that GNMDS differ qualitatively as well as quantitatively from major depressive disorder, especially as defined in younger cohorts. Although some elders with nonmajor depression do present with "traditional" symptoms such as dysphoria, geriatric patients are far more likely than younger patients to present with somatic, cognitive, and functional difficulties that are not immediately recognizable as having a primary affective etiology

(Devanand et al., 1994). In combination with the inherently subtle presentation of a "subthreshold" depressive phenomenon, such qualitative differences give rise to a number of diagnostic challenges.

As discussed in Chapter 3, a substantial number of geriatric patients who exhibit symptoms of depression in the absence of subjective low mood or dysphoria nevertheless show remission of these symptoms when treated with antidepressants. This observation has supported the hypothesis that a syndrome lacking specifically depressed or dysphoric mood can nonetheless represent a variant of major depressive disorder (Roy et al., 1984). Somatic complaints figure prominently in the profile of geriatric depressive symptoms, with a primary somatic focus occurring twice as often as a dysphoric presentation (Judd et al., 1997).

Elderly patients with nonmajor depressive symptoms, too, often focus on somatic and cognitive concerns, with the result that many first seek treatment for physiological rather than psychological complaints. Patients with major and nonmajor depressive disorders, as a consequence, utilize nonpsychiatric medical services at an increased rate. They are most likely to turn first to primary care providers for assistance (Oxman and Sengupta, 2002). Because many symptoms of depression are identical to systemic effects of medical illness (including fatigue, diminished energy, loss of appetite, and psychomotor slowing), it is possible for both patients and clinicians to overlook a depressive etiology.

In combination with a somatic symptom focus, the absence of a subjective experience of sadness can make diagnosis particularly difficult. In addition, when geriatric patients do experience subjective dysphoria, there are often qualitative differences as compared to a younger cohort. Dysphoria among elders, for example, is often expressed as hopelessness rather than as sadness (Gallo et al., 1997). Clinical manifestations of geriatric nonmajor depression also differ from those in younger populations in that elders are vulnerable to more prevalent and more pronounced DRCI.

Although GNMDS patients with DRCI can easily be mistaken for cognitively impaired patients without depression, some known clinical differences can aid clinicians in making a correct diagnostic differentiation. Patients with DRCI as opposed to a primary cognitive disturbance are more often very distressed by their forgetfulness, reporting their symptoms with a great amount of concern. Clinicians should note that many of these patients become so anxious about their abilities that they in fact fail to perform well on formal memory tests. However, these same patients may be able to describe specific and detailed accounts of memory lapses, which illustrates *preserved* rather than disturbed memory functioning.

In contrast to the extensive research exploring cognitive effects of geriatric major depression, less research effort has been devoted to the cognitive dysfunction associated with nonmajor depression. Preliminary unpublished observations presented recently by Lavretsky and Kumar (2002), however, suggest that patients with minor depression do experience cognitive difficulties, with performance on neuropsychological tasks falling between that of normal control subjects and patients with major depression. In particular, subjects fulfilling criteria for minor depression have been shown to demonstrate decrements in processing speed, working memory, verbal recall, and executive functioning (Lavretsky and Kumar, 2002).

Laboratory investigations—including serological screening assays and neuroimaging—may help determine whether a GNMDS is primary or is instead a secondary expression of an underlying abnormality, especially for a patient who lacks any significant psychiatric history and/or is affected by concurrent medical illness. The same range of tests described in Chapter 3 with respect to the medical differential diagnosis of major depressive disorder can be applied to the assessment of GNMDS.

Neuropsychological evaluation provides a standardized, systematic means for assessing an individual's cognitive performance relative to a normal reference population. Test findings can be used to detect the presence and/or extent of cognitive dysfunction and to delineate diagnosis-specific profiles of impairment. Serial neuropsychological evaluations can be used to characterize cognitive changes over time, thereby helping to differentiate depression-related cognitive impairment from deficits caused by other mechanisms such as a neurodegenerative dementia.

COMPLICATIONS OF GNMDS

Nonmajor depressive syndromes are associated with significant levels of morbidity, contributing to increased psychosocial and functional impairment, diminished quality of life, and resultant disability (Judd and Akiskal, 2002; Lyness et al., 2002). "Disability" refers to problems in day-to-day living caused by either physical or mental health problems and is defined as either (1) the discrepancy between an individual's abilities and environmental demands (Gill et al., 1999), or (2) the discrepancy between an individual's abilities and his or her personal standards (Deeg et al., 1995). In either case, minor depression is known to inflate that discrepancy among elders, contributing to unnecessarily diminished functioning. Even minor levels of depressive symptomatology, as reported by Judd and Akiskal (2000), are associated with diminished functioning: As the severity of depressive symptoms increased, there were direct and concomitant increases in disability levels. When the same subjects were symptom-free, psychosocial dysfunction diminished or disappeared (Judd and Akiskal, 2000).

When compared to subjects diagnosed with major depressive disorders, GNMDS subjects show less disability (Jaffe et al., 1994). In contrast, the level of disability associated with GNMDS exceeds that accompanying many common and debilitating medical conditions such as hypertension, diabetes, and

TABLE 4 GNMDS Outcomes: Representative Studies

Study	Study design	Sample	Depressive subtype	Results
Beekman et al., 1997	Cross-sectional association study of depression and disability	646 community-dwelling older adults, age 55–85 years	Major and minor depression	Associations of major and minor depression with disability and well-being remained significant after controlling for chronic disease and functional limitations; adequate treatment was often not administered, even in subjects with major depression; major and minor depression were associated with increased use of nonmental health services
Penninx et al., 2001	Longitudinal follow-up of the community sample	2847 community-dwelling persons age 55–85; 450 subjects with and 2397 subjects without cardiac disease	Major depression (DSM-III) and minor depression (CES < 17)	Depression increased risk of cardiac mortality in subjects with and without cardiac disease; excess cardiac mortality was more than twice as high for major depression than for minor depression

Penninx et al., 2000	Longitudinal follow-up of a community sample (4.5 years)	3107 older persons (age 55–85)	Major depression (DSM-III) and minor depression (CES < 17)	At baseline, 12.8% had minor depression and 2% had major depression; minor depression was associated with a significantly greater decline in functional status and performance, as well as with increased risk of death in men; major depression increased risk of functional decline and death in men and women
Penninx et al., 1998	Epidemiological follow-up of community samples (the established populations for epidemiological studies of elderly subjects)	4,825 persons age 71 years and older, followed up at 3 and 6 years	Chronic depression (CES-D) based on cutoff criteria	When present at least 6 years, depression was associated with a generally increased risk of cancer after controlling for age, sex, race, disability, hospital admissions, alcohol intake, and smoking

Source: Adapted from Lavretsky and Kumar, 2002.

arthritis (Wells et al., 1989). In addition, when the increased prevalence of nonmajor depressive syndromes is taken into account, the complications of geriatric minor depression have a cumulative impact on the older population far in excess of those caused by major depressive disorder (Lyness et al., 1999). Representative outcome studies such as those summarized in Table 4 indicate the severity of morbidity associated with GNMDS.

Although dysthymic disorder and other nonmajor depressive conditions are known to be associated with high-risk health behaviors that increase mortality rates, investigators have also questioned whether these conditions have a primary adverse effect on mortality as well. Pulska and colleagues (1998) found an increased risk of death in dysthymic as opposed to nondysthymic elders; however, when age, sex, marital status, education, smoking, physical health status, and functional status were controlled, they found no evidence that dysthymic disorder conferred an independent increase in mortalitiy rates. Instead, they determined that the higher mortality in their dysthymic elders was incidental to a higher co-occurrence of somatic disease and disabilities in that cohort. However, this study did not address the tendency of dysthymic elders to magnify the effects of existing illness or disability on self-report measures.

In support of a primary mortality-increasing effect of GNMDS, a well-controlled controlled study performed by Hybels et al. (2002) examined over 3600 elders and determined that men but not women with nonmajor depression exhibited increased odds of mortality. This study came soon after similar findings by Penninx and colleagues (1999), summarized in Table 5. Although a number of possible explanations for a primary effect of GNMDS on mortality have been posited, no clear mechanism has been proposed to explain such differential gender effects. Perhaps this difference is simply an artifact of differential self-reporting, since men report fewer depressive symptoms than women at the same degree of functional impairment (Angst and Dobler-Mikola, 1984). Male subjects may have been more severely depressed, in other words, than female subjects classified at a similar level of depressive symptomatology. This discrepancy in degree of depression could then be reflected in differential degrees of influence on mortality rates. Future studies could shed light on this issue by controlling for self-report biases.

MANAGEMENT OF GNMDS

At present, the evidence base for the treatment of GNMDS by any modality is limited, especially in patients with comorbid medical and/or neurological disorders. The situation is particularly problematic with respect to pharmacological treatment, given the fact that most GNMDS patients are treated within primary care settings, where pharmacotherapy tends to be the favored treatment modality when treatment is provided at all (Williams et al., 2000).

TABLE 5 Mortality Rates Among Elders with No Depression, Minor Depression, or Major Depression

Population	Death rate per 1000 person-years
Total population	
No Depression	39.5
Minor Depression	71.4
Major Depression	60.7
Men	
No Depression	51.5
Minor Depression	116.4
Major Depression	69
Women	
No Depression	27.7
Minor Depression	48.4
Major Depression	58.2

Source: Adapted from Penninx et al., 1999.

Clinical trials involving young and middle-aged subjects with dysthymic disorder have demonstrated good response to antidepressant medication. In one large study of pure dysthymic disorder, for example, over 400 subjects were randomly assigned to sertraline, imipramine, or placebo treatment for 12 weeks (Thase et al., 1996). Remission criteria were strict, requiring that subjects no longer met the DSM-IIIR symptom criteria for dysthymic disorder at the end of the 12-week trial. Remission criteria, nonetheless, were met by 50% of sertraline-treated subjects and 44% of imipramine-treated subjects, compared to 28% of placebo-treated subjects. In a post hoc analysis of 340 subjects, the sertraline and imipramine treatment groups were divided by age (age 50 or older and under age 50) and response rates were similar between older and younger subgroups (Thase et al., 1996).

Only a few prospective trials have investigated the effects of antidepressant treatment on GNMDS. In one open-label study of fluvoxamine, geriatric subjects with minor depression and disabling subthreshold depression demonstrated amelioration of depressive symptoms and measurable improvements in functioning (Rapaport and Judd, 1998). In an open-label trial of sertraline involving 12 nursing home residents who met DSM-IV criteria for minor depression, 75% of subjects demonstrated remission by the sixth week of treatment (Rosen et al., 2000).

A prospective study of fluoxetine treatment of geriatric dysthymic disorder was reported by Nobler and colleagues (1996). The subjects in this study were adults of at least 60 years of age with primary dysthymic disorder and Mini-Mental State Examination scores greater than 24. Very few of these subjects had previously received adequate medication trials; in fact, 40% of them reported no prior treatment despite having been symptomatic for a mean duration of 12.5 years at the time dysthymic disorder was diagnosed. Fluoxetine treatment was initiated after a 2-week placebo washout and continued at a dose of 20 mg/d for 3 weeks. For nonresponders, dosage was increased to 40 mg/day for the next 5 weeks. Sixty percent of the subjects met the criteria for response at the end of the 8-week trial, and fluoxetine was generally well tolerated (Nobler et al., 1996).

Williams and colleagues (2000) performed a rather comprehensive prospective randomized, placebo-controlled, double-blind study of the treatment of minor depression and dysthymic disorder in older adults in a primary care setting. Of the 415 subjects with minor depression (n = 204) or dysthymic disorder (n = 211) initially enrolled, 311 (74.9%) completed the study. Subjects were randomly assigned to receive one of the following: (1) paroxetine 10 mg/d, titrated to a maximum of 40 mg/day (n = 137); (2) placebo (n = 140); or (3) Problem Solving Treatment–Primary Care (PST-PC), a behaviorally based psychotherapy designed specifically for primary care administration (n = 138) (Williams et al., 2000). Each subject was offered six visits, either for medication management (paroxetine and placebo groups) or psychotherapy (PST-PC). Outcomes were measured on the 20-item Hopkins Symptom Checklist Depression Scale (HSCL-D-20), Hamilton Depression Rating Scale (HDRS), and Medical Outcomes Study Short-Form 36 (SF-36) physical and mental components. Paroxetine subjects had greater symptom resolution than placebo subjects (mean HSCL-D-20 score difference 0.21, $p < 0.01$). Paroxetine showed beneficial effects on depressive symptoms that were similar for subjects with either dysthymic disorder or minor depression. Subjects treated with PST-PC, however, did not show any significant benefits compared to placebo-treated subjects.

Burrows and colleagues (Burrows et al., 2002) performed a randomized double-blind, placebo-controlled study of paroxetine treatment of nonmajor depression in elderly nursing home residents with nonmajor depression. Results were disappointing: paroxetine failed to demonstrate statistically significant superiority over placebo (as assessed by Hamilton Depression Rating Scale and Cornell Scale for Depression). A trend toward worsening cognitive impairment was also noticed in the paroxetine group (Burrows et al., 2002).

In one of the few published long-term maintenance studies of the treatment of dysthymic disorder or double depression, subjects were entered into an acute and continuation phase of open treatment with desipramine (Kocsis et al., 1996). Responders were randomly selected to either continue active drug treatment or taper to placebo, and followed during a 2-year maintenance phase. Results revealed an 11% relapse rate in the active medication group compared to a 52% relapse rate in the placebo group, demonstrating the efficacy of long-term maintenance treatment in adult subjects with dysthymic disorder (Kocsis et al., 1996).

Despite the high prevalence of depressive symptomatology among geriatric patients with neurodegenerative or posttraumatic disorders, there have also been few randomized placebo-controlled trials of antidepressant treatment in these populations. Desipramine, in other studies, reduced depressive symptoms in subjects with major depressive disorder and multiple sclerosis or traumatic brain injury (Rummans et al., 1999). We could identify no study that has exclusively or specifically investigated treatment of geriatric nonmajor depressive syndromes comorbid with these disorders. Several ongoing collaborative trials, however, are investigating the relative effectiveness of pharmacological and nonpharmacological treatments of depressive syndromes, including nonmajor depressive syndromes, in the primary care setting (Lavretsky and Kumar, 2002). It is hoped that their findings will better inform GNMDS management strategies.

Electroconvulsive therapy (ECT) is recognized as a powerful intervention in geriatric major depressive disorder, but no studies have specifically addressed its efficacy in treating GNMDS. In one of the few studies investigating the use of ECT for double depression, Prudic and colleagues (1993) compared ECT response in subjects with double depression (n = 25; mean age 50) to that of subjects with major depressive disorder alone (n = 75; mean age 60). Short-term clinical response rates, both in percentage of responders and in group mean symptomatic improvements, were similar in both groups. Subjects with double depression, however, tended to have more residual symptomatology and tended toward higher relapse rates. Given the differences observed between geriatric and nongeriatric dysthymic disorders—and by implication between geriatric and nongeriatric double depression—the applicability of these results to GNMDS is questionable. More GNMDS-specific research is needed.

Double depression—the combination of dysthymic disorder and major depressive episodes—is associated with a poorer response to antidepressant pharmacotherapy or ECT and with a greater likelihood of relapse than measured in subjects with either dysthymic disorder or major depressive disorder alone (Kocsis, 1998; Lavretsky and Kumar, 2002; Williams et al., 2000). Analogously, GNMDS patients who have experienced major depressive episodes might be expected to respond less robustly to pharmacotherapy or ECT. This is an area for further study that has not yet been systematically investigated. The effects of *behavioral and psychotherapeutic treatments*—though these are probably less frequently offered than pharmacotherapy to GNMDS patients in actual clinical settings—have been examined in a few studies. The value of reported findings are limited in some cases, however, by methodological issues such as lack of controls or randomization (Oxman and Sengupta, 2002). Some elders, however, might prefer nonpharmacological approaches. Furthermore, the strong association between late-onset depressive syndromes and adverse life events suggests that the majority of GNMDSs reflect at least a contribution from psychosocial factors and difficulties adapting to external events. As such, late-life depressive syndromes may be especially amenable to nonpharmacological treatment strategies aimed at helping patients cope more successfully with losses, stressors, or transitions. A comprehensive psychotherapeutic approach might involve both instruction in practical methods for coping with such stresses and empathic recognition of the patient's irreversible losses coupled with support for acceptance and adaptation.

Interestingly, nonpharmacological approaches to treatment of minor depression were found to produce effects of greater magnitude than seen with pharmacological treatments, according to a comprehensive review of randomized clinical trials authored by Oxman and Sengtupta (2002). The two nonpharmacological treatments employed in the reviewed studies were cognitive-behavioral therapy (CBT), which focuses on challenging self-defeating beliefs and increasing beneficial behaviors, and interpersonal therapy (IPT), which focuses upon relationships, security, and personal growth. In an earlier study, Miranda and Munoz (1994) utilized CBT to treat elders with minor depression; they too reported a significant decrease in symptomatology at the end of 4 months of treatment. Benefits persisted at 12-month follow-up. In the Williams et al (2000) study described previously, the nonpharmacological treatment (PST-PC) produced no measurable improvement in dysthymic elders, but the PST-PC treatment in this study involved only 3½ hours of therapy over the course of 11 weeks and therefore the lack of subject response may simply reflect insufficient treatment exposure. Altogether, studies of nonpharmacological treatments for GNMDS elders suggest that such treatments hold promise; however, studies of sufficient design, scope, and symptom focus to provide definitive data remain to be done.

CONCLUSIONS

There is growing evidence to suggest that late-life depressive syndromes are distinct from depressive disorders in younger adults, differing in potential etiological mechanisms, comorbidities, and clinical manifestations. Although dysthymic disorder and other nonmajor depressive conditions have long been recognized, inadequate attention has been paid to the particular ways in which these disorders manifest among elders. GNMDSs are the most frequently occurring depressive syndromes in later life; they merit increased clinical notice. GNMDSs are associated with significant medical, functional, and psychosocial morbidities, and they seem to respond favorably to behavioral, psychotherapeutic, and psychopharmacological interventions. Their wider recognition and more aggressive treatment can be expected to benefit many affected elders.

REFERENCES

Akiskal HS. Towards a definition of dysthymia: boundaries with personality and mood disorders. In: Burton SW, Akiskal HS, eds. Dysthymic Disorder. London: Gaskell, 1990: 1–12.

American Psychiatric Association. Diagnostic and Statistical Manual of Mental Disorders. Washington, DC: American Psychiatric Press, 1994.

Angst, J, Dobler-Mikola A. Do the diagnostic criteria determine the sex ratio in depression? J Affect Disord 1984; 7:189–198.

Ballard CG, O'Brien JT, Swann AG, Thompson P, Neill D, McKeith IG. The natural history of psychosis and depression in dementia with Lewy bodies and Alzheimer's disease: persistence and new cases over 1 year of follow-up. J Clin Psychiatry 2001; 62:46–49.

Bandura A. Self-efficacy mechanism in human agency. American Psychologist 1982; 37: 122–147.

Beekman AT, Deeg DJ, Braam AW, Smit JH, Van Tilburg W. Consequences of major and minor depression in later life: a study of disability, well-being and service utilization. Psychol Med 1997; 27:1397–1409.

Beekman AT, Deeg DJ, Smit JH, van Tilburg W. Predicting the course of depression in the older population: results from a community-based study in the Netherlands. J Affect Disord 1995; 34:41–49.

Beekman AT, Geerlings SW, Deeg DJ et al. The natural history of late-life depression: a 6-year prospective study in the community. Arch Gen Psychiatry 2002; 59(7): 605–611.

Benson DF, Davis RJ, Snyder BD. Posterior cortical atrophy. Arch Neurol 1988; 45: 789–793.

Blazer D. Depression in the elderly. N Engl J Med 1989; 320:164–166.

Blazer D. Depression in Late Life. St. Louis, MO: Mosby Yearbook, 1994:9–16.

Blazer D, Hughes DC, George LK. The epidemiology of depression in an elderly community population. Gerontologist 1987; 27:281–287.

Brown RG, Marsden CD. How common is dementia in Parkinson's disease? Lancet 1984; 2:1262–1265.

Burrows AB, Salzman C, Satlin A et al. A randomized placebo-controlled trial in nursing home residents with non-major depression. Depress Anxiety 2002; 15(3):102–110.

Caine ED, Lyness JM, King DA. Clinical and etiological heterogeneity of mood disorders in elderly patients. In: Schneider LS, Reynolds CE, Lebowits BD et al., eds. Diagnosis and Treatment of Major Depression in Late Life. Washington DC: American Psychiatric Press, 1994:23–53.

Campbell S, Stephens, S, Ballard C. Dementia with Lewy bodies: clinical features and treatment. Drugs Aging 2001; 18:397–407.

Deeg DJH, Dardaun JWPF, Fozard JL. Health, behavior, and aging. In: Birren JE, Schaie KW, eds. Handbook of the Psychology of Aging. San Diego: Academic Press, 1995.

Devanand DP, Kim MK, Paykina N, Sackeim HA. Adverse life events in elderly patients with major depression or dysthyic disorders and in healthy-control subjects. Am J Geriatr Psychiatry 2002; 10:265–274.
Devanand DP, Nobler MS, Singer T, Kiersky JE, Turret N, Roose SP, Sackeim HA. Is dysthymia a different disorder in the elderly? Am J Psychiatry 1994; 151:1592–1599.
Eaton WW, Weissman MM, Anthony JJ et al. Problems in the definition and measurement of prevalence and incidence of psychiatric disorders. In: Eaton WW, Kessler LG, eds. Epidemiologic Field Methods in Psychiatry: The NIMH Epidemiologic Catchment Area Program. New York: Academic Press, 1985.
Ernst C, Angst J. Depression in old age: is there a real decrease in prevalence? A review. Eur Arch Psychiatry Clin Neurosci 1995; 245:272–287.
Flint AJ. The complexity and challenge of non-major depression in late life. Am J Geriatr Psychiatry 2002; 10:229–232.
Gallo JJ, Rabins PV, Lyketsos CG, Tien AY, Anthony JC. Depression without sadness: functional outcomes of nondysphoric depression in later life. J Am Geriatr Soc 1997; 45:570–578.
Geiselmann B, Bauer M. Subthreshold depression in the elderly: qualitative or quantitative distinction? Compr Psychiatry 2000; 41:32–38.
Gill TM, Robison JT, Williams CS, Tinetti ME. Mismatches between the home environment and physical capabilities among community-living older persons. J Am Geriatr Soc 1999; 47:88–92.
Hughes DC, George LK, Blazer DZ. Age differences in life events qualities: multivariate controlled analyses. American Journal of Community Psychology 1988; 16:161–174.
Hybels CF, Pieper CF, Blazer DG. Sex differences in the relationship between subthreshold depression and mortality in a community sample of older adults. Am J Geriatr Psychiatry 2002; 10:283–291.
Jaffe A, Froom, J, Galambos N. Minor depression and functional impairment. Arch Fam Med 1994; 3:1081–1086.
Judd LL, Akiskal HS. The clinical and public health relevance of current research on subthreshold depressive symptoms to elderly patients. Am J Geriatr Psychiatry 2002; 10:233–238.
Judd LL, Akiskal HS, Maser JD, Zeller PJ, Endicott J, Coryell W, Paulus MP, Kunovac JL, Leon AC, Mueller TI, Rice JA, Keller MB. A prospective 12-year study of subsyndromal and syndromal depressive symptoms in unipolar major depressive disorders. Arch Gen Psychiatry 1998; 55:694–700.
Judd LL, Akiskal HS, Paulus MP. The role and clinical significance of subsyndromal depressive symptoms (SSD) in unipolar major depressive disorder. J Affect Disord 1997; 45:5–18.
Judd LL, Akiskal HS, Zeller PJ, Paulus M, Leon AC, Maser JD, Endicott J, Coryell W, Kunovac JL, Mueller TI, Rice JP, Keller MB. Psychosocial disability during the long-term course of unipolar major depressive disorder. Arch Gen Psychiatry 2000; 57:375–380.
Judd LL, Kunovac JL. Bipolar and unipolar depressive disorders in geriatric patients. In:

Brunello N, Langer SZ, Racagni G, eds. Mental Disorders in the Elderly: New Therapeutic Approaches, vol. 13. Basel, Switzerland: Karger, 1998:1–10.

Judd LL, Paulus MP, Wells KB, Rapaport MH. Socioeconomic burden of subsyndromal depressive symptoms and major depression in a sample of the general population. Am J Psychiatry 1996; 153:1411–1417.

Keller MB, Hirschfeld RM, Hanks D. Double depression: a distinctive subtype of unipolar depression. J Affect Disord 1997; 145(1–2):65–73.

Keller MB, Shapiro RW. "Double depression": superimposition of acute depressive episodes on chronic depressive disorders. Am J Psychiatry 1982; 139(4):483–442.

Kessler RC, Zhao S, Blazer DG, Swartz M. Prevalence, correlates, and course of minor depression and major depression in the National Comorbidity Survey. J Affect Disord 1997; 45:19–30.

Klein DN, Taylor EB, Harding K, Dickstein S. Double depression and episodic major depression: demographic, clinical, familial, personality, and socioenvironmental characteristics and short-term outcome. Am J Psychiatry 1988; 145:1226–1231.

Kocsis JH. Geriatric dysthymia. J Clin Psychiatry 1998; 59(suppl 10):13–15.

Kocsis JH, Friedman RA, Markowitz JC, Leon AC, Miller NL, Gniwesch L, Parides M. Maintenance therapy for chronic depression: a controlled clinical trial of desipramine. Arch Gen Psychiatry 1996; 53:769–776.

Lavretsky H, Kumar A. Clinically significant non-major depression: old concepts, new insights. Am J Geriatr Psychiatry 2002; 10:239–255.

Lyness JM, Caine ED, King DA, Conwell Y, Duberstein PR, Cox C. Depressive disorders and symptoms in older primary care patients: one-year outcomes. Am J Geriatr Psychiatry 2002; 10:275–282.

Lyness JM, King DA, Cox C, Yoediono Z, Caine ED. The importance of subsyndromal depression in older primary care patients: prevalence and associated functional disability. J Am Geriatr Soc 1999; 47:647–652.

Markowitz JC, Moran ME, Kocsis JH, Frances AJ. Prevalence and comorbidity of dysthymic disorder among psychiatric outpatients. J Affect Disord 1992; 24:63–71.

Mazure CM, Maciejewski PK, Jacobs SC, Bruce ML. Stressful life events interacting with cognitive/personality styles to predict late-onset major depression. Am J Geriatr Psychiatry 2002; 10:297–304.

McCullough JP, Klein DN, Keller MB et al. Comparison of DSM-III-R chronic major depression superimposed on dysthymia (double depression): validity of the distinction. J Abnorm Psychol 2000; 109(3):419–427.

McHugh PR. The neuropsychiatry of basal ganglia disorders: a triadic syndrome and its explanation. Neuropsychiatry, Neuropsychology, and Behavioral Neurology 1989; 2:239–247.

Meyers BS. Depression and dementia: comorbidities, identification, and treatment. J Geriatr Psychiatry Neurol 1998; 11:201–205.

Miranda J, Munoz R. Intervention for minor depression in primary care patients. Psychosom Med 1994; 56:136–141.

Mulsant BH, Ganguli M. Epidemiology and diagnosis of depression in late life. J Clin Psychiatry 1999; 60(suppl 20):9–15.

Nobler MS, Devanand DP, Kim MK, Fitzsimons LM, Singer TM, Turret N, Sackeim

HA, Roose SP. Fluoxetine treatment of dysthymia in the elderly. J Clin Psychiatry 1996; 57:254–256.
Oxman TE, Sengupta A. Treatment of minor depression. Am J Geriatr Psychiatry 2002; 10:256–264.
Pahkala K, Kivela SL, Laippala P. Social and environmental factors and dysthymic disorder in old age. J Clin Epidemiol 1992; 45:775–783.
Penninx BW, Beekman AT, Deeg DJ, van Tilburg W. [Effects of depression on physical health and mortality in the elderly: longitudinal resuls of the LASA research]. Tijdschr Gerontol Geriatr 2000; 31:211–218.
Penninx BW, Beekman AT, Honig A, Deeg DJ, Schoevers RA, van Eijk JT, van Tilburg W. Depression and cardiac mortality: results from a community-based longitudinal study. Arch Gen Psychiatry 2001; 58:221–227.
Penninx BW, Geerlings SW, Deeg DJ, van Eijk JT, van Tilburg W, Beekman AT. Minor and major depression and the risk of death in older persons. Arch Gen Psychiatry 1999; 56:889–895.
Penninx BW, Guralnik JM, Pahor M, Ferrucci L, Cerhan JR, Wallace RB, Havlik RJ. Chronically depressed mood and cancer risk in older persons (see comments). J Natl Cancer Inst 1998; 90:1888–1893.
Pincus HA, Davis WW, McQueen LE. 'Subthreshold' mental disorders: a review and synthesis of studies on minor depression and other 'brand names.' Br J Psychiatry 1999; 174:288–296.
Prudic J, Sackeim HA, Devanand DP et al. The efficacy of ECT in double depression. Depression 1993; 1:38–44.
Pulska T, Pahkala K, Laippala P, Kivela SL. Survival of elderly Finns suffering from dysthymic disorder: a community study. Soc Psychiatry Psychiatr Epidemiol 1998; 33:319–325.
Rapaport MH, Judd LL. Minor depressive disorder and subsyndromal depressive symptoms: functional impairment and response to treatment. J Affect Disord 1998; 48: 227–232.
Raskind MA. The clinical interface of depression and dementia. J Clin Psychiatry 1998; 59(suppl 10):9–12.
Remick RA, Sadovnick AD, Lam RW, Zis AP, Yee IM. Major depression, minor depression, and double depression: are they distinct clinical entities? Am J Med Genet 1996; 67:347–353.
Rollman BL, Reynolds CF 3rd. Minor and subsyndromal depression: functional disability worth treating. J Am Geriatr Soc 1999; 47:757–758.
Rosen J, Mulsant BH, Pollock BG. Sertraline in the treatment of minor depression in nursing home residents: a pilot study. Int J Geriatr Psychiatry 2000; 15:177–180.
Rovner BW, Casten RJ. Activity loss and depression in age-related macular degeneration. Am J Geriatr Psychiatry 2002; 10:305–310.
Roy R, Thomas M, Matas M. Chronic pain and depression: a review. Compr Psychiatry 1984; 25:96–105.
Rummans TA, Lauterbach EC, Coffey CE, Royall DR, Cummings JL, Salloway S, Duffy J, Kaufer D. Pharmacologic efficacy in neuropsychiatry: a review of placebo-controlled treatment trials. A report of the ANPA Committee on Research. J Neuropsychiatry Clin Neurosci 1999; 11:176–189.

Sapolsky RM, Krey LC, McEwen BS. Prolonged glucocorticoid exposure reduces hippocampal neuron number: implications for aging. J Neurosci 1985; 5:1222–1227.

Speck CE, Kukull WA, Brenner DE, Bowen JD, McCormick WC, Teri L. Pfanschmidt ML, Thompson JD, Larson EB. History of depression as a risk factor for Alzheimer's disease. Epidemiology 1995; 6:366–369.

Stefansson JG, Lindal E, Bjornsson JK, Guomundsdottir A. Lifetime prevalence of specific mental disorders among people born in Iceland in 1931. Acta Psychiatr Scand 1991; 84:142–149.

Thase ME, Fava M, Halbreich U, Kocsis JH, Koran L, Davidson J, Rosenbaum J, Harrison W. A placebo-controlled, randomized clinical trial comparing sertraline and imipramine for the treatment of dysthymia. Arch Gen Psychiatry 1996; 53:777–784.

Vali FM, Walkup J. Combined medical and psychological symptoms: impact on disability and heatlh care utilization of patients with arthritis. Med Care 1998; 36:1073–1084.

Weissman MM, Leaf PJ, Bruce ML, Florio L. The epidemiology of dysthymia in five communities: rates, risks, comorbidity, and treatment. Am J Psychiatry 1988; 145: 815–819.

Wells KB, Stewart A, Hays RD, Burnam MA, Rogers W, Daniels M, Berry S, Greenfield S, Ware J. The functioning and well-being of depressed patients: results from the Medical Outcomes Study. JAMA 1989; 262:914–919.

Williams JW Jr, Barrett J, Oxman T, Frank E, Katon W, Sullivan M, Cornell J, Sengupta A. Treatment of dysthymia and minor depression in primary care: a randomized controlled trial in older adults. JAMA 2000; 284:1519–1526.

Zlotnick C, Shea MT, Pilkonis PA, Elkin I, Ryan C. Gender, type of treatment, dysfunctional attitudes, social support, life events, and depressive symptoms over naturalistic follow-up. Am J Psychiatry 1996; 153:1021–1027.

5

Bereavement and Depression in Late Life

Kelly Harless
University of California, San Diego, La Jolla, California, U.S.A.

Sidney Zisook
University of California, San Diego, La Jolla, and Veterans Affairs San Diego Healthcare System, San Diego, California, U.S.A.

INTRODUCTION

Bereavement is a darkness impenetrable to the imagination of the unbereaved. One can debate the merits of Iris Murdoch's (1919–1999) words, but one thing is for sure: the loss of a loved one and the painful feelings that ensue comprise an excruciating yet inevitable event in the human experience. The term *bereavement* refers to a specific kind of loss, that through death. And although it may be defined quite succinctly, bereavement and its sequelae are far from simple. When presented with a bereaved patient, the clinician faces a number of questions: Is the patient experiencing normal grief or a pathological depression? Should these symptoms be treated or left to resolve on their own, in what many believe to be a restorative process? And if intervention is appropriate, which therapeutic domain maximizes the probability of a successful outcome? These issues, perplexing in any clinical encounter, pose an additional set of challenges when the patient is elderly, as the loss may be accompanied by a host of factors associated with aging, such as poor health, impaired cognitive abilities, declining income, decreasing independence, and the loss of social and occupational roles to name a few.

BEREAVEMENT REACTION

Bereavement reaction, more commonly known as grief, is most readily understood as the emotional, cognitive, and behavioral responses to loss. It is a normal reaction, accompanying and following bereavement, which involves a complex array of psychological, physiological, and behavioral responses. Many investigators (Bowlby, 1980, 1981; Devaul et al., 1979; Horowitz, 1986) have described the grief process in terms of stages that bereaved individuals pass through as they accept and adjust to the loss of a loved one. These stages are typically described as an initial period of disbelief and denial, followed by a time of intense emotional discomfort as the reality of the loss registers with the bereaved. This second, intermediate stage may include crying spells and a myriad of feelings, including anguish, guilt, anxiety, fear, and apathy. The bereaved may become socially withdrawn in an attempt to avoid interactions that may arouse painful memories. Somatic disturbances may appear in the form of gastrointestinal complaints, problems with sleep and appetite, chest pain, heart palpitations, dyspnea, dizziness, tremulousness, and other distressing symptoms. The grief process culminates in a period of reorganization and recovery as the bereaved comes to terms with the loss. These stages—although helpful in delineating the journey from numbness to acute anguish to reconciliation and, ultimately, the ability to accept and cope with the loss—are best viewed as highly variable from person to person (Shuchter and Zisook, 1993) and fluid even within the individual. To the extent that such staging prescribes an expected or "normal" trajectory or that full resolution is either always possible or even desirable, the concept is oversimplified and misleading.

COMPLICATED GRIEF

Given the highly individualized nature of grief, how does the clinician determine whether a particular bereavement reaction is complicated or even pathological when, in fact, there is no single set of responses one can designate as "normal"? Why is it that some individuals experience the pain of loss while managing to function in their day-to-day lives, while others are devastated to the point of incapacitation or even death? (Cleiren, 1991). Two major categories of complications exist: [1] those that arise from the grief process itself and [2] medical and psychiatric disorders that occur or worsen in the context of bereavement. The first category may describe an insufficient or abbreviated bereavement reaction or, alternatively, one that is overly intense or protracted. The second category encompasses a host of ailments that may be precipitated by the death of a loved one and that pose significant health risks for the bereaved individual. Both categories warrant further exploration and boast a number of issues relevant to late-life bereavement.

Complications Arising from the Grief Process

Absent, Delayed, or Inhibited Grief

Clinicians are often confronted with relatives or friends of the bereaved expressing concern over the lack of grief displayed by the survivor, particularly when the bereaved is elderly. Such attenuated grief reactions most often occur when the relationship with the deceased has been extremely dependent and/or ambivalent (Parkes and Weiss, 1983; Raphael and Maddison, 1976), the relationship lacked a deep quality of attachment, or the bereaved suffers from a major psychiatric disorder that has inhibited the grief process. While many believe that the overt expression of grief is healthy and even therapeutic and the absence of such a reaction indicates pathology (Deutsch, 1937), more recent data fail to support this premise. The older individual who keeps his or her grief "bottled up" will not burst, as loved ones may fear. In fact, studies suggest that absent, delayed, or inhibited grief reactions are relatively common in older persons (Parkes, 1965). Stern et al. (1951) noted the apparent absence of grief in middle-aged and older bereaved individuals. Based on the number of somatic illnesses reported in this group, Stern suggested that the affective disturbance of grief in these individuals somehow converts into somatic complaints. Still other investigators (Cumming and Henry, 1961) submit that individuals undergo a process of "disengagement" at approximately age 65 and that, "with age occurs a mutual severing of ties between a person and others in his society." The loss of a spouse in this older group, suggests the theory, poses less trauma than for its younger counterpart. Parkes (1965) concludes that, while the inhibition of grief may be characteristic of the old, the long-term effects of this attenuation are unknown.

Hypertrophic Grief

Because grief is, by its very definition, a state of extreme emotional anguish, clinicians cannot easily determine when a bereavement reaction is exaggerated or overly intense—i.e., hypertrophic. Nor has hypertrophic grief been fully described or studied, although some investigators contend that such grief reactions correlate significantly with later distress and sometimes with major depression (Clayton, 1990; Parkes, 1972; Zisook and Shuchter, 1991a), and that hypertrophic grief is relatively uncommon in the elderly (Zisook et al., 1990b).

Recently, investigators have begun describing a related syndrome called *traumatic grief* (Prigerson et al., 1999; Shear et al., 2001; and Horowitz et al.,

1997). This condition is characterized by persistent, intense grief; yearning, pining, and longing for the deceased; recurrent intrusive images of the death; and a distressing admixture of avoidance and preoccupation with reminders of the loss. Positive memories regarding the deceased are either blocked or excessively sad. Traumatic grief has been associated with concomitant (Prigerson et al., 1985) and subsequent mental and physical morbidity (Prigerson et al., 1997). It has been reported that if recently bereaved individuals meet criteria for traumatic grief by 6 months, then by 13 months they are at increased risk for changes in smoking, eating, depression, and high blood pressure. By 25 months, such individuals express suicidal ideation more often and demonstrate an increased risk to develop heart trouble and new cases of cancer (Prigerson et al., 1999). One study of bereaved individuals with traumatic bereavement reported improvement in grief intensity as well as in associated depressive symptoms with either nortriptyline or paroxetine (Zygmont et al., 1998).

Chronic Grief

Little agreement exists about the time course of normal grief following bereavement. Typically, the frequency and intensity of the initial pangs of grief begin to lessen by the third or fourth month following the loss, but several investigators have found that symptoms of depression often remain as long as 1 year (Bornstein et al., 1973; Zisook and Shuchter, 1991a) or 2 years (Lund et al., 1985; Harlow et al., 1991; Zisook and Shuchter, 1993). Parkes (1971) concluded that the process of grieving often continues for more than 13 months, while other investigators (Goin, 1979; Zisook, 1987) suggest that the grieving process may never end for a significant proportion of otherwise normally bereaved individuals. Chronic grief may constitute the most common form of complication (Parkes, 1965).

A prolonged duration of the bereavement process is not sufficient to determine whether an individual suffers from chronic, pathological grief. Rather, the clinician should consider the nature of the grief experience and its impact on the bereaved, in addition to its duration, in evaluating an individual who has suffered a loss. Is the grief overwhelming, accompanied by dysphoria, and characterized by an unyielding preoccupation with and idealization of the deceased? Is the intensity of the sorrow unmitigated by time? Investigators have not reached a consensus regarding how long grief must last to be deemed chronic; however, persistent and pervasive grief lasting more than 1 year and characterized by the features described above requires clinical attention. Careful consideration should be given to whether the grief process has been impeded by another psychiatric disorder, such as major depression, anxiety disorder, or posttraumatic stress disorder. Clinicians should determine whether criteria for one or more of these syndromes are met and target treatment accordingly. Risk factors for chronic grief are loss of a child (Raphael, 1983), a dependent relationship with the deceased (Parkes, 1983), or an unnatural death (Rynaearson, 1987b). The condition is frequently reported in young and middle-aged adults, most often in women and adolescents. Prognosis for this condition is guarded and treatment may be protracted and difficult.

Complications Arising from Medical and Psychiatric Disorders

Medical Morbidity and Mortality

According to most investigators, the presence of pre-existing health problems constitutes the greatest risk factor for declining health after bereavement. Given the higher incidence of medical morbidity in the older population, it is not surprising that the elderly evince a particular vulnerability to such complications after the loss of a spouse. Thompson et al. (1984) have suggested that this group (especially older women) suffers an exacerbation in existing conditions and develops new illnesses in the months immediately following the bereavement, although other studies suggest these effects are transient and disappear by 30 months follow-up (Gallager-Thompson et al., 1983). One explanation for this phenomenon lies in the increased caretaking burden wives assume as they care for their dying husbands (Hutchin, 1993; Moss et al., 1993) while neglecting their own health.

Stroebe and Stroebe (1993) conducted a comprehensive review of the mortality of bereavement and concluded that the vast majority of studies support an excess mortality rate in bereaved versus nonbereaved individuals. Since most studies focus on the effects of spousal bereavement, the findings pose particular relevance to the elderly population, as the likelihood of becoming widowed between the ages of 65 and 74 is 8.9% for men and 36.6% for women. The risk of widowhood increases dramatically after age 74 to 23.4% for men and 65.8% for women (U.S. Bureau of Census, 1991). Several large studies demonstrate higher mortality rates for individuals who have lost spouses than for their married counterparts (Cox and Ford, 1964; Helsing and Szklo, 1981; Kaprio et al., 1987; Kraus and Lilienfeld, 1959; Levav et al., 1988; Rees and Lutkins, 1967). Interestingly, the group at greatest risk of dying (relative to their peers) following spousal bereavement comprises younger widows (Helsing and Szklo, 1981; Jones, 1987; Kaprio et al., 1987; Mellstrom et al., 1982), although one study (Bowling and Charlton, 1987) demonstrates that the oldest old persons might be at relatively higher risk compared to controls. Widowers appear to be at greatest risk within the first 6 months of bereavement (Helsing and Szklo, 1981; Rees and Lutkins, 1967; Young et al., 1963); this period of risk may be delayed 1 or 2 years in widows (Cox and Ford, 1964; Helsing and Szklo, 1981). Other risk factors include moving into a chronic care facility (Helsing and Szklo,

1981), social isolation and lack of social support (Bowling and Charlton, 1987; Gallagher-Thompson et al., 1993; Helsing and Szklo, 1981), living alone or not remarrying (for widowers) (Helsing and Szklo, 1981), sudden deaths for widowers or widows under the age of 50, and death from a chronic illness for widowers between 50 and 64 years (Stroebe and Stroebe, 1993). One well-known study (Levav et al., 1988) of survivors of Israeli soldiers suggested that divorced or widowed mothers who lose a son in war are at higher risk for increased mortality.

No consistent pattern emerges for the cause of excess mortality during bereavement (Stroebe and Stroebe, 1993). Some of the most compelling data implicate death from suicide (Kaprio et al, 1987; MacMahon and Pugh, 1965). Other investigators suggest that accidents (Helsing and Szklo, 1981; Jones 1987; Mellstrom et al., 1982) and heart disease (Jones et al., 1984) may be significant contributors to higher mortality rates in bereaved individuals; but cancer, liver cirrhosis, diabetes, and infectious diseases may also correlate.

Psychiatric Morbidity

A variety of psychiatric disorders may worsen or emerge in the context of a severe life stressor such as bereavement. Some of the most common conditions include substance abuse, anxiety disorder, posttraumatic stress disorder, subsyndromal depression, and major depressive disorder. Although the list of potential psychiatric complications extends far beyond these and the impact of any condition should never be dismissed, the issues delineated below constitute those most commonly observed in clinical encounters with bereaved individuals and warrant further discussion.

Substance Abuse. Individuals who have lost a spouse are at high risk for increased substance use, including alcohol, tobacco (Blankfield, 1983; Klerman and Izen, 1977; Osterweis et al., 1984), and drugs (primarily sedatives and hypnotics) (Maddison and Viola, 1968). Clayton (1979) found a higher incidence of alcohol use in a sample of older widows and widowers compared to married controls. Many studies suggest that such increases occur in people with preexisting alcohol problems. Valanis et al. (1987), for example, noted no new cases of heavy or problem drinking in widowed individuals. Similarly, Zisook et al. (1990b) measured changes in alcohol consumption in middle-aged and elderly widowed individuals (mean age 61 years) and found that approximately equal numbers increased (30%) and decreased (26%) the number of days per month they drank. However, when looking at the quantity of alcohol consumed, Zisook reported that more widows and widowers increased (34%) than decreased (10%) their quantity of alcohol consumption. Risk factors for increased drinking included the amount of drinking prior to bereavement, being male, a history of depression, dissatisfaction with social and emotional supports, and experiencing a depressive episode soon after the death.

Anxiety Disorder. Parkes (1964) found that an array of symptoms typically associated with anxiety often accompany grief. Restlessness, tension, insomnia, headaches, and irritability may characterize the first year of spousal bereavement. Parkes further noted that panic attacks often punctuate the first several months of bereavement. Clayton (1968, 1974) suggested an increased prevalence of anxiety symptoms in widows in comparison to their married counterparts. Widows reported an increased frequency of anxiety attacks, insomnia, weight loss, fatigue, decreased concentration, poor memory, shortness of breath, palpitations and blurred vision. Maddison and Viola (1968) similarly reported increased nervousness, panic feelings, fears, insomnia, and trembling in widows 1 year after losing their husbands. Jacobs et al. (1990) found that more than 40% of bereaved spouses reported at least one type of anxiety disorder based on the modified Structured Clinical Interview for DSM-III. There were higher than expected rates for panic and for generalized anxiety disorders during the first year, for agoraphobia in the first 6 months, and for social phobia in the latter 6 months.

According to Zisook et al. (1990a, 1993), older widows and widowers used more over-the-counter "nerve pills," as well as more prescribed antianxiety medications and hypnotics. This group also demonstrated higher risk rates of several anxiety symptoms during the first 7 months of spousal bereavement, elevated scores on Hopkins Symptom Checklist scales of anxiety, somatization, interpersonal sensitivity, and obsessions compared to community norms. Individuals at greatest risk for continued high anxiety 7 months after bereavement tended to be female, younger, and of lower socioeconomic status. Additional risk factors included lack of environmental support, presence of unresolved grief, and increased depression and anxiety symptom intensity soon after the loss. The risks for panic and generalized anxiety disorders were highest among those who had a previous history of anxiety disorders.

Related to the syndrome of traumatic grief described above, several investigators have reported that bereavement, especially after a violent and untimely death, may precipitate an actual episode of posttraumatic stress disorder (PTSD) (Horowitz, 1986; Zisook et al., 1998). Indeed, in the first published epidemiological study of PTSD using the criteria of the *Diagnostic and Statistical Manual of Mental Disorders*, 4th ed. (DSM-IV) (APA, 1994), Breslau et al. reported that the sudden and unexpected death of a loved one accounted for more PTSD than any other stressor (1998). Rynearson (1981, 1984, 1987a, 1987b, 1990) and Parkes (1993) have compared the reactions to such traumatic losses as suicide, homicide, or other forms of unnatural death to PTSD. Rynearson noted that people bereaved by a homicide event report symptoms typically associated with a posttraumatic stress syndrome: intrusive, vivid, and repetitive images of the death; impaired cognitive processes; nightmares, heightened arousal; hypervigilance; and avoidance. Zisook et al. reported that almost 10% of recently bereaved widows and widowers experienced PTSD, even after an expected death following a chronic illness (1998). According to Middleton et al. (1993), grief complicated by PTSD can be differentiated from other bereavement reactions by hyperarousal, avoidance, nightmares and intrusive, recurrent, or traumatic images that often reflect the scene of the death. Few data exist on whether or when bereavement is likely to lead to PTSD in the elderly; more work is warranted in this area.

Subsyndromal Depression. In evaluating clinically relevant manifestations of bereavement-related depression, one must include the minor and subsyndromal depressions—in addition to the more familiar major depression—in the equation (Zisook et al., 1997). As defined in the DSM-IV appendix, minor depressive episodes differ from major depressive episodes primarily in the number of depressive symptoms—fewer than five. Subsyndromal depression has been defined in many ways: The definition of Judd et al. requires two or more depressive symptoms, lasting for 2 weeks or more, in the absence of a minor or major depression. He found that subsyndromal syndromes often correlate with marked disability and precede a full major depressive syndrome (Judd et al., 1996). Indeed, these attenuated forms of depression occur more frequently than do major depressive syndromes. Such subsyndromal depressions may be quite common in elderly persons and may be associated with substantial suffering and morbidity (Blazer 1994; Blazer and George, 1987; Broadhead et al., 1990). Unfortunately, despite its prevalence in this vulnerable population, the condition often goes unrecognized (Pasternak et al., 1994; Zisook et al., 1994).

During the first 2 years of spousal bereavement, minor and subsyndromal depressions may be prodromes of major depression, may represent residual symptoms and/or syndromes as a major depression is improving, or even reflect the aftermath of a partially remitted major depression. It is also possible that these depressions constitute independent mood disturbances or forms of attenuated depression important in their own right. Often, widows and widowers shift back and forth between phases of no depression, subsyndromal depression, minor depression, and major depression. An individual who experiences a major depressive episode 6 to 8 weeks after his or her spouse dies can expect to spend roughly 38% of the next 2 years in a major depressive state, 38% to experience either minor or subsyndromal depression, and only 24% to remain depression-free. These percentages are similar to rates reported for nonbereaved depressed populations (Judd et al., 1998). And these minor and subsyndromal manifestations of depression are not innocuous. Widows and widowers with minor and subsyndromal manifestations of depression experience psychosocial morbidity roughly midway between those with no depression and those with major depression (Zisook et al., 1997).

Major Depression. Clinicians often equate grief with depression when in fact they are two distinct phenomena with overlapping features. Bereaved individuals often manifest symptoms of grief that are commonly associated with major depression: crying, insomnia, dysphoria, anorexia, restlessness, fatigue, poor memory, loss of interest, and difficulty in concentrating (Weller, et al., 1991; Clayton, 1990; Bruce, et al., 1990; Zisook and Shuchter, 1993; Gallagher-Thompson et al., 1993; Harlow et al., 1991; Zisook et al., 1991). Indeed, as a symptom, depression is considered a fundamental aspect of normal grief and bereavement. Clayton (1979, 1990) reported that over half of all widowed persons experience crying spells, sleep disturbances, low mood, loss of appetite, fatigue, and/or poor memory at some point during the first year of bereavement. Others (Lund et al., 1993; Zisook and Shuchter, 1991) have reported that widows and widowers experience a far greater number of depressive symptoms than do married individuals. Specifically, one-third of all widows and widowers expressed feelings of loneliness, feeling blue, insomnia, diminished interests, thoughts of death or dying, and hopelessness for as long as 2 years following the death of their spouses.

According to the DSM-IV, a diagnosis of major depression applies when either (not necessarily both) depressed mood or loss of interest in normal activities is present most of the time for at least 2 weeks. In addition, several other symptoms must coexist during the same period, the syndrome must create either marked distress or psychosocial impairment, and it must not be causally related to medications, drugs or general medical illness. However, when the syndrome occurs in the context of bereavement, DSM-IV conventions extend the 2-week requirement and dictate a diagnosis of bereavement if any or all symptoms of a depressive episode occur within 2 months of the loss (APA, 1994). The only exception to this mandate occurs when certain markers of depression severity (e.g., psychomotor retardation, morbid feelings of worthlessness, or suicidal ideation) prevail. After the first 2 months have elapsed, the diagnosis of major depression is relatively straightforward; symptoms that emerge during the first 2 months pose a more complex diagnostic dilemma. Such episodes are common, occurring in 29–58% of widows and widowers 1 month after their spouse's death (Clayton et al., 1972; Gilewski et al., 1991; Harlow et al., 1991); they can be disabling, and often are chronic (Zisook and Shuchter, 1993).

Interestingly, major depression is the only Axis I disorder whose condition is negated by bereavement. If, for example, a person develops a panic disorder, no one would repudiate the diagnosis if the individual also happened to be bereaved. In addition, no other stressors aside from bereavement nullify the diagnosis of major depression. As an illustration, consider an individual recently divorced, disabled, or impoverished who manifests symptoms of depression. An astute clinician would recognize the stressor as precipitant to a major depression in a vulnerable person, not simply dismiss the depressive symptoms as a product of the situation (Zisook and Shuchter, 1997).

Until recently, few studies on bereavement focused on elderly persons and issues surrounding the loss of a loved one in late life. In the late 1970s, the

National Institute on Aging established bereavement and aging as priorities and funded three controlled, prospective, longitudinal studies that looked at depression and its risk factors after late-life bereavement (Lund et al., 1993). Investigations followed that examined depressive reactions in late-life bereavement (Bruce et al., 1990; Goldberg et al., 1988; Harlow et al., 1991; McHorney and Mor, 1988; Norris and Murrell, 1990; Zisook and Shuchter, 1991b). In general, these studies reveal that there are more similarities than differences between the depressive reactions experienced by older versus younger individuals. As in younger individuals, the risk for depressive symptoms and syndromes in late life is substantial (Breckenridge et al., 1986; Bruce et al., 1990; Gallagher-Thompson et al., 1983; Harlow et al., 1991) and remain greater than the risk for married controls for at least 2 years beyond the death of a loved one (Harlow et al., 1991; Zisook and Shuchter, 1993). On the other hand, several investigators have found that the frequency and intensity of depressive symptoms and syndromes after late-life bereavement may be less than in younger individuals (Faletti et al., 1989; McHorney and Mor, 1988; VanZandt et al., 1989). Zisook and Shuchter (1993) found that risk for major depressive syndrome in older widows and widowers is less than their younger counterparts only for the first year; by the end of the second year of bereavement, the frequency of major depressive syndrome in widows and widowers over 65 years of age is identical to the frequency in those under 65 years. Therefore, it may not be that older widows and widowers are less distressed or depressed than younger ones but rather that it takes somewhat longer for them to experience the full impact of bereavement.

There are also more similarities than differences in the nature of the bereavement-related depression in late life compared with other forms of major depression. Gallagher-Thompson et al. (1982) and Breckenridge et al. (1986) emphasized that the depressions experienced by late-life widows and widowers tend to be milder than other major depressive syndromes and that self-deprecation is rarely observed in bereavement reactions. Similarly, Bruce et al. (1990) found bereavement increased the risk for dysphoria and major depressive syndrome and that, except for fewer reports of guilt or worthlessness, the major depressive syndrome experienced by widows and widowers roughly parallels other major depressive syndromes in terms of symptomatology. One sleep study found abnormal sleep architecture in depressed elderly widows, further supporting the similarities between a major depressive syndrome associated with loss and a non-bereavement-related depression (Reynolds et al., 1992).

Not all bereaved individuals experience a major depressive syndrome after their loss; individuals undergoing a severe life stressor often display amazing adaptive capacities (Pollock, 1987; Shuchter and Zisook, 1993; Silverman, 1972). But because risk for developing a major depressive syndrome after bereavement is substantial and the morbidity of untreated depression so great, it is important to identify risk factors. In general, no consistent findings on risk factors that relate to gender emerge. Some studies found that older widows are at higher risk (Bruce et al., 1990; Gallagher-Thompson et al., 1983) and other studies reported that older widowers are most vulnerable (Richards and McCallum, 1979), but most studies have not found substantial differences between bereaved men and women (Clayton, 1990; Feinson, 1986; Zisook and Shuchter, 1991a). Loss of a spouse may pose a greater risk than most other types of losses (Norris and Murrell, 1990). Poor prior physical and mental health (McHorney and Mor, 1988; Nuss and Zubenko, 1992) and prebereavement depression (Norris and Murrell, 1990) or dysphoria (Bruce et al., 1990) are additional risk factors. A particularly traumatic loss, such as a suicide, may be especially likely to result in persistent depressive syndromes (Gilewski et al., 1991). The protective role of social supports in attenuating the risks for depression associated with late-life bereavement appears to be especially important (Dimond et al., 1987; Goldberg et al., 1988; Norris and Murrell, 1990; Nuss and Zubenko, 1992). Other investigators have identified early intense reactions soon after the loss (Farberow et al., 1987; Lund et al., 1985; Parkes and Weiss, 1983; Zisook and Shuchter, 1991a) and early depressive reactions (Dimond et al., 1987; Gilewski et al., 1991; Zisook and Shuchter, 1991a) as powerful predictors of later depression. Additional risk factors include financial problems, global stress (Norris and Murrell, 1990), recent disability (Goldberg et al., 1988), and subsequent losses in widowers (Siegel and Kuykendall, 1990). Using a stepwise, logistic regression procedure, Zisook and Shuchter (1993) identified a six-variable model that correctly classified 91% of widows and widowers in terms of major depressive syndrome two years after loss. The six variables are [1] presence of a major depressive syndrome soon after the loss, [2] intense symptoms of depression soon after the death, [3] family history of major depression, [4] increased alcohol consumption soon after the loss, [5] poor physical health around the time of the death, and [6] a sudden and unexpected death.

TREATMENT OF BEREAVEMENT-RELATED DEPRESSION SYNDROMES

To Treat or Not to Treat?

Just as a clinician would treat any other Axis I disorder that emerges in the context of bereavement, so too should one assess the need for treatment when symptoms of depression occur after the loss of a loved one. Even subsyndromal depressive syndromes occurring in the context of bereavement can be chronic, associated with poor functioning, and replete with risk factors for major depressive episodes, raising questions of whether and how these minor variants of depression should be treated (Zisook et al., 1994).

Although there are overwhelming data to support treating major depressive episodes, less is known about the risk-to-benefit ratios of treating minor and subsyndromal depression. What is known is that minor depressions are associated with significant morbidity (Rollman and Reynolds, 1999) and respond to antidepressant medications (Stewart et al., 1992). Therefore, minor episodes of depression should be treated if they significantly interfere with function, impede the normal flow of grief, or persist without showing signs of spontaneously abating. Whether to treat subsyndromal symptoms is even more controversial, as subsyndromal symptoms of depression also are associated with biopsychosocial morbidity (Judd et al., 1996) but fail to demonstrate a clear response to treatment. Subsyndromal symptoms warrant treatment only when they clearly are an early manifestation of a more robust major depressive episode (i.e., prodromal symptoms) or represent residual symptoms after partial remission from a major depressive episode. In the latter situation, ample data suggests that such residual symptoms correlate with prolonged functional impairment and are strong predictors of imminent recurrent full-blown episodes (Judd et al., 1998).

Major depressive disorders, even when the episode's onset falls near the time of death of a loved one, have been associated with chronicity, recurrence, impaired interpersonal and occupational functioning, feelings of worthlessness, suicidal ideation, medical morbidity, and poor overall adjustment to widowhood. Such depressive episodes add to the already substantial pain, suffering and poor functioning associated with bereavement, and also have biological underpinnings similar to other nonbereavement major depressions. They predict prolonged biopsychosocial impairment (Zisook et al., 1994). Thus, they appear to be at last as clinically significant as other major depressive episodes not associated with bereavement and, just as any major depressive episode is worthy of treatment, so too are those syndromes associated with bereavement.

There are increasing but still too limited data on the efficiency of psychopharmacology, psychotherapy, or both for the treatment of major depression associated with bereavement in the elderly. However, there is little reason to think that such depressions will not respond to adequate treatment, as most studies consistently support the effectiveness of the treatment studied. Psychopharmacological trials suggest that such interventions are safe and effective and that treatment of depression does not interfere with grief. Indeed, studies suggest that depression interferes with grief and that the treatment of depression facilitates the work of grief. However, they also found that grief resolution requires more than short-term medication treatment (Pasternak et al., 1998). Alternative or augmenting treatment options include a wide range of psychotherapies. Both cognitive and interpersonal therapies, for example, have been found effective for the acute treatment of mild to moderate major depressive episodes. A more thorough discussion of the two most common treatment modalities, psychopharmacological intervention and psycotherapy, follow.

Psychopharmacological Intervention

Unfortunately, the optimal place for antidepressant medications in the treatment of bereavement-associated depression remains largely uncharted by controlled data. In general, these depressions are underdiagnosed and undertreated, and even recognized psychopharmacology experts have traditionally recommended caution (Klein and Blank, 1969; Hollister, 1972). Two open studies with tricyclic antidepressants support the safety and efficacy of these medications for bereavement-related major depressive syndromes (Jacobs et al., 1987; Pasternak et al., 1991), while noting that residual grief symptoms remained even after 6–8 weeks of antidepressant therapy. Perhaps early treatment for those depressive syndromes seen within months of the death of a loved one helps prevent some of the prolonged suffering, morbidity, and even mortality associated with bereavement.

In the only randomized, placebo-controlled study on bereavement-related major depression, Reynolds and colleagues (1999) found that nortriptyline was more effective than placebo in achieving remission of major depressive episodes, that interpersonal therapy was not more effective than placebo, and that the combination of medication and psychotherapy was more effective than either treatment alone. Zisook et al. (2001) recently reported the results of an open-label preliminary study showing that bupropion sustained-release effectively reduces both depressive symptoms and grief intensity in widows and widowers meeting criteria for major depressive syndromes within 2 months of their loss. Thus, the available data overwhelmingly support the acute treatment of bereavement-related depression, perhaps as early as 6–8 weeks after the loss, and certainly anytime thereafter.

There is no reason to think that any one class of antidepressant medications is more effective than others for the treatment of bereavement-related depression. As with treating other, non-bereavement-related depressions, selection should be based on past or family history of response or, to a lesser extent, on clinical subtype. In the absence of information on past history or specific subtypes known to be preferentially responsive to a particular class of medications, side effects and toxicity guide the choice of medications. Of course, the issues surrounding the pharmacological treatment of older, nonbereaved individuals also apply when treating older, depressed patients who have lost a loved one. Clinicians should consider prescribing lower doses of antidepressant medications in this population than in their younger counterparts. Concerns surrounding polypharmacy are relevant in this group, as the elderly often take multiple medications for various ailments. Special attention should be paid to compliance issues: older individuals may suffer from visual or hearing losses and not perceive instructions properly, or they may have problems with memory and easily forget when and how much medication should be taken. Clinicians should, whenever possible, involve family members or other caregivers in treating older bereaved individuals.

Psychotherapy

Although several published treatment studies support the usefulness of psychotherapy for various aspects of bereavement related difficulties (Horowitz et al., 1984; Walls and Meyers, 1985; Kleber and Brom, 1987; Sireling et al., 1988; Kavanaugh, 1990; Volkan, 1971; Melges and DeMaso, 1980; Rando, 1984; Paul and Grosser, 1965), very few data are available to specifically address psychotherapeutic treatment of bereavement-related depression in the elderly. A small case report series suggests the potential effectiveness of interpersonal psychotherapy for bereavement related depression following loss of a spouse in late life (Miller et al., 1994). We have advocated a psychotherapeutic approach that addresses both grief and depression and includes the following components:

1. Establish a supportive relationship with the bereaved individual and possibly his or her family.
2. Obtain a detailed assessment of the bereaved's relationship to the deceased as it began and evolved over time, the events and associated feelings surrounding the death, the impact of the loss, social support, other stressors, and background and family issues.
3. Probe the psychological, behavioral, and cognitive responses to the death.
4. Assess coping strategies, encouraging flexibility and "healthy" responses while discouraging less healthy coping strategies (e.g., alcohol or drugs).
5. Accept the person's pain and anguish without offering false platitudes or offering empty reassurance.
6. Help the person accept his or her own idiosyncratic responses without feeling guilty for not grieving in a conventional manner or as others tell them is "normal."
7. Help facilitate acceptance of the loss as the person is ready while simultaneously fostering the development of adaptive symbolic and psychological ties to the deceased.
8. Explore ongoing relationships with key friends and relatives.
9. Attend to psychological, social, and medical needs as necessary.
10. Some individuals may need help attending requirements of everyday life, such as paying bills, housekeeping, or child care; others may need help with grief-specific tasks necessitated by the loss, such as funeral arrangements and tracking important papers and documents.
11. Consider referral to social services or grief support services.
12. Apply the "first aid" principle of care (i.e., if it's wet, dry it; if it's dry, wet it).

13. For unflappable avoidance or numbness, consider evocative techniques such as guided imagery, visiting the grave, or writing letters.
14. For pervasive preoccupation with painful images, consider treatment aimed at anxiety reduction and distraction.
15. Help the bereaved person to understand that grief is a lifelong process, but that people nevertheless learn to go on.
16. Treatment goals must take into account that depression is often chronic, recurrent, and pleiomorphic in its manifestations over time.
17. Understand that grief work is exhausting and demanding, often for the therapist as well as the patient.

An Integrative Model for Treatment

Most bereaved individuals do not require professional help. Their arduous journey through the grief process will ultimately culminate in an acceptable level of adjustment to a life without their loved one. Some, however, will find themselves facing a potentially serious psychiatric disorder as they try to cope with their loss. When confronted with such an individual, the clinician must decide whether and which interventions—psychotherapeutic, psychopharmacological, or a combination of the two—are appropriate. The major factors that determine when and how to treat are past history; time since death; and the intensity, duration, and pervasiveness of the depressive syndrome.

Past History

The more vulnerable the person is, the sooner after the loss active treatment should begin. The risk of developing a major depressive syndrome more than doubles if the person has had only one episode of major depression before the death of a spouse; if a person has had two or more previous episodes, the risk is more than sixfold greater than if the person was never before depressed (Zisook and Shuchter, 1993). Thus, for a patient with a history of recurrent major depressive episodes, treatment should begin by the time the death of a loved one is considered imminent. Such a person is vulnerable to an exacerbation or relapse of the depressive illness after the death and prevention is warranted. If first seen after the death, a bereaved person with a history of recurrent depression should be either observed closely or started on prophylactic treatment. The decisions regarding which treatment or combination of treatments will be best for each unique person are based on the patient's preferences; the severity, duration, proximity, and treatment-response of previous depressions; the likelihood of the patient's promptly initiating treatment should depression develop; the intensity of grief and depressive symptoms at the time of the initial evaluation; and the general medical health of the patient. In other words, the risk factors previously described help to guide treatment.

Time Since Death

Compared with the past history and the nature of the depressions, time since death is a relatively minor factor. The question is not so much how long to wait before treating but rather under what circumstances one should wait. If there is no past or family history of major depression and the syndrome is relatively mild in terms of severity, reactivity, and impairment, treatment may be delayed for at least the first 2 months if not longer. The clinician may then initiate treatment with educational-supportive psychotherapy, using the same general guidelines as one would for nonbereavement depressions. If the depression does not fully respond to psychotherapeutic interventions, antidepressant medications should be given. Aggressive treatment of minor or subsyndromal depressive syndromes during the first few months of bereavement is rarely necessary. However, the farther the patient is from loss, the more therapeutic intervention may be warranted, even in these subthreshold variants. The more vulnerable the person is in terms of past or family history and the more intense or autonomous the symptoms are, the earlier in the course of bereavement is intervention justified. Suicidal or melancholic symptoms, for example, require prompt intervention regardless of the proximity to bereavement (or any other psychosocial stressor for that matter).

Nature of Symptoms

As in all other depressions, the decision of when and how to treat is dependent on the intensity, autonomy, duration, and pervasiveness of the syndrome. The more severe and autonomous the depression is, the more likely it is that somatic treatment is necessary. Even in the absence of previous episodes or immediately after the death of a loved one, if depressive symptoms are severe, present in the absence of grief triggers, and associated with suicidal ideation or melancholic features, aggressive pharmacological treatment should prevail. Conversely, if the depressive symptoms and the impairment are mild, seem most pronounced around reminders of the deceased, and are not associated with significant impairment, suicidal thoughts, or melancholic features, education and support may be all that is necessary. If the bereaved person does not have close friends or a supportive social milieu, a support group might be helpful for this type of mild depression. For depression between these two extremes, combinations of somatic and psychotherapeutic interventions are indicated.

No single form of psychotherapy or antidepressant medication is currently designated the "best" treatment for bereavement-related depression, and few studies exist which focus on the treatment of older bereaved individuals. Cognitive-behavioral and interpersonal therapy have both proved effective for treating depression; indeed there are no strong data demonstrating that either of these forms of therapy is superior to the other. Similarly, all classes of antidepressant medications are about equally effective, but differences in their side-effect profiles usually dictate which medication is best suited for an individual patient. It is important to address the individual's specific needs and resources, as well as the availability of various treatment modalities, in deciding the best approach. A paradigm that includes education, supportive psychotherapy and medication management maximizes the probability of successful treatment (Zisook and Shuchter, 1996).

CONCLUSION

Grief and depression are by no means identical and constitute two separate albeit intertwined, phenomena. Despite—or perhaps because of—the pain, disability, and life disruption associated with bereavement, many individuals experience enormous growth and development throughout the grief process. Perhaps Thomas Mann (1875–1955) was right when he stated, "*A man's dying is more the survivors' affair than his own.*" For although the shattering impact of losing a loved one should never be minimized, many individuals emerge from the experience with a renewed sense of who they are and with an expanded repertoire of competencies. On the other hand, a substantial minority of bereaved individuals may find their loss precipitating the onset, persistence, or exacerbation of a psychiatric disorder. In such cases, the problem should not be ignored, rationalized, or minimized. Psychiatric disturbances that emerge in the context of bereavement, including depressive syndromes, warrant full clinical attention. Sadness, unhappiness, loneliness, and other dysphoric experiences commonly characterize "normal grief," but major depression does not. Bereavement-related depressions respond just as well to treatment, as do other non-bereavement-related depressions. More studies are needed in the area of late-life bereavement; a particular dearth of literature exists in the area of treatment strategies geared toward this population. An integrative approach combining patient support, family education, psychotherapy, and pharmacological therapy is ideal.

REFERENCES

American Psychiatric Association (APA). Diagnostic and Statistical Manual of Mental Disorders, 4th ed. Washington, DC: American Psychiatric Association, 1994.

Blankfield A. Grief and alcohol. Am J Drug Alcohol Abuse 9:435–446, 1983.

Blazer DG. Epidemiology of depressive disorders in late life, In: Schneider LS, Reynolds CF, Lebowitz BD, et al., eds. Diagnosis and Treatment of Depression in Late Life: Results of the NIMH Consensus and Development Conference. Washington, DC: American Psychiatric Press, 1994, pp 9–20.

Blazer DG, George LK. The epidemiology of depression in an elderly community population. Gerontologist 27:281–287, 1987.

Bornstein PE, Clayton PJ, Halikas JA, et al. The depression of widowhood after thirteen months. Br J Psychiatry 122:561–566, 1973.
Bowlby J. Attachment and Loss. Loss: Sadness and Depression. Vol 3. New York: Basic Books, 1980/1981.
Bowling A, Charlton J. Risk factors for mortality after bereavement: a logistic regression analysis. J R Coll Gen Pract 37:551–554, 1987.
Breckenridge JN, Gallagher D, Thompson LW, et al. Characteristic depressive symptoms of bereaved elders. J Gerontol 41:163–168, 1986.
Breslau N, Kessler RC, Chilcoat HD, Schultz LR, Davis GC, Andreski P. Trauma and posttraumatic stress disorder in the community: the 1996 Detroit Area Survey of Trauma. Arch Gen Psychiatry 55:626–632, 1998.
Broadhead WE, Blazer DG, George LK, et al. Depression, disability days, and days lost from work in a prospective epidemiologic survey. JAMA 264:2524–2528, 1990.
Bruce M, Kim K, Leaf P, et al. Depressive episodes and dysphoria resulting from conjugal bereavement in a prospective community sample. Am J Psychiatry 147:608–611, 1990.
Clayton PJ. Mortality and morbidity in the first year of bereavement. Arch Gen Psychiatry 30:747–750, 1974.
Clayton, PJ. The sequelae and nonsequelae of conjugal bereavement. Am J Psychiatry 136:1530–1534, 1979.
Clayton PJ. Bereavement and Depression. J Clin Psychiatry 51:34–40, 1990.
Clayton PJ, Desmarais L, Winokur G. A study of normal bereavement. Am J Psychiatry 125:168–178, 1968.
Clayton PJ, Halikas JA, Maurice WL. The depression of widowhood. Br J Psychiatry 120:71–76, 1972.
Cleiren MPHD. Adaptation After Bereavement. Leiden: DSWO Press, 1991.
Cox, PR, Ford JR. The mortality of widows shortly after widowhood. Lancet 1:163–164, 1964.
Cumming E, Henry WR. Growing Old. New York, Basic Books, 1961.
Deutsch H. Absence of grief. Psychoanal Q 6:12–22, 1937.
DeVaul RA, Zisook S, Faschingbauer TR. Clinical aspects of grief and bereavement. Primary Care 6:391–402, 1979.
Dimond MF, Lund DA, Caserta MS. The role of social supporting the first two years of bereavement in an elderly sample. Gerontologist 27:599–604, 1987.
Faletti MV, Gibbs JM, Clark C, et al. Longitudinal course of bereavement in older adults. In: Lund DA, ed. Older Bereaved Spouses: Research with Practical Applications. New York: Taylor & Francis/Hemisphere, 1989, pp 37–51.
Farverow NL, Gallagher DE, Gilewski MJ, et al. An examination of the early impact of bereavement on psychological distress in survivors of suicide. Gerontologist 27: 592–598, 1987.
Feinson, MC. Aging widows and widowers: are there mental health differences? Int J Aging Hum Dev 23:241–255, 1986.
Gallagher-Thompson DE, Breckenridge JN, Thompson LW. Similarities and differences between normal grief and depression in older adults. Essence 5:127–140, 1982.
Gallagher-Thompson DE, Breckenridge J, Thompson LW, et al. Effects of bereavement

on indicators of mental health in elderly widows and widowers. J Gerontol 38: 565–571, 1983.

Gallagher-Thompson D, Futerman A, Farberow N, et al. The impact of spousal bereavement on older widows and widowers. In: Stroebe MS, Stroebe W, Hansson RO, eds. Handbook of Bereavement: Theory, Research and Intervention. Cambridge, UK: Cambridge University Press, 1993, pp 227–239.

Gilewski MJ, Farberow NL, Gallagher DE, et al. Interaction of depression and bereavement on mental health in the elderly. Psychol Aging 6:67–75, 1991.

Goin Mk, Burgoyne RW, Goin JM. Timeless attachment to a dead relative. Am J Psychiatry 136:988–989, 1979.

Goldberg EL, Comstock GW, Harlow SD. Emotional problems and widowhood. J Gerontol 3:5206–5208, 1988.

Harlow SD, Goldberg EL, Comstock GW. A longitudinal study of the prevalence of depressive symptomatology in elderly widowed and married women. Arch Gen Psychiatry 48:1065–1068, 1991.

Helsing KJ, Szklo M. Mortality after bereavement. Am J Epidemiol 114:41–52, 1981.

Hollister L. Psychotherapeutic drugs in the dying and bereaved. J Thanatol 2:623–629, 1972.

Horowitz MJ. Stress Response Syndromes. Northvale, NJ: Aronson, 1986.

Horowitz MJ, Marmar C, Weiss DS, et al. Brief psychotherapy of bereavement reactions. Arch Gen Psychiatry 41:438–448, 1984.

Horowitz MJ, Siegel, B, et al. Diagnostic criteria for complicated grief disorder. Am J Psychiatry 154(7):904–910, 1997.

Hutchin S. The distress of care giving. Presented at the 146th annual meeting of the American Psychiatric Association, San Francisco, CA, May 22–27, 1993.

Jacobs SC, Nelson JC, Zisook S. Treating depression of bereavement with antidepressants: a pilot study. Psychiatr Clin North Am 10:501–510, 1987.

Jacobs SC, Hansen F, Kasl S, et al. Anxiety disorders in acute bereavement: risk and risk factors. J Clin Psychiatry 51:267–274, 1990.

Jacobs SC, and Zisook, S. Treatment of major depression during bereavement. Geriatr Psychopharmacol 6:115–126, 1998.

Jones DR. Heart disease mortality following widowhood: some results form the OPCS longitudinal study. J Psychosom Res 31:325–333, 1987.

Jones DR, Goldblatt PO, Leon DA. Bereavement and cancer: some results using data on deaths of spouses form the Longitudinal Study of the Office of Population Censuses and Surveys. Br Med J 298:461–464, 1984.

Judd LL, Akiskal HS, Maser JD, Zeller PJ, Endicott J, Coryell W, Paulus MP, Kunovac JL, Leon AC, Mueller TI, Rice JA, Keller MB. A prospective 12-year study of subsyndromal and syndromal depressive symptoms in unipolar major depressive disorder. Arch Gen Psychiatry 55:694–700, 1998.

Judd LL, Paulus MP, Wells KB, Rapaport MH. Socioeconomic burden of subsyndromal depressive symptoms and major depression in a sample of the general population. Am J Psychiatry 153:1411–1417, 1996.

Kaprio J, Koskenvuo M, Rita H. Mortality after bereavement: a prospective study of 95,647 widowed persons. AM J Public Health 77:283–287, 1987.

Kavanaugh DG. Towards a cognitive-behavioral intervention for adult grief reactions. Br J Psychiatry 157:373–383, 1990.

Kleber RJ, Brom D: Psychotherapy and pathological grief: controlled outcome study. Israeli J Psychiatry Rel Sci 24:99–109, 1987.

Klein DF, Blank HR. Psychopharmacological treatment of bereavement and its complications. In: Kutscher AH, ed. Death and Bereavement. Springfield, IL: Charles C Thomas, 1969:299–305.

Kraus AS, Lilienfeld AM. Some epidemiological aspects of the high mortality rate in the young widowed group. J Chronic Dis 10:207–217, 1959.

Levav I, Friedlander Y, Kark J, et al. An epidemiologic study of mortality among bereaved patients. N Engl J Med 319:457–461, 1988.

Lund DA, Dimond MF, Caserta MS, et al. Identifying elderly with coping difficulties after two years bereavement. Omega 16:213–223, 1985.

Lund DA, Caserta MS, Dimond MF. The course of spousal bereavement in later life. In: Stroebe MS, Stroebe W., Hansson RO, eds. Handbook of Bereavement: Theory, Research and Intervention. Cambridge, UK: Cambridge University Press, 1993, pp 240–254.

MacMahon B, Pugh TF. Suicide in the widowed. Am J Epidemol 81:23–31, 1965.

Maddison D, Viola A. The health of widows in the year following bereavement. J Psychosom Res 12:297–306, 1968.

McHorney CA, Mor V. Predictors of bereavement depression and its health services consequences. Med Care 26:882–893, 1988.

Melges FT, DeMaso DR. Grief resolution therapy: reliving, revising, and revisiting. Am J Psychotherapy 34:51–61, 1980.

Mellstrom D, Nilsson A, Oden A, et al. Mortality among the widowed in Sweden. Scand J Soc Med 10:33–41, 1982.

Middleton W, Raphael B, Martinek N, et al. Pathological grief reactions, In: Stroebe MS, Stroebe W, Hansson RO, eds. Handbook of Bereavement: Theory, Research and Intervention. Cambridge, UK: Cambridge University Press, 1993, pp 44–61.

Miller MD, Frank E, Cornes C, et al. Applying interpersonal psychotherapy to bereavement-related depression following loss of a spouse in late-life. J Psychother Pract Res 3:149–162, 1994.

Moss MS, Moss SZ, Rubinstein R, et al. Impact of elderly mother's death on middle age daughters. Int J Aging Hum Dev 37:1–22, 1993.

Norris FH, Murrell SA. Social Support, life events, and stress as modifiers of adjustment to bereavement by older adults. Psychol Aging 5:429–436, 1990.

Nuss WS, Zubenko GS. Correlates of persistent depressive symptoms in widows. Am J Psychiatry 149:346–351, 1992.

Osterweis M, Solomon F, Green M, eds. Bereavement Reactions, Consequences, and Care. Washington, DC: National Academy Press, 1984.

Parkes CM. The effects of physical and mental health: a study of the medical records of widows. Br Med J 2:274–279, 1964.

Parkes CM. Bereavement and mental illness. Br J Med Psychol 38:388–397, 1965.

Parkes CM. Psycho-social transitions: a field for study. Soc Sci Med 5:101–115, 1971.

Parkes CM. Bereavement Studies of Grief in Adult Life, 2nd ed. New York: International Universities Press, 1972.

Parkes CM. Psychiatric problems following bereavement by murder or manslaughter. Br J Psychiatry 162:49–54, 1993.
Parkes CM, Weiss RS. Recovery from Bereavement. New York: Basic Books, 1983.
Pasternak RE, Reynolds CF III, Schlernitzauer M, et al. Acute open-trial nortriptyline therapy of bereavement-related depression in late life. J Clin Psychiatry 52:307–310, 1991.
Pasternak RE, Reynolds CF, Miller MD, et al. The symptom profile and two-year course of subsyndromal depression in spousally bereaved elders. Am J Geriatr Psychiatry 2:210–219, 1994.
Paul N, Grosser G. Operational mourning and its role in conjoint family therapy. Community Ment Health J 1:339–345, 1965.
Pollock GH. The mourning liberation process in health and disease. Psychiatr Clin North Am 10:345–354, 1987.
Prigerson HG, Shear MK, Jacobs SC, et al. Consensus criteria for traumatic grief: a preliminary empirical test. Br J Psychiatry 174:67–73, 1999.
Prigerson HG, Bierhals AJ, Kasl SV, et al. Traumatic grief as a risk for mental and physical morbidity. Am J Psychiatry 154:616–623, 1997.
Prigerson HG, Bridge J, Maciejewski PK. Influence of traumatic grief on suicidal ideation among young adults. Am J Psychiatry 156:1994–1995, 1999.
Rando, TA. Grief, dying and death: clinical interventions for caregivers. Champaign, IL: Research Press, 1984.
Raphael B. Preventive intervention with the recently bereaved. Arch Gen Psychiatry 34: 1450–1454, 1977.
Raphael B. Mourning and prevention of melancholia. Br J Med Psychol 41:303–310, 1978.
Raphael B. The Anatomy of Bereavement. New York: Basic Books, 1983.
Raphael B, Maddison D. The care of bereaved adults. In: Hill OW, ed. Modern Trends in Psychosomatic Medicine. London: Butterworth, 1976.
Rees W, Lutkins S. Mortality of bereavement. Br Med J 4:13–16, 1967.
Reynolds C, Hoch CC, Buysse DJ, et al. Electroencephalographic sleep in spousal bereavement and bereavement-related depression in late-life. Biol Psychiatry 31:69–82, 1992.
Reynolds CF, Miller MD, Pasternak RE, Frank E, Perel MJ, Cornes C. Treatment of bereavement-related major depression episodes in later life: a controlled study of acute and continuation treatment with nortriptyline and interpersonal psychotherapy. Am J Psychiatry 156:202–208, 1999.
Richards JG, McCallum J. Bereavement in the elderly. NZ Med J 89:201–204, 1979.
Rollman BL, Reynolds CF. Minor and subsyndromal depression: functional disability worth treating. J Am Geriatr Soc 47:757–758, 1999.
Rynearson EK. Suicide internalized: existential sequestrum. Am J Psychiatry 138:84–87, 1981.
Rynearson EK. Bereavement after homicide: a descriptive study. Am J Psychiatry 141: 1452–1454, 1984.
Rynearson EK. Psychotherapy of pathologic grief: revisions and limitations. Psychiatr Clin North Am 10:487–500, 1987a.
Rynearson EK. Psychological adjustments to unnatural dying. In: Zisook S, ed. Biopsy-

chosocial Aspects of Bereavement. Washington, DC: American Psychiatric Association, 1987b.
Rynearson EK. Pathologic grief: the queen's croquet ground. Psychiatr Ann 20:295–303, 1990.
Shear MK, Frank E, et al. Traumatic grief treatment: a pilot study. Am J Psychiatry 158(9):1506–1508, 2001.
Shuchter SR, Downs N, Zisook S. Biologically Informed Psychotherapy for Depression. New York: Guilford Press, 1996.
Shuchter SR, Zisook S. The course of normal grief. In: Stroebe MS, Stroebe W, Hansson RO, eds. Handbook of Bereavement: Theory, Research and Intervention. Cambridge, UK: Cambridge University Press, 1993, pp 23–43.
Siegel JM, Kuykendall DH. Loss, widowhood, and psychological distress among the elderly. J Consult Clin Psychol 58:519–524, 1990.
Silverman PR. Widowhood and prevention intervention. Family Coordinator 21:95–102, 1972.
Sireling L, Cohen D, Marks I. Guided mourning for morbid grief: a replication. Behav Ther 29:121–132, 1988.
Stern K, Williams GM, Prados M. Grief reactions in later life. Am J Psychiatry 108: 289–294, 1951.
Stewart JW, Quitkin FM, Klein DF. The pharmacotherapy of minor depression. Am J Psychother 1:23–36, 1992.
Stroebe MS, Stroebe W. The mortality of bereavement: a review. In: Stroebe MS, Stroebe W, Hansson RO, eds. Handbook of Bereavement: Theory, Research and Intervention. Cambridge, UK: Cambridge University Press, 1993, pp 175–195.
Thompson LW, Breckenridge JN, Gallagher D, et al. Effects of bereavement on self-perception of physical health in elderly widows and widowers. J Gerontol 39: 309–314, 1984.
US Bureau of the Census. Current Population Reports. Series P-20, No. 450, 1991.
Valanis B, Yeaworth RC, Mullis MR. Alcohol use among bereaved and nonbereaved older persons. J Gerontol Nurs 13:26–32, 1987.
VanZandt S, Mou R, Abbott R. Mental and physical health of rural bereaved and nonbereaved elders: a longitudinal study. In: Lund A, ed. Older Bereaved Spouses: Research with Practical Applications. New York: Hemisphere, 1989, pp 25–35.
Volkan VD. "Regrief" therapy. In: Schoenberg G, Gerber IE, Wiener A, et al, eds. Bereavement: Its Psychosocial Aspects. New York: Columbia University Press, 1971, pp 334–350.
Walls N, Meyers AW. Outcome in group treatments for bereavement: experimental results and recommendations for clinical practice. Int J Mental Health 13:126–147, 1985.
Weller RA, Weller EB, Fristad MA, et al. Depression in recently bereaved prepubertal children. Am J Psychiatry 148:1536–1540, 1991.
Young M, Benjamin B, Wallis C. Mortality of widowers. Lancet 2:254–256, 1963.
Zisook S. Unresolved grief. In: Zisook S, ed. Biopsychosocial Aspects of Bereavement. Washington, DC: American Psychiatric Association, 1987, pp 23–34.
Zisook S, Mulvihill M, Shuchter SR. Widowhood and anxiety. Psychiatr Med 8:99–116, 1990a.

Zisook S, Paulus M, Shuchter SR, Judd LL. The many faces of depression following spousal bereavement. J Affect Disord 45:85–95, 1997.
Zisook S, Shuchter SR. Treatment of the depressions of bereavement. Am Behav Sci 44: 782–797, 2001.
Zisook S, Shuchter SR. Grief and bereavement. Comp Rev Geriatr Psychiatry 18:529–562, 1998.
Zisook S, Shuchter SR. Bereavement. Curr Psychiatr Ther 34:248–252, 1997.
Zisook S, Shuchter SR. Psychotherapy of the depression in spousal bereavement. Psychother Pract 2(4):31–45, 1996.
Zisook S, Shuchter SR. Major depression associated with widowhood. Am J Geriatr Psychiatry 1:316–326, 1993.
Zisook S, Shuchter SR. Uncomplicated bereavement. J Clin Psychiatry 54:365–372, 1993.
Zisook S, Shuchter SR. Depression through the first year after the death of a spouse. Am J Psychiatry 148:1346–1352, 1991a.
Zisook S, Shuchter SR. Early psychological reaction to the stress of widowhood. Psychiatry 54:320–323, 1991b.
Zisook S, Shuchter SR, Dunn L. Grief and depression: diagnostic and treatment challenges. Primary Psychiatry 8(5):37–38, 51–53, 2001.
Zisook S, Shuchter SR, Mulvihill M. Alcohol, cigarette and medication use during the first year of widowhood. Psychiatr Ann 20:318–326, 1990b.
Zisook S, Shuchter SR, Pedrelli P, Sable J, Deaciue SC. Acute, open-trial of bupropion SR therapy in bereavement. J Clin Psychiatry 62:227–230, 2001.
Zisook S, Shuchter SR, Sledge P. Diagnostic and treatment considerations in depression associated with late-life bereavement. In: Schneider LS, Reynolds CF, Lebowitz BD, Friedhoff AJ, eds. Diagnosis and Treatment of Depression in Late Life: Results of the NIH Consensus Development Conference. Washington, DC: American Psychiatric Press, 1991, pp 419–435.
Zisook S, Shuchter SR, Sledge PA, et al. Aging and bereavement. J Geriatr Psychiatry Neurol 6:137–143, 1993.
Zisook S, Shuchter SR, Sledge PA, et al. The spectrum of depressive phenomena after spousal bereavement. J Clin Psychiatry 55(suppl 4):29–36, 1994.
Zygmont M, Prigerson HG, Houck PR, et al. A post hoc comparison of paroxetine and nortriptyline for symptoms of traumatic grief. J Clin Psychiatry 59:241–245, 1998.

6

Depression and Medical Illness

Abi V. Rayner and James G. O'Brien
University of Louisville, Louisville, Kentucky, U.S.A.

OVERVIEW

Medical illness, as Lyness and colleagues (1996) have noted, is "the most consistently identified factor associated with the presence of late life depression and is the most powerful predictor of poor depressive outcome" (1). Conversely, depression is a major risk for onset or progression of a range of medical illnesses. When medical illness is complicated by depression, morbidity and mortality are increased (3). Distress is magnified and quality of life is decreased. Each condition independently requires treatment in order to ameliorate these effects.

Clinicians and family members often mistakenly attribute depressive symptoms to concurrent medical disorders or functional changes associated with aging. This position, however, leads to a nihilistic attitude toward treatment. There is no support for the view that an older adult with chronic illness "*should* be depressed." On the contrary, depression among the medically ill elderly is underrecognized and undertreated. A conservative estimate concludes that 15% to 40% of patients followed with comorbid medical illness will have some element of depression (10,16). Studies of medical inpatients with depressive symptoms demonstrate a significant adverse impact of mood alteration on survival, rehospitalization, outpatient visits, nursing home placement, and length of stay.

Diagnosing depression in the presence of medical illness, however, can be a complicated process. It is often impossible to disentangle the relative contributions of depression and medical illnesses to a patient's distress. Furthermore, there is a complex interplay between medical and psychiatric factors. Medical illnesses can increase depression both directly, through neurohumoral effects, and indirectly, through impaired role functioning and resultant demoralization. Depression, similarly, can aggravate medical illnesses through both direct and indirect routes. Acceptance of ill health as a normative aspect of aging and illness, resulting in adoption of a "sick role," can contribute further to a condition of "excess disability." The outcome can be a positive feedback loop or "reciprocal spiraling" (6) mechanism in which depression and medical illness mutually exacerbate each other, ultimately producing greater dysfunction than would be accounted for by either component of illness alone (7).

RECOGNIZING DEPRESSION IN MEDICALLY ILL INDIVIDUALS

> Mrs. O, a 79-year-old retired teacher, is accompanied by her daughter to an office visit for back pain. She has been diagnosed with hypertension and diabetes. Her daughter is angry and says about her mother, "She complains all the time. She won't go to church. She wasn't even dressed when I went to pick her up." The slightly disheveled elderly mother sits, unmoving, with poor eye contact. "I don't know why I am here. I am OK. She pushes too hard. I just need you to give me something to help me sleep and make my bowels move."

Often, the presentation of depression in an older adult resembles that in this vignette. Mrs. O reports concerns about her bodily functioning, specifically sleep and bowels, more readily than she describes her apparent emotional withdrawal and possible depressed mood. Many older adults will dismiss depressive symptoms, attributing them to their known medical illnesses. Others may underreport depressive symptoms as a result of a negative attitude toward psychiatric illness. Further questioning—including inquiry about subjective sense of well-being—can help to detect superimposed depression.

Although depressive states that accompany medical illnesses range along a continuum from subsyndromal symptom clusters to full-blown major depressive disorder, much of the depression in medically ill older adults fails to meet full criteria for major depressive disorder. As discussed in Chapter 4 of this book and elsewhere, even the less florid depressive conditions diminish a person's sense of well-being and increase the risk of medical deterioration or complications (8). Patients suffering from minor or subsyndromal depressions, for example, experience lower quality of life, visit physicians more frequently, and require more hospitalization than nondepressed adults.

Further obfuscating the recognition of depressive states, some elderly medical patients describe what has been termed "minor depression without mood disorder," a condition characterized by apathy and self-neglect rather than by a typically sad or depressed mood. Whether such patients experience a variant constellation of symptoms or simply deny and underreport the more typical symptoms, clinicians may be less likely to diagnose and treat a mood disorder as an entity separable from the concurrent medical illness (11). The presence of self-deprecating remarks, loss of interest and energy, and diminished participation in hobby and leisure activities may reveal the presence of a mood disturbance that should be independently targeted for treatment.

Even florid depressive symptoms may be obscured by concurrent medical illnesses with symptomatically overlapping clinical presentations. Loss of energy, sleep disturbances, poor concentration, psychomotor changes, or loss of appetite can be nonspecific symptoms representative either of depression or medical illness (13). Since the presence of such symptoms identifies a group of patients at high risk for persistent depression, some clinicians choose a more inclusive diagnostic approach when ambiguous symptoms are present. Attributing all complaints to a proposed mood disorder, however, can underplay the importance of the contribution of concomitant medical illness or of preexisting functional deficits to the patients clinical picture. The presence of diminished quality of life in a medically ill individual, moreover, is not unusual and does not by itself justify the diagnosis of a mood disorder (7).

One factor that helps determine the presence of depression in a medically ill patient is the relative timing of onset of symptoms. For example, a stroke patient may first begin to show apathy, withdrawal, and low mood at the time of the stroke or much later, after rehabilitation is well under way. Depressive symptoms occurring at the time of the stroke may well be linked to the focal loss, whereas those occurring after rehabilitation are often associated with psychosocial factors. Such a distinction may be important in treatment planning.

Because so few depressed elderly are ever seen by a mental health specialist, recognition of depression often falls to the primary care clinician. Depression that is missed in the primary care setting may simply go untreated. To supplement the clinical interview, a variety of structured screening tools are available. Two that have proven useful in primary care settings are the two question case finding instrument (14,15) and the GDS-4 (16).

DEPRESSION AND MEDICAL ILLNESS: DEVELOPING A CONCEPTUAL FRAMEWORK

Various theories have been advanced to describe the interactions of physiological and psychosocial factors in patients suffering from concurrent medical illnesses and depressive symptoms. The interplay of physiological and psychosocial factors has been modeled using field theory, which provides a useful approach for understanding and describing these interactions as well as for testing hypotheses and designing interventions, as illustrated in Figure 1.

Among the physiological factors of importance in linking medical and depressive illnesses, much attention has been directed toward disturbances in the functioning of corticotropin-releasing hormone (CRH) and the hypothalamic–pituitary–adrenocortical (HPA) axis. The integration of hormonal, autonomic, and behavioral responses to stress appears to be mediated by CRH stimulation of the HPA axis, which causes both behavioral changes (arousal, increased attention, and vigilance) and physiological changes (including increased blood pressure and heart rate, and alteration of immune response). Glucocorticoid secretion, which exerts a negative feedback on CRH release, is dysregulated in depression and other stress-exacerbated disease states. Old age may reduce the sensitivity of this negative feedback system, further strengthening the link between many age-associated diseases and depression. Dysregulated glucocorticoid secretion may thus link some "chronic illness" or "disability" states with depression (18–20). Indeed, excessive glucocorticoid levels have been associated with hypertension, diabetes, and coagulation abnormalities. Recently, the roles of cytokines IL-1b (2) and IL-6 (20) in cortisol production, inflammation, and the immune system have also been studied. Further investigations may suggest treatment approaches that target this endocrine dysregulation (Figure 2).

In addition to such physiological factors, psychosocial and socioeconomic variables also affect health status in depression and medical illness. Poor outcome, for example, is associated with diminished treatment compliance (22) (see Chapter 9). Attitudes and beliefs such as a nihilistic view of intervention or acceptance of the "disabled" role may worsen prognosis. Lower socioeconomic status is strongly correlated with increased disability, increased health service use, and mortality. Indeed, analysis of the specific indicators suggests that lower educational and income levels significantly influence patients' response to chronic diseases.

DEPRESSION AND SPECIFIC ILLNESSES

The relationships between depression and several specific chronic illnesses have been investigated. We will review research on depression and cardiovascular disease, cerebrovascular disease, dementia, cancer, and diabetes.

Cardiovascular Disease

The interaction between depression and cardiovascular disease appears to be bidirectional. Depression increases the risk for cardiovascular disease, and cardiovascular pathology in turn increases the risk for depression.

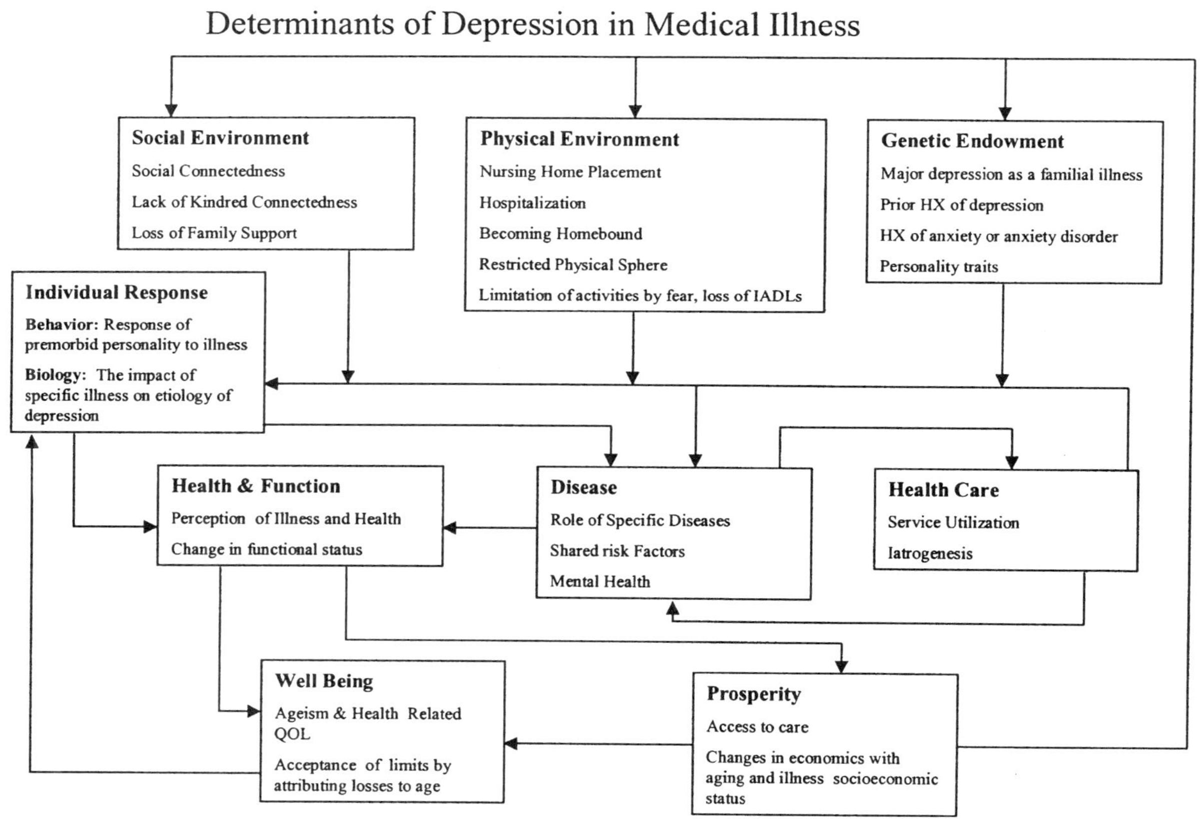

FIGURE 1 A model of the determinants of health demonstrates the interplay of multiple influences on the depression in medical illness. It allows a descriptive framework in which to test the hypothesis and design interventions. (Adapted from Evans RG, Stoddard GL. Producing health: consuming health care. Social Science and Medicine 31:1347–1363, 1990.)

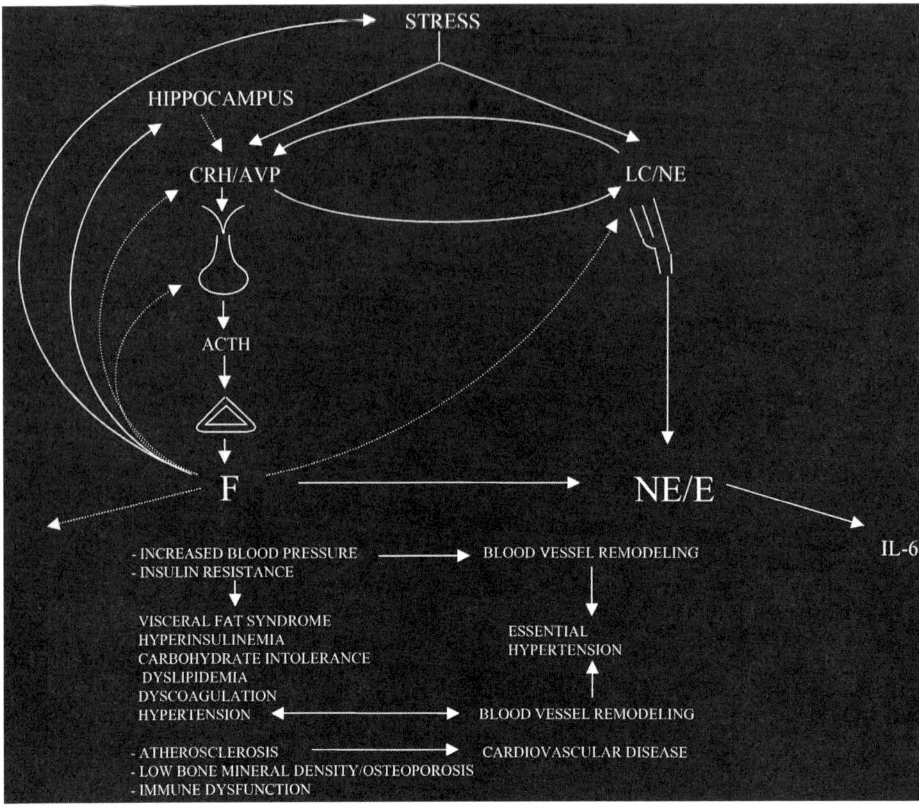

FIGURE 2 A schematic representation of the stress system. The CRH/AVP neurons are reciprocally connected with the noradrenergic neurons of the LC/NE system in a positive reverberatory circuit. The HPA axis is controlled by several negative feedback loops, which tend to normalize the time-integrated secretion of cortisol, yet glucocorticoids stimulate the amygdala and hence the fear center. Activation of the HPA axis leads to suppression of the GH/IGF-1, LH/testosterone/estradiol, and TSH/T_3 axes; activation of the sympathetic system increases IL-6 secretion. Chronic increases in cortisol, catecholamines, and IL-6 and chronic suppression of the GH/IGF/1, LH/T, and TSH/T_3 axes lead to visceral obesity, hypertension, atherosclerosis, osteoporosis, and immune dysfunction and their sequelae, resulting in increased morbidity and mortality. Symbols: *Solid lines* indicate stimulation; *interrupted lines* indicate inhibition. Abbreviations: *HPA*, hypothalamic–pituitary–adrenal; *CRH*, corticotropin-releasing hormone; *AVP*, arginine-vasopressin; *LC/NE*, locus ceruleus/norepinephrine system; *GH*, growth hormone; *IGF-1*, insulin-like growth factor–1; *LH*, luteinizing hormone; *T*, testosterone; *TSH*, thyrotropin; T_3, triiodothyronine; *F*, cortisol; *NE*, norepinephrine; *E*, epinephrine; *IL-6*, interleukin-6. (Reprinted with permission from Chrousos GP, Gold PW. A healthy body in a healthy mind—and vice versa—the damaging power of "uncontrollable" stress. J Clin Endocrinol Metab 83:1842–1845, 1998.)

A substantial literature now associates depression with exacerbation of cardiovascular disease, including hypertension, coronary artery disease (CAD), and congestive heart failure (CHF). Depressive complaints—in prospective studies of patients with cardiovascular risk factors—are strong predictors of myocardial infarction, stroke, congestive heart failure, and death. This association remains consistent even when logistic regression and modeling theory are used to control for confounders.

Multiple studies have demonstrated that the presence of depressive symptoms after myocardial infarction increases comorbidity, including chest pain, angina, hospitalizations, myocardial infarction, and stroke (3). In one study (25), presence of depression at the time of myocardial infarction doubled the risk of death over the first year, and continued to influence survival over a 5-year period in an apparent dose/response curve (see Figure 3). Risk of death was 25% to 43% higher over a 5-year period in patients with high levels of depression.

Furthermore, depression has been shown to increase the risk for congestive heart failure, hypertension, coronary heart disease, and peripheral vascular

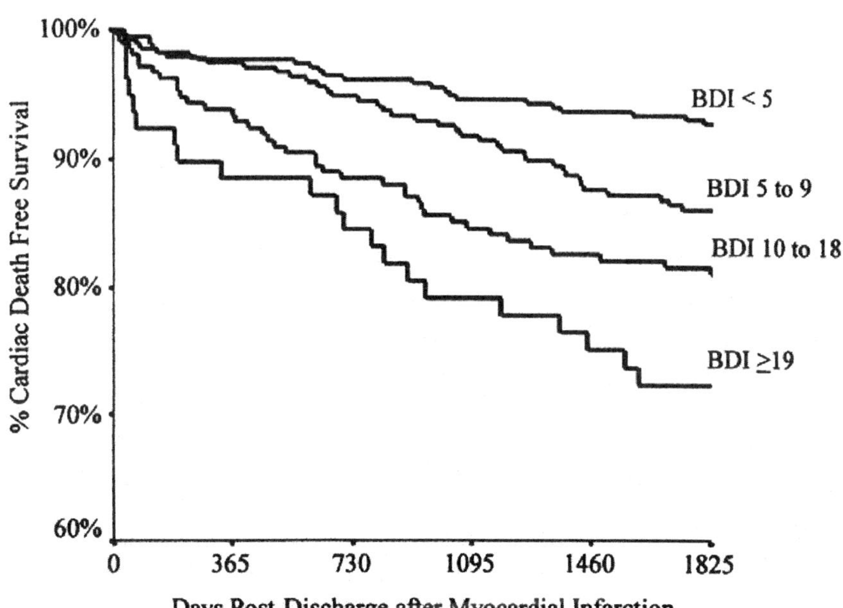

FIGURE 3 Five-year risk of cardiac mortality in relation to initial severity and one-year changes in depression symptoms after myocardial infarction. (Reprinted with permission from Lespérance F, Frasure-Smith N, Talajic M, Bourassa MG. Five-year risk of cardiac mortality. Circulation 105(9):1049–1053, 2002.)

disease (36,26). In several studies, baseline depressive characteristics have predicted subsequent heart attack as strongly as other risk factors (12,27,28). In a study of patients with hypertension, the presence of depression was associated with the development of congestive heart failure even after controlling for other risk factors (29).

Just as depression can contribute to cardiovascular disease, cardiovascular disease can cause or exacerbate depression (31). The risk of depression as measured 1 week after myocardial infarction, for example, was increased by about 24% in one study. Another study, examining patients hospitalized for congestive heart failure, identified severe depression in 85% (35). Depression predicted elevated cortisol levels and worse health perceptions. Interestingly, much of the evidence that cardiovascular disease exacerbates depression has been developed using questionnaires about psychological symptoms that rely heavily on the CES-D and other interviews that may overemphasize negative symptoms and loss of power. In one study, for example, CES-D items of "I felt that everything I did was an effort" and "I could not get going" were independently predictive of mortality (12). Further investigation is warranted, therefore, into the specific effects of cardiovascular disease on depressive symptomatology.

It is difficult to assess the relationship between depression and cardiovascular disease without factoring in anxiety. Depression is often accompanied by anxiety, and anxiety symptoms and disorders have each been strongly correlated with disability (7). Anxiety may have a direct negative impact on the symptoms of congestive heart failure, resulting in an increased heart rate, shortened diastole, and further compromise of cardiac output. The increased cardiovascular symptoms may in turn exacerbate anxiety in a positive feedback loop (31). Furthermore, anxiety symptoms reduce both adherence to a treatment regimen and response to antidepressant treatment.

Cerebrovascular Disease

Cerebrovascular disease bears a relationship to depression that is clearly significant yet is still far from completely understood. Clinical observations have linked stroke and depression for decades. Even with MRI (32,37) and PET (38) imaging techniques, however, a neuroanatomical or physiological cause-and-effect relationship between cerebral insult and depression has been difficult to establish. EEG and neuroimaging approaches—including quantitative analysis of specific abnormalities—have been disappointing in detecting specific loci or predicting specific amounts of volume loss that would predict the development of depression.

Distinguishing between early and late mood effects of stroke may be meaningful. "Early depression" as an illness occurring at the time of the "brain attack" has been characterized clinically and neuroanatomically to some degree.

Its development appears to arise primarily in conjunction with destructive lesions in the basal ganglia and frontal lobes, although the data are far from compelling.

Certainly, stroke victims with significant residual deficits have a risk/benefit analysis that strongly supports an aggressive approach. "Late depression" can develop months after the stroke. Since careful studies of function following stroke suggest limited improvement after three months (40), this late depression may represent bereavement over functional loss, reduced independence, and altered social status (41). Late poststroke depression appears strongly related to changes in social support. Premorbid personality traits and prior depression or family history of depressive disorders may also play important roles. "Disability" itself may influence the neurohormonal pathway and induce depression that further reduces functional status. When decreased performance capacity becomes evident more than several months after a stroke, it is therefore important to consider the possibility of comorbid depression with significant psychosocial components. Cumulative insults may result in development of late, presumably vascular dementia. This mandates aggressive management of vascular risk factors to prevent further ischemic injury (42). In general, a proactive approach with supportive psychotherapy and antidepressant medication appears warranted when feasible.

Depression, apathy, and vegetative signs at the time of stroke have important prognostic implications (39). Inability to cooperate with rehabilitation as a result of depression may significantly reduce optimum function. The additive effect that occurs when depressive symptoms join with cognitive deficits further complicates recovery. Clear distinctions between physical, cognitive, and emotional aspects of stroke may be impossible. Some evidence supports the use of antidepressants or stimulant agents to increase participation in rehabilitation.

Depression not only interferes with recovery; it can also contribute to the risk for stroke. In one cohort, depression appeared to increase the risk of stroke threefold when the confounding contribution of diabetes, hypertension, heart disease, and tobacco use were taken into account (43). In another study, the risk of death from stroke measured prospectively in a community cohort was increased by 54% in depressed compared to nondepressed patients, even when this comparison controlled for the contributions of other illnesses and poor health habits such as alcohol use, smoking, and obesity (44).

Conversely, cerebrovascular disease may contribute to depression (45). In patients with risk factors for heart disease, for example, the presence of increased brain white matter changes—which are associated with hypertension and coronary artery disease—add to the likelihood that depression will be found as well (32). "Vascular depression," described in detail in Chapter 7, is the hypothetical clinical syndrome that reflects lesions in the white matter. It is a distinctive clinical state characterized by apathy, withdrawal, and impaired executive functions rather than the type of "depressed" mood often found in younger patients.

The high rate of depression observed following coronary artery bypass surgery may initiate or accelerate the destructive process that is hypothesized to produce vascular depression. A cascade of small microembolisms may occur in bypass patients, producing postoperative delirium, depression, or dementia (47). Clinically, some of these patients may have also shown antecedent cognitive or behavioral impairments that continue to progress in a pattern indistinguishable from Alzheimer's disease. The relationship of microangiopathy to neurobehavioral pathology remains incompletely resolved; while it is considered important (48), skepticism exists as to whether there is indeed a separate and distinct vascular dementia (49,50).

Dementia

Depression, defined in various ways, is justly regarded as a risk factor for dementia (51,52). People whose first episode of major depression develops in later life, for example, show an unexpectedly high incidence of subsequent dementia. Those at highest risk for dementia are those with vegetative depressive symptoms such as loss of interest, decreased energy, poor concentration, and psychomotor agitation or retardation (53). Impaired executive function with depression has also been identified as a risk factor for subsequent dementia. Even complaints of memory impairment in the setting of depression are correlated with an increased dementia risk. The intermediate link between depression and dementia may involve white matter changes and the neuropathological changes of Alzheimer's disease. The risk of dementia in patients with early-onset, recurrent major depression in one study was not elevated, nor were such microvascular changes or Alzheimer's lesions more frequent (55).

Depression associated with cognitive complaints historically was described as "pseudodementia" and regarded as reversible (see Chapter 3). This condition, now usually termed "dementia syndrome of depression," may represent an intermediate state combining aspects of depression and dementia. We know from prospective studies that most of these patients will eventually be identified as having mild cognitive impairment or dementia. Identifying mild cognitive impairment or the early stages of dementia in a depressed patient, however, can be difficult (54). Dysphoric mood, decreased concentration and attention, and reduced activities are frequent concomitants of both early dementia and depression. Thus these symptoms may misleadingly suggest depression but arise from a different cause. Furthermore, complaints of weight loss, psychomotor retardation, and diminished concentration have not discriminated between depressed and demented patients (56). Whether the pathophysiology of depression and dementia overlap—for example, through HPA dysregulatory effects—

remains to be further investigated. Perhaps a shared pathophysiology will explain the overlap of symptom complexes.

A potentially helpful strategy in discriminating between demented patients with and without depression are the observations offered by close family and caregivers. Depression diagnosed in this way can be termed "attributive depression" (53). On the basis of reports from collateral sources (family members, close friends, or care providers), such patients are considered potential candidates for antidepressant treatment even when they themselves deny experiencing depression. Treating such patients—provided valid consent can be obtained—is considered appropriate because the demented patient may lack sufficient insight and memory to make an accurate report of his or her symptoms. Care must be taken, however, not to overdiagnose depression in patients whose dementing illness is the primary cause of prominent behavioral symptoms. Prominent behavioral symptoms, for example, are the hallmark of frontotemporal dementia (64), and fluctuating behavioral symptoms characterize Lewy body disease. In his illness metaphor approach, Tariot (65) identifies a group of those with late behavioral manifestations, including "negativistic, irritable behavior or dysphoric anxious mood," as "reminiscent of depression." He recommends antidepressant therapy as first-line pharmacotherapeutic agents in this subgroup. The approach is appealing from a clinical standpoint and offers a matrix for decision making that appears to have the most face validity. When unsuccessful, however, clinical gains may still be achieved with alternate approaches, including the use of cholinesterase inhibitors. Atypical antipsychotics and/or mood stabilizing medications can be useful in the treatment of agitated behaviors (66).

The threshold should be for an empirical antidepressant trial in demented patients who may be depressed, because the potential clinical benefits associated with treatment are significant (59). In the subset of depressed patients with mild cognitive impairment or early dementia, treatment often improves mood and may in addition improve concentration. Patients typically report improved sense of well-being, energy, and sleep. Even a dramatic response to treatment, however, may fail to halt the progress of a dementing illness. It remains unknown whether independent treatment of depressive symptoms will have some impact on the course of the dementing process, but it is worth exploring. The recent development of consensus criteria for diagnosing depression in Alzheimer's disease will help guide efforts to identify the characteristics of the syndrome that predict response to treatment (61,62).

Cancer

Cancer, a class of medical illness comprising conditions with a broad range of severity, can be a source of depression. Though younger lives are often affected by cancer, approximately 60% of all cases occur in elderly individuals. Because of the anxiety surrounding this group of illnesses, a diagnosis of cancer represents perhaps the most dreaded disease to many individuals and may cause greater emotional disturbance than many diseases with a poorer actual prognosis, such as congestive heart failure. In addition to this psychological effect, the physical effects of cancers and the requirements of their treatment can disrupt all aspects of daily life, including family, work, finances, and friendships (67). Depression occurs frequently in cancer patients. It is difficult, however, to calculate exact prevalences because of wide variations in definitions, screening instruments utilized, location of participants, and stage of disease across studies. Pancreatic cancer has possibly the highest rate of associated depressive illness, reaching 50% in some studies. Pain may be a confounder in this disease. In a review by Green and Austin (73) of cases of pancreatic cancer, 71% of patients had symptoms of a "depression-related" disorder and, of interest, 33% of the patients reported that psychiatric symptoms preceded the physical symptoms. The preexistence of mood disturbance in pancreatic cancer has suggested that intrinsic physiological effects—not simply an emotional reaction to the diagnosis—plays a role in associated depression. The mechanism or mechanisms by which cancer might produce depressive symptoms are not well understood. One theory postulates that cytokines play a role in the pathophysiology of mood disorders. Cytokines have an essential function in host defense but also serve as messengers communicating between the brain and the neuroendocrine system. Musselman (21) noted increased levels of interleukin-6 (IL-6) in cancer patients with depression compared to healthy controls or to cancer patients without depression.

In addition to direct physical effects, psychosocial factors are important contributors to the depression and anxiety that often follows a diagnosis of cancer. Depression and anxiety often begin with a cancer diagnosis and continue throughout treatment (68). There is ample evidence to suggest that a patient's initial adaptation to a diagnosis of cancer diagnosis is significantly influenced by preexisting psychosocial factors that patients bring to their cancer experience (69). Precipitants of stress and depression include fear of pain and suffering, disability, dependence, and possibly being disfigured by surgery. A patient's emotional response to cancer is often influenced by medical factors such as the cancer's location, the stage of illness and type of treatments required, the clinical course of the disease, and the degree of associated pain; by psychological factors including prior mental health and adjustment, emotional maturity, flexibility, and ability to modify plans; and by social factors including quality and quantity of emotional and practical support offered by family, friends and coworkers (70). One can readily appreciate how an older individual with a newly discovered malignancy and limited social supports may be at high risk for depression.

In a study of older women suffering from lung, breast, or colon cancer, Kurtz and colleagues (71) identified symptom severity as being the primary factor affecting mental health in these cancer patients. Loss of function, physical symptoms, and social isolation may be more potent precipitants of the stress and depression than the nature of the cancer, including prognosis. In an additional study of 211 adults over age 65 diagnosed with lung cancer, Kurtz (72) used the CES-D and identified severe depression in 38.9% of this study group. Social functioning, disease severity, and an absence of radiation treatment were significant predictors of depressive symptomatology. Not receiving the radiation treatment might have represented a poorer prognosis and less hope. Other contributing factors to the onset of a cancer-associated depressive syndrome include chemotherapy, surgery, radiotherapy and paraneoplastic syndromes. Intrinsic factors interacting with these cancer-related variables included coping skills, self-control, personal history of depression, and the presence of alcohol or substance abuse.

Failure to recognize and treat depression as a frequent concomitant of cancer robs the older victim of an opportunity to optimize the quality of life during the terminal phase of illness.

Diabetes

Depression and type 2 diabetes, each debilitating on its own, appear to have a potent adverse impact on quality of life for older adults when present comorbidly. Diabetes mellitus has now achieved almost epidemic status among the elderly, affecting up to 25%. Eaton et al. (74) identified depression as a risk factor for the development of type 2 diabetes mellitus. In a longitudinal study in East Baltimore that assessed diabetes and depression, the relative risk for depression in the diabetic probands was 2.23 (95% CI 0.90-5.55). Other studies have suggested that diabetes can increase the risk for depression as well. Wing and colleagues (75), for example, reported depressive symptomatology occurring more commonly among type 2 diabetic subjects than among members of a control group.

Depression—and stressful life events or chronic psychological distress (77)—undermines control of blood sugar and adversely affects the sympathoadrenal system, dysregulating the hypothalamopituitary adrenal axis and increasing glucose intolerance, while increased glucose intolerance in turn acts through the neuroendocrine system to affect mood state (75).

Suicide and Medical Illness

Because of the intimate relationship between depression and suicide, the impact of medical illness on suicide risk demands consideration. Specific medical illnesses have been associated with an increased risk of suicide (79), but the association of these diseases with depression may be the most important source of risk. Interestingly, few terminally ill patients without depression commit suicide (although reporting bias may result in an underestimate of the frequency of such suicides). Furthermore, some of the specific illnesses that are associated with increased rates of suicide are confounded by their associations with alcoholism, depression, or lower socioeconomic level. Among the diseases related in this ambiguous way to suicide risk, the research literature has directed attention to liver disease with cirrhosis, carcinoma (particularly of the head and neck), traumatic spinal cord injury, and peptic ulcer disease. A further way in which medical illness can increase suicide risk arises from the impairments of functional capacity and independence associated with many medical illnesses. The careful work on patients requesting physician-assisted suicide in Oregon has revealed the importance of patients' sense of control over their environments. Reduction of suffering, adequate palliative care, and increased control of pain have been demonstrated to dramatically reduce patients' stated wishes for suicide. For a broader discussion of suicide in late-life depression, the reader is referred to Chapter 13.

TREATMENT

A recent expert consensus panel concluded that patients with concurrent medical and psychiatric illness in general should receive independent treatment for each disorder. The tools most useful in treating depression in these patients are psychotherapy, pharmacotherapy with antidepressants, and electroconvulsive therapy (ECT). These treatment modalities are reviewed in detail elsewhere in this book; their use will be summarized briefly here.

Regarding psychotherapy, it is important to reiterate the extent to which medical illnesses compromise physical and role functioning. Working through the associated life changes that these alterations require can be facilitated by individual or group psychotherapies. Even terminally ill patients in palliative care have been shown to benefit from such therapeutic support (92). Studies of psychotherapy in depressed elders are reviewed in Chapter 11.

For most patients with comorbid medical illnesses and depression, however, treatment takes place in a primary care setting and relies heavily on the use of antidepressants. The optimal choices of agent, dosage, and duration have been subjects of considerable research and discussion.

One clear and consistent finding is that antidepressants are superior to placebo in the treatment of elderly depressed patients. Meta-analysis of treatment trials of depression in the elderly by the Cochrane collaboration strongly favored use of antidepressants for those identified with a depressive syndrome (24). This assessment specifically excluded demented patients, however, and did not separately analyze findings from those subjects with comorbid medical illness. Various depressive syndromes were included, with better results among patients with major depression. Patients demonstrated similar degrees of benefit from treatment with all three major classes of drugs.

Studies in older adults with chronic disease are more limited. A different publication from the Cochrane collaborative (84) targeted medical illness and depression but did not stratify the assessment by age. Diagnosis of depression varied, including clinical assessments and structured interviews or checklists. Multiple illnesses were grouped in the analysis, and response to treatment appeared to be independent of the primary disease and similar to that in the healthy population. Each class of antidepressant produced benefits of similar magnitude.

In the absence of clear superiority of other antidepressant groups, the expert consensus panel made a general recommendation that SSRIs—particularly those with better-tolerated side effects and limited drug–drug interactions—appear to be reasonable first-line choices (87). SSRIs appear to be safe even in patients with significant concurrent cardiovascular or cerebrovascular disease. Clinically significant alterations in blood pressure or cardiac arrhythmias are unusual. Selection of agents may be further individualized on the basis of co-prescribed medications, level of agitation or retardation, appetite, and sleep difficulties. Though evidence-based support for such practices is limited, clinicians often choose a more activating drug for an anergic patient, an appetite-enhancing drug for an anorexic patient, or a more sedating drug for the insomniac patient.

Despite general consensus regarding the first-line use of SSRIs, clinicians must not become too complacent about their side effects and tolerability. The Cochrane meta-analysis, for example, showed that approximately the same number of subjects discontinued treatment with SSRIs as with TCAs. Further, treatment with antidepressants did not in general improve the control of concurrent medical disorders. Another study showed a surprising absence of significant difference in the rates of falls among elderly patient groups treated with SSRIs or TCAs.

Optimal dosing strategies remain to be fully worked out. Treatment-emergent side effects may be minimized by initiating antidepressant treatment at low doses and titrating slowly. A proactive approach with discussion of likely side effects and their management, as well as a realistic understanding of the delay in efficacy for mood symptoms, is important to compliance. Early follow-up to assess tolerability and willingness to continue a therapeutic trial may be helpful.

In the elderly, the optimal target dose for antidepressants remains uncertain and difficult to generalize. Trials favor use of the full recommended doses for younger adults, but age-associated alterations in pharmacokinetics and pharmacodynamics and concomitant medication suggest dose reductions. In the patient with good treatment response, reduced maximal doses are justified when effective. In a treatment-resistant patient, however, doses similar to those recommended in younger people are often warranted.

Telephone follow-up 1 to 2 weeks after initiating treatment is helpful in reinforcing the need for continued medication and checking for adverse effects. Reassessment of response after a period of 4 to 6 weeks at therapeutic dosage provides an opportunity to gauge the degree of response and assess adherence to the treatment plan. Treatment goals include improved mood, improved sense of well-being, restoration of optimism, and improved control of concurrent medical diseases as a result of increased level of functioning. Those patients with significant comorbid anxiety appear to respond less well (89). They may require more support to prevent discontinuing therapy and require higher doses for adequate response (90).

Antidepressant responders should be continued on antidepressants for a minimum of 6 to 12 months with appropriate interim monitoring visits and reassessment. With sustained remission of depressive symptoms, a joint decision can be made regarding further therapy, ideally with family input to prepare for early recognition of subtle mood changes in a patient that may have limited insight. There seems to be little adverse effect in continuing pharmacotherapy in a patient at high risk for recurrence. A strong argument can be made for extended maintenance therapy to prevent relapse, recurrence, and chronicity in this group (91). Maintenance therapy should be continued at the same dose that achieved remission.

For those patients in whom depressive symptoms are life threatening, ECT should be considered as a choice even for first-line therapy. It is generally well tolerated. Acceptable rates of complications (primarily atrial arrhythmias) are documented even in the very frail elderly with multiple illnesses (including coronary heart disease) and the "old-old" (93). This must be balanced with significant mortality associated with severe depression and suicide. Maintenance antidepressant therapy after remission with ECT appears superior to observation for recurrence for both depression and suicide. ECT is discussed in greater detail in Chapter 10.

Finally, in treating depression among medically ill seniors, certain questions remain. In the presence of medical illness, how should a clinician modify the usual diagnostic criteria for depression that justify treatment? Which diagnostic criterion or screening instrument is most valuable with such patients? What criteria should be used to define treatment response? How many empirical trials are appropriate in the nonresponder? Who should be considered for ECT? How should persistent depressive symptoms be treated in ECT nonresponders? In patients identified clinically as less likely to respond (e.g., elderly depressives with vascular changes on MRI), what threshold must be crossed in order to warrant a trial of therapy? Further work will need to be done to answer these questions and to elucidate further the nature of the relationship between various medical illnesses and mood symptoms, the natural history of depression in medically ill elders, and the optimal approach to treatment (94).

REFERENCES

1. Lyness JM, Bruce ML, Koenig HG, Parmelee PA, Schulz R, Lawton MP, Reynolds CF III. Depression and medical illness in late life: report of a symposium. J Am Geriatr Soc 44:198, 1996.
2. Lebowitz BD, Pearson JL, Schneider LS, Reynolds CF III, Alexopoulos GS, Bruce ML, Conwell Y, Katz IR, Meyers BS, Morrison MF, Mossey J, Niederehe G, Parmelee P. Diagnosis and treatment of depression in late life: consensus statement update. JAMA 278:1186–1190, 1997.
3. Koenig HG, Kuchibhatla M. Use of health services by medically ill depressed elderly patients after hospital discharge. Am J Geriatr Psychiatry 7:48–56, 1999.
4. Blazer DG, Hybels CF, Peiper CF. The association of depression and mortality in elderly persons: a case for multiple, independent pathways. J Gerontol A Biol Sci Med Sci 56A:M505–M509, 2001.
5. Lyness JM, Duberstein PR, King DA, Cox C, Caine ED. Medical illness burden, trait neuroticism, and depression in older primary care patients. Am J Psychiatry 155:969–971, 1998.
6. Bruce ML. Depression and disability in late life: directions for future research. Am J Geriatr Psychiatry 9:102–112, 2001.
7. Lenze EJ, Rogers JC, Martire LM, Mulsant GH, Rollman BL, Dew MA, Schulz R, Reynolds CF III. The association of late-life depression and anxiety with physical disability. Am J Geriatr Psychiatry 9:113–135, 2001.
8. Van den Berg MD, Oldehinkel AJ, Bouhuys AL, Brilman EI, Beekman ATF, Ormel J. Depression in later life: three etiologically different subgroups. J Affect Disord 65:19–26, 2001.
9. Saz P, Dewey ME. Depression, depressive symptoms and mortality in persons aged 65 and older living in the community: a systematic review of the literature. Int J Geriatr Psychiatry 16:622–630, 2001.
10. Beck DA, Koenig HG. Minor depression: a review of the literature. Int J Psychiatry Med 26:177–209, 1996.
11. Lyness JM, Cox C, Curry J, Conwell Y, King DA, Caine ED. Older age and the underreporting of depressive symptoms. J Am Geriatr Soc 43:216–221, 1995.
12. Schulz R, Beach SR, Ives DG, Martire LM, Ariyo AA, Kop WJ. Association between depression and mortality in older adults: the Cardiovascular Health Study. Arch Intern Med 160:1761–1768, 2000.
13. Montano CB. Primary care issues related to the treatment of depression in elderly patients. J Clin Psychiatry 60(suppl 20):45–51, 1999.
14. Whooley MA, Avins AL, Miranda J, Browner WS. Case-finding instruments for depression: two questions are as good as many. J Gen Intern Med 12:439–445, 1997.
15. Whooley MA, Simon GE. Primary Care: managing depression in medical outpatients. N Engl J Med 343:1942–1950, 2000.

16. Parashos IA, Stamouli S, Rogakou E, Theodotou R, Nikas I, Mougias A. Recognition of depressive symptoms in the elderly: what can help the patient and the doctor. Depress Anxiety 15:111–116, 2002.
17. Hotopf M, Chidgey J, Addington-Hall J, Ly KL. Depression in advanced disease: a systematic review. Part 1. Prevalence and case finding. Palliat Med 16:81–97, 2002.
18. Makino S, Hashimoto K, Gold PW. Multiple feedback mechanisms activating corticotropin-releasing hormone system in the brain during stress. Pharmacol Biochem Behav 73:147–158, 2002.
19. Gold PW, Goodwin FK, Chrousos GP. Clinical and biochemical manifestations of depression: relation to the neurobiology of stress [erratum appears in N Engl J Med 319:1428, 1988]. N Engl J Med 319:413–420, 1988.
20. Chrousos GP, Gold PW. A healthy body in a healthy mind—and vice versa—the damaging power of "uncontrollable" stress. J Clin Endocrinol Metab 83:1842–1845, 1998.
21. Musselman DL, Miller AH, Porter MR, Manatunga A, Gao F, Penna S, Pearce BD, Landry J, Glover S, McDaniel JS, Nemeroff CB. Higher than normal plasma interleukin-6 concentrations in cancer patients with depression: preliminary findings. Am J Psychiatry 158:1252–1257, 2001.
22. DiMatteo MR, Lepper HS, Croghan TW. Depression is a risk factor for noncompliance with medical treatment. Meta-analysis of the effects of anxiety and depression on patient adherence. Arch Intern Med 160:2101–2107, 2000.
23. Blazer DG. Depression in the elderly: myths and misconceptions. Psychiatr Clin North Am 20:111–119, 1997.
24. Wilson K, Mottram P, Sivanranthan A, Nightingale A. Antidepressants versus placebo for the depressed elderly: Cochrane Depression Anxiety and Neurosis Group. In: Cochrane Database of Systemic Reviews. Issue 2, 2002.
25. Lespérance F, Frasure-Smith N, Talajic M, Bourassa MG. Five-year risk of cardiac mortality in relation to initial severity and one-year changes in depression symptoms after myocardial infarction. Circulation 105:1049–1053, 2002.
26. Okwumabua JO, Baker FM, Wong SP, Pilgram BO. Characteristics of depressive symptoms in elderly urban and rural African Americans. J Gerontol A Biol Sci Med Sci 52:M241–M246, 1997.
27. Ford DE, Mead LA, Chang PP, Cooper-Patrick L, Wang N-Y, Klag MJ. Depression is a risk factor for coronary artery disease in men: the precursors study. Arch Intern Med 158:1422–1426, 1998.
28. Hippisley-Cox J, Fielding K, Pringle M. Depression as a risk factor for ischaemic heart disease in men: population based case-control study. BMJ 316:1714–1719, 1998.
29. Abramson J, Berger A, Krumholz HM, Vaccarino V. Depression and risk of heart failure among older persons with isolated systolic hypertension. Arch Intern Med 161:1725–1730, 2001.
30. SHEP Cooperative Research Group. Prevention of stroke by antihypertensive drug treatment in older persons with isolated systolic hypertension: final results of the Systolic Hypertension in the Elderly Program (SHEP). JAMA 265:3255–3264, 1991.

31. MacMahon KMA, Lip GYH. Psychological factors in heart failure: a review of the literature. Arch Intern Med 162:509–516, 2002.
32. Steffens DC, Helms MJ, Krishnan KRR, Burke GL. Cerebrovascular disease and depression symptoms in the cardiovascular health study. Stroke 30:2159–2166, 1999.
33. Frasure-Smith N, Lesperance F, Talajic M. Depression following myocardial infarction. Impact on 6-month survival [erratum appears in JAMA 271:1082, 1994]. JAMA 270:1819–1825, 1993.
34. Frasure-Smith N, Lespérance F, Talajic M. Depression and 18-month prognosis after myocardial infarction [erratum appears in Circulation 97:708, 1998]. Circulation 91:999–1005, 1995.
35. Zuccala G, Cocchi A, Carbonin P. The impact of depression on self-perceived health status. J Am Geriatr Soc 43:198–199, 1995.
36. Murberg TA, Bru E, Svebak S, Tveteras R, Aarsland T. Depressed mood and subjective health symptoms as predictors of mortality in patients with congestive heart failure: a two-year follow-up study. Int J Psychiatry Med 29:311–326, 1999.
37. Longstreth WT Jr, Manolio TA, Arnold A, Burke GL, Bryan N, Jungreis CA, Enright PL, O'Leary D, Fried L. Clinical correlates of white matter findings on cranial magnetic resonance imaging of 3301 elderly people: the Cardiovascular Health Study. Stroke 27:1274–1282, 1996.
38. de Asis JM, Stern E, Alexopoulos GS, Pan H, Van Gorp W, Blumberg H, Kalayam B, Eidelberg D, Kiosses D, Silbersweig DA. Hippocampal and anterior cingulate activation deficits in patients with geriatric depression. Am J Psychiatry 158:1321–1323, 2001.
39. Krishnan KRR. Depression as a contributing factor in cerebrovascular disease. Am Heart J 140:S70–S76, 2000.
40. Kwiatkowski TG, Libman RB, Frankel M, Tilley BC, Morgenstern LB, Lu M, Broderick JP, Lewandowski CA, Marler JR, Levine SR, Brott T. Effects of tissue plasminogen activator for acute ischemic stroke at one year: National Institute of Neurological Disorders and Stroke Recombinant Tissue Plasminogen Activator Stroke Study Group. New England Journal of Medicine 340:1781–1787, 1999.
41. Angeleri F, Angeleri VA, Foschi N, Giaquinto S, Nolfe G, Saginario A, Signorino M. Depression after stroke: an investigation through catamnesis. J Clinical Psychiatry 58:261–265, 1997.
42. Alexopoulos GS. The treatment of depressed demented patients. J Clin Psychiatry 57(suppl 14):14–20, 1996.
43. Larson SL, Owens PL, Ford D, Eaton W. Depressive disorder, dysthymia, and risk of stroke: thirteen-year follow-up from the Baltimore epidemiologic catchment area study. Stroke 32:1979–1983, 2001.
44. Everson SA, Roberts RE, Goldberg DE, Kaplan GA. Depressive symptoms and increased risk of stroke mortality over a 29-year period. Arch Intern Med 158: 1133–1138, 1998.
45. Lyness JM, King DA, Conwell Y, Cox C, Caine E. Cerebrovascular risk factors and 1-year depression outcome in older primary care patients. Am J Psychiatry 157:1499–1501, 2000.
46. Baldwin RC, O'Brien J. Vascular basis of late-onset depressive disorder. Br J Psychiatry 180:157–160, 2002.

47. Newman MF, Kirchner JL, Phillips-Bute B, Gaver V, Grocott H, Jones RH, Mark DB, Reves JG, Blumenthal JA. Longitudinal assessment of neurocognitive function after coronary-artery bypass surgery. New England Journal of Medicine 344:395–412, 2001.
48. Thomas AJ, Ferrier IN, Kalaria RN, Woodward SA, Ballard C, Oakley A, Perry RH, O'Brien JT. Elevation in late-life depression of intercellular adhesion molecule-1 expression in the dorsolateral prefrontal cortex. Am J Psychiatry 157:1682–1684, 2000.
49. Groves WC, Brandt J, Steinberg M, Warren A, Rosenblatt A, Baker A, Lyketsos CG. Vascular dementia and Alzheimer's disease: is there a difference? A comparison of symptoms by disease duration. J Neuropsychiatry Clin Neurosci 12:305–315, 2000.
50. Stewart R. Vascular dementia: a diagnosis running out of time. Br J Psychiatry 180:152–156, 2002.
51. Cervilla JA, Prince M, Joels S, Mann A. Does depression predict cognitive outcome 9 to 12 year later? Evidence from a prospective study of elderly hypertensives. Psychol Med 30:1017–1023, 2000.
52. Jorm AF. History of depression as a risk factor for dementia: an updated review. Aust NZ J Psychiatry 35:776–781, 2001.
53. Rubin EH, Veiel LL, Kinscherf DA, Morris JC, Storandt M. Clinically significant depressive symptoms and very mild to mild dementia of the Alzheimer type. Int J Geriatr Psychiatry 16:694–701, 2001.
54. Blair BD. Frequently missed diagnosis in geriatric psychiatry. Psychiatr Clin North Am 21:941–971, 1998.
55. O'Brien J, Thomas A, Ballard C, Brown A, Ferrier N, Jaros E, Perry R. Cognitive impairment in depression is not associated with neuropathologic evidence of increased vascular or Alzheimer-type pathology. Biol Psychiatry 49:130–136, 2001.
56. Purandare N, Burns A, Craig S, Faragher, Scott K. Depressive symptoms in patients with Alzheimer's disease. Int J Geriatr Psychiatry 16:960–964, 2001.
57. Lowery K, Mynt P, Aisbett J, Dixon T, O'Brien J, Ballard C. Depression in the carers of dementia sufferers: a comparison of the carers of patients suffering from dementia with Lewy bodies and the carers of patients with Alzheimer's disease. J Affect Disord 59:61–65, 2000.
58. Hagedoorn M, Sanderman R, Ranchor AV, Brilman EI, Kempen GIJM, Ormel J. Chronic disease in elderly couples: are women more responsive to their spouses' health condition than men? J Psychosom Res 51:693–696, 2001.
59. Thorpe L, Groulx B. Depressive syndromes in dementia. Can J Neurol Sci 28 (suppl 1):S83–S95, 2001.
60. Katz IR. Diagnosis and treatment of depression in patients with Alzheimer's disease and other dementias. J Clin Psychiatry 59(suppl 9):38–44, 1998.
61. Olin JT, Katz IR, Meyers BS, Schneider LS, Lebowitz BD. Provisional diagnostic criteria for depression of Alzheimer disease: rational and background. J Geriatr Psychiatry 10:129–141, 2002.
62. Olin JT, Schneider LS, Katz IR, Meyers BS, Alexopoulos GS, Breitner JC, Bruce ML, Caine ED, Cummings JL, Devanand DP, Krishnan KRR, Lyketsos CG, Lyness JM, Rabins PV, Reynolds CF III, Rovner BW, Steffens DC, Tariot PN, Lebo-

witz BD. Provisional diagnostic criteria for depression of Alzheimer disease. Am J Geriatr Psychiatry 10:125–128, 2002.
63. Ballard C, Neill D, O'Brien J, McKeith IG, Ince P, Perry R. Anxiety, depression and psychosis in vascular dementia: prevalence and associations. J Affect Disord 59:97–106, 2000.
64. Bathgate D, Snowden JS, Blackshaw A, Neary D. Behaviour in frontotemporal dementia, Alzheimer's disease and vascular dementia. Acta Neurol Scand 103:367–378, 2001.
65. Tariot PN. Treatment strategies for agitation and psychosis in dementia. J Clin Psychiatry 57(suppl 14):21–29, 1996.
66. Rojas-Fernandez CH, Lanctôt KL, Allen DD, MacKnight C. Pharmacotherapy of behavioral and psychological symptoms of dementia: time for a different paradigm? Pharmacotherapy 21:74–102, 2001.
67. Weisman AD. Early diagnosis of vulnerability in cancer patients. Am J Med Sci 271:187–196, 1976.
68. Kaasa S, Malt U, Hagen S, Wist E, Moun T, Kvikstad A. Psychological distress in cancer patients with advanced disease. Radiother Oncol 27:193–197, 1993.
69. Zabora J, Brintzenhofeszoc K, Curbow B, Hooker C, Piantadosi S. The prevalence of psychological distress by cancer site. Psycho-Oncology 10:19–28, 2001.
70. Massie MJ, Holland JC. Overview of normal reactions and prevalence of psychiatric disorders. In JC Holland, H Rowland, eds. Handbook of Psycho-Oncology: Psychological Care of the Patient with Cancer. New York: Oxford University Press, 1989.
71. Kurtz ME, Kurtz JC, Stommel M, Given CW, Given B. Predictors of physical functioning among geriatric cancer patients with small cell or non–small cell lung cancer 3 months after diagnosis. Support Care Cancer 7:328–331, 1999.
72. Kurtz ME, Kurtz JC, Stommel M, Given CW, Given B. Predictors of depressive symptomatology of geriatric patients with lung cancer—a longitudinal analysis. Psycho-Oncology 11:12–22, 2002.
73. Green A, Austin C. Psychopathology of pancreatic cancer: a psychobiologic probe. Psychosomatics 34:208–221, 1993.
74. Eaton WW, Armenian H, Gallo J, Pratt L, Ford DE. Depression and risk for onset of type II diabetes: a prospective population-based study. Diabetes Care 19:1097–1102, 1996.
75. Wing RR, Marcus MD, Blair EH, Epstein LH, Burton LR. Depressive symptomatology in obese adults with type II diabetes. Diabetes Care 13:170–172, 1990.
76. Gary TL, Crum RM, Cooper-Patrick L, Ford D, Brancati FL. Depressive symptoms and metabolic control in African-Americans with type 2 diabetes. Diabetes Care 23:23–29, 2000.
77. Björntorp P, Holm G, Rosmond R. Hypothalamic arousal, insulin resistance and type 2 diabetes mellitus. Diabet Med 16:373–383, 1999.
78. Grandinetti A, Kaholokula JK, Chang HK. Delineating the relationship between stress, depressive symptoms, and glucose intolerance. Diabetes Care 23:1443–1444, 2000.
79. Harris EC, Barraclough BM. Suicide as an outcome for medical disorders. Medicine (Baltimore) 73:281–296, 1994.

80. Szanto K, Gildengers A, Mulsant BH, Brown G, Alexopoulos GS, Reynolds CF III. Identification of suicidal ideation and prevention of suicidal behaviour in the elderly. Drugs Aging 19:11–24, 2002.
81. Raue PJ, Alexopoulow GS, Bruce ML, Kilmstra S, Mulsant BH, Gallo JJ, PROSPECT Study Group. Int J Geriatr Psychiatry 16:560–569, 2001.
82. Goldsmith SK, Pellmar TC, Kleinman, Bunney WE, eds. Committee on Pathophysiology and Prevention of Adolescent and Adult Suicide, Board on Neuroscience and Behavioral Health. Institute of Medicine Report, June 17, 2002. Available at http://www.nap.edu/books/0309083214/html/ [accessed July 15, 2002].
83. Lyness JM, Conwell Y, King DA, Cox C, Caine ED. Age of onset and medical illness in older depressed inpatients. International Psychogeriatrics 7:63–73, 1995.
84. Gill D, Hatcher S. Antidepressants for depression in medical illness. Cochrane Depression Anxiety and Neurosis Group. In: Cochrane Database of Systematic Reviews. Issue 2, 2002.
85. Januzzi JL Jr, Stern TA, Pasternak RC, DeSanctis RW. The influence of anxiety and depression on outcomes of patients with coronary artery disease. Arch Intern Med 160:1913–1921, 2000.
86. Leipzig RM, Cumming RG, Tinetti ME. Drugs and falls in older people: a systematic review and meta-analysis: I. Psychotropic drugs. J Am Geriatr Soc 47:30–39, 1999.
87. Lyketsos CG, Sheppard JE, Steele CD, Kopunek S, Steinberg M, Baker AS, Brandt J, Rabins PV. Am J Psychiatry 157:1686–1689, 2000.
88. Evans DL, Staab JP, Petitto JM, Morrison MF, Szuba MP, Ward HE, Wingate B, Luber MP, O'Reardon JP. Depression in the medical setting: biophyschological interactions and treatment considerations. J Clin Psychiatry 60(suppl 4):40–55, 1999.
89. Lenze EJ, Mulsant BH, Shear MK, Alexopoulos GS, Frank E, Reynolds CF III. Comorbidity of depression and anxiety disorders in later life. Depress Anxiety 14: 86–93, 2001.
90. Doraiswamy PM. Contemporary management of comorbid anxiety and depression in geriatric patients. J Clin Psychiatry 62(suppl 12):30–35, 2001.
91. Reynolds CF III, Alexopoulos GS, Katz IR, Lebowitz BD. Chronic depression in the elderly: approaches for prevention. Drugs Aging 18:507–514, 2001.
92. Lander M, Wilson K, Chochinov HM. Depression and the dying older patient. Clin Geriatr Med 16:335–356, 2000.
93. Tew JD Jr, Mulsant BH, Haskett RF, Prudic J, Thase ME, Crowe RR, Dolata D, Begley AE, Reynolds CF III, Sackeim HA. Acute efficacy of ECT in the treatment of major depression in the old-old. Am J Psychiatry 156:1865–1870, 1999.
94. Wulsin LR. Does depression kill? Arch Intern Med 160:1731–1732, 2000.

7

Vascular Depression

P. Murali Doraiswamy
Duke University Medical Center, Durham, North Carolina, U.S.A.

Yvette Sheline
Washington University, St. Louis, Missouri, U.S.A.

INTRODUCTION

The concept of vascular depression in psychiatric research is analogous to the use of the term *vascular dementia*. Vascular dementia is a syndrome and the term encompasses a variety of vascular disorders (e.g., stroke, vasculitis, angiopathy) that as an end result can cause dementia. Likewise, the term *vascular depression* was proposed to synthesize research findings that implicate a growing role for cerebrovascular disease in the pathophysiology of a subset of patients with late-life depression. Although the term *vascular depression* is relatively new, the concept of arteriosclerotic depression dates back many decades. In 1905, Gaupp diagnosed 45 elderly patients as having depression secondary to arteriosclerosis, with symptoms characterized by persistent apathy and depressed mood. Post (1) noted that the cerebrovascular brain damage was more prevalent in elderly depressed patients than that reported in surveys of the elderly population, with a close temporal association between cases with cerebrovascular accident and the onset of affective disorder. This suggested that cerebrovascular pathology played an etiological role in affective illness. Studies indicate that 20–50% of patients with stroke develop the symptoms of major depression (2). The modern conceptualization of vascular depression arose from magnetic resonance imaging (MRI) studies of depressed subjects conducted in the last 10 years.

MRI STUDIES IN DEPRESSION

Areas of increased signal intensity in the periventricular and deep white matter are frequently observed in the brains of many older individuals on T2-weighted MRI (Fig. 1). These are referred to in this chapter as T2 hyperintensities (T2H) but have also been referred to in the literature as small vessel disease, leukoencephalopathy, or leukoariosis. Hyperintensities can be classified into major groups by location and tissue type: for example, frontal deep white matter (FD-WMH), and subcortical gray matter (SCGMH) hyperintensities. These hyperintensities may occur at rates of up to 60% in healthy elderly patients (3), in whom their significance is unknown (4).

The earliest reports of T2H in major depression came from Krishnan et al. (5) and Coffey et al. (6). In an expanded study, Coffey et al. (7) found that moderate and severe periventricular hyperintensities, as well as large and confluent deep white matter hyperintensities (DWMH), were far more common in 51 depressed patients compared with 22 matched controls. The age-adjusted odds ratio for PVH was 5.32. Lesions of the basal ganglia were present in 51% of depressed patients and 5% of controls. The occurrence of PVH, DWMH, and basal ganglial lesions was associated with risk factors for cerebrovascular disease, but these vascular risk factors were more relevant in depressed patients relative to control subjects, creating a potential confound. Lesions of the deep gray nuclei and large PVH or DWMH were not seen in any of the control subjects, indirectly suggesting that the site and size of the lesions may be important in predicting vulnerability to depression. Subsequent studies comparing patients with unipolar depression as well as bipolar disorder have found a higher rate and severity of T2H in comparison to non-ill individuals (8). Specifically, increased T2H in elderly subject groups with depression has been a well-replicated finding (9–14). This result has also been reported in studies that included younger subjects (7,15), though negative findings with younger groups have been reported as well (16,17). Many of these studies were conducted with hospitalized patients, raising the question of generalizability of the findings to a community sample.

Recently, Steffens et al. (18) have shown a relationship between depression and T2H in a population-based study, the Cardiovascular Health Study (CHS). In a sample of 3660, they examined the association between MRI lesions and depressive symptoms measured by using a modified version of the Centers for Epidemiological Studies Depression (CES-D) scale. They controlled for a

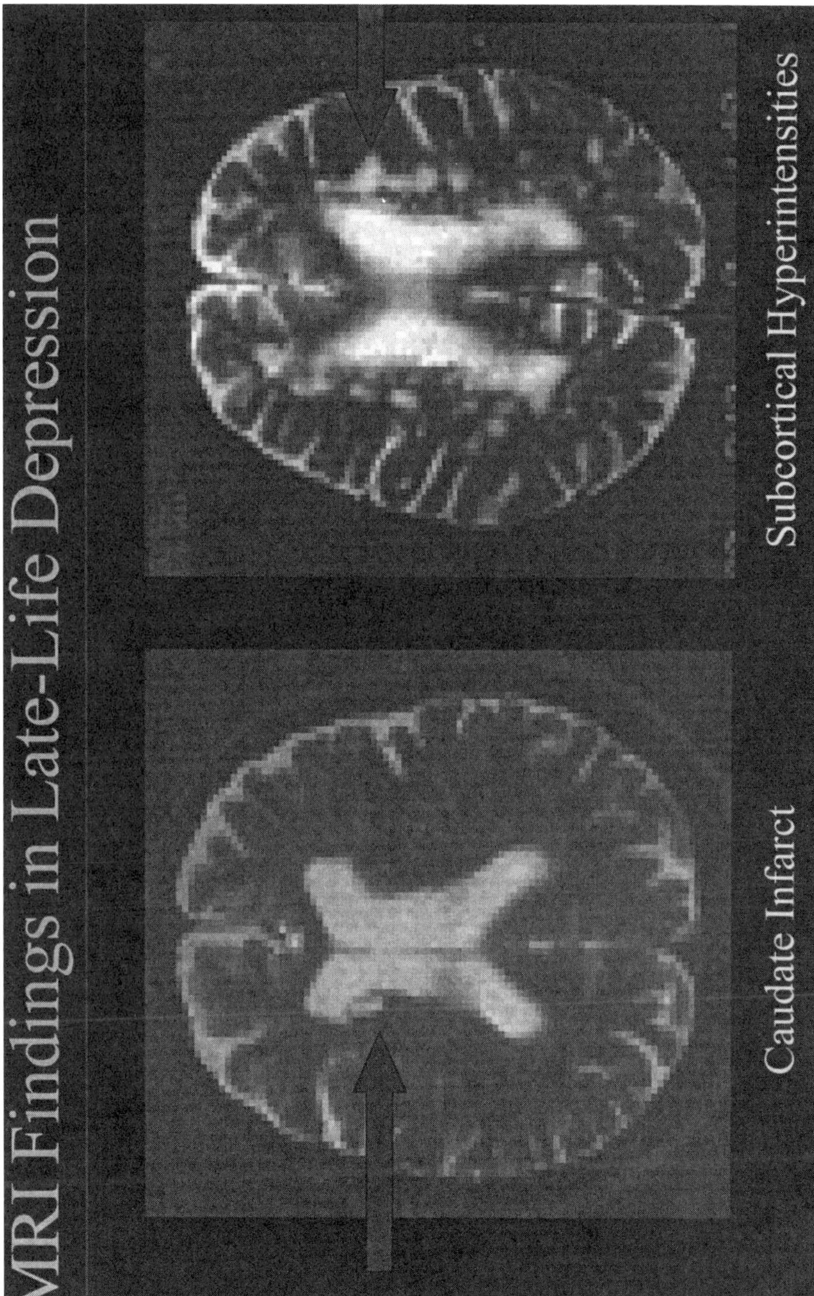

FIGURE 1 MRI findings in late-life depression.

variety of demographic and medical variables as well as functional status and modified Mini-Mental State Exam score. They found that number of small (less than 3 mm) basal ganglial lesions and severity of DWMH were significantly associated with reported depressive symptoms. In subsequent logistic regression models, number of basal ganglia lesions remained a significant predictor (odds ratio 1.4, $p = 0.004$) after controlling for non-MRI variables (age, gender, race, hypertension, cardiovascular disease, ADL (activities of daily living) score, IADL (instrumental ADL) score, cognitive score, and severity of white matter lesions.

Another recent study used a novel MRI technique (arterial spin tagging) to evaluate cerebral perfusion in 19 elderly patients with coronary artery disease (CAD) (19). These patients were then further subdivided into those with and without major depression. Depressed CAD patients did not differ in age, gender, cognition, or medical comorbidity from the nondepressed CAD group. MRI showed that perfusion in left-sided frontal and subcortical regions in the depressed CAD patients was relatively lower than that in nondepressed CAD patients (Fig. 2). Despite limitations such as a small sample size and indirect estimates of flow, these findings suggest that left-sided hypoperfusion may underlie late-life depression in patients with vascular risk factors. A larger study is under way at Duke to confirm these initial findings and test the effects of treatment on cerebral tissue perfusion.

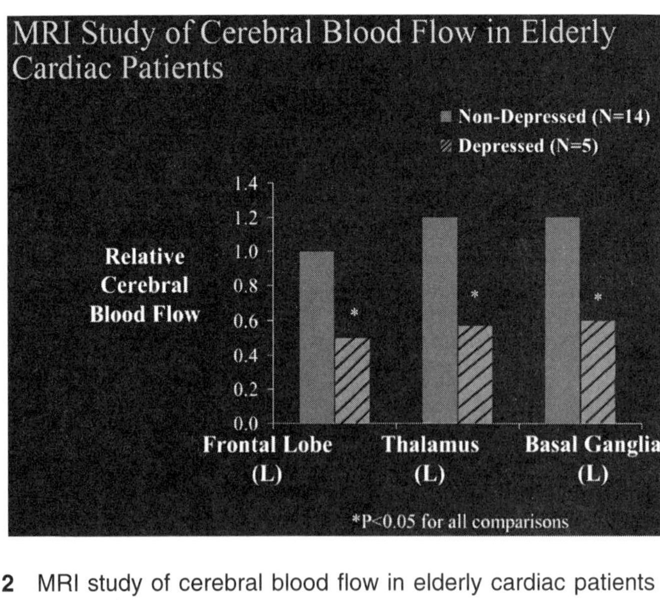

FIGURE 2 MRI study of cerebral blood flow in elderly cardiac patients ($p < 0.05$ for all comparisons).

CLINICAL CORRELATES OF MRI CHANGES

In late-life depression, clinical correlates of MRI-defined T2H have included older age, vascular risk factors, and late-onset depressive illness (7,20). Fujikawa et al. (21,22) found a higher rate of "silent" cerebral infarctions (T2H) in late- compared to early-onset major depressive disorder. In a small sample, we found that a higher rate of caudate subcortical gray matter hyperintensities and large DWMH distinguished late-onset from early-onset unipolar depression (23). Large (>10 mm in diameter) DWMH were observed in 6 of 10 (60%) patients with late-onset depression (LOD) compared with only 1 of 9 (11%) patients with early-onset depression (EOD). In addition, caudate hyperintensities were found in 6/10 (60%) of LOD patients compared with only 1 of 9 (11%) EOD patients. Of 10 LOD patients, 9 had either a caudate hyperintensity and/or a large DWMH while only 1 EOD patient had either of these structural changes. Given that frontal-basal ganglia pathways are believed to be important in mood regulation, these new lines of evidence indirectly suggest that frontal and subcortical gray matter hyperintensities play a role in the development of some late-onset depression. MRI-defined vascular depression is based on the presence of characteristic MRI changes in key brain regions (Fig. 1) in subjects with appropriate presentation of depression. These studies suggest that the frontal lobes and basal ganglia may be involved in the pathophysiology of affective disorder.

Vascular depression is hypothesized to result from silent cerebral infarctions in end arterioles (21). These, in turn, may interrupt the functioning of the frontal-subcortical circuits that are critically involved in the regulation of mood and executive function. Thus, in vulnerable subjects, the presence of vascular risk factors may lead to silent or overt ischemic changes. Such changes could then interrupt mood circuits, which may then interact with negative life events to precipitate depression. This may be one potential mechanism by which vascular changes may lead to late-life depression (24). While most T2H are thought to reflect small infarcts (25), it should be borne in mind that other pathology has been suggested (26,27).

NEUROPSYCHOLOGICAL CORRELATES OF VASCULAR DEPRESSION

Recent data suggests that there may be specific pattern of deficits in vascular depression, predominantly affecting frontal lobe functioning and also producing slowing (24,28,29). In normal subjects, the associations between T2H and cognitive test performance are unclear, and there may be threshold effects for lesion volume. Studies utilizing patient populations have typically yielded patterns of impairment consistent with the subcortical dementias. In a group of elderly patients with mixed vascular risk factors, there were significant associations with four neuropsychological measures, all relying upon executive control (30). In a similar group of subjects, Gupta et al. (31) reported impairment on 13 of 17 neuropsychological instruments evaluating executive control, recent memory, constructional praxis, and speeded psychomotor integration. In a group composed purely of hypertensive patients, van Sweiten et al. (32) observed impairment on five instruments assessing executive control and recent memory.

Disturbances in neuropsychological function, including planning, sequencing, organizing, and abstraction are common in depression and are characteristic of prefrontal dysfunction (11). White matter hyperintensities found in patients with depression and prefrontal dysfunction predicted a more chronic course in geriatric depression (15). One measure of prefrontal dysfunction, the Mattis Dementia Initiation-Perseveration (IP) Subscale, has been shown to be associated with poor response and greater relapse/recurrence rates (33–35). The IP domain consists of word generation, manual sequencing and graphomotor copying tasks. Alexopoulos (34) found that patients with lower IP scores were significantly less likely to achieve remission during an acute antidepressant trial. In this study, the majority of patients were treated with nortriptyline (>30 ng/mL) and nontricyclic agents were administered to patients who did not qualify for treatment with tricyclic agents. Of patients who responded to antidepressant treatment, 80% fell in the normal range on the IP scale (>34), whereas half of those who failed to respond to antidepressant treatment had scores <30 on the IP scale. These findings have formed the basis of "clinically defined vascular depression" in which executive dysfunction is proposed to be a sign of frontal subcortical brain changes (e.g., Ref. 36).

MRI HYPERINTENSITIES AND RISK FOR DEMENTIA

Recently Steffens et al. (37) studied 182 nondemented elderly (60 years of age or older) subjects with major depression in the Duke Mental Health Center Clinical Research Center study. Patients were assessed every 3 months for 1–5 years. Of these subjects, 26 met critiera for dementia at follow-up. Older age, lower baseline cognitive scores, older age at onset of depression, and higher volume of MRI-measured gray matter hyperintensities were associated with the diagnosis of dementia (Alzheimer's disease, vascular dementia, or both) at follow up. In survival analyses, gray matter lesion volume was associated with an approximately twofold greater risk for subsequent dementia. Other studies have linked late-life depression to risk for dementia and also suggested an interactive effect with apolipoprotein E genotype. Taken together, these pilot findings raise the hypothesis that "vascular depression" may increase the risk for subsequent dementia. A prospective longitudinal study is under way at Duke to further confirm these findings.

TREATMENT OUTCOMES OF VASCULAR DEPRESSION

Hickie et al. (15) reported that deep white matter hyperintensities predicted poorer outcome with heterogeneous pharmacological regimens or electroconvulsive therapy (ECT). Their sample size was small, however, patients were treated with a variety of medications and/or ECT. Simpson et al. (38) showed that basal ganglia lesions predicted poor response to monotherapy, ECT and lithium augmentation. Fujikawa (22) suggested that patients with lesions took longer to recover and had more adverse experiences. O'Brien et al. (39) found that patients with severe T2H had poorer outcome with antidepressant treatment in a naturalistic 32-month follow-up study.

Krishnan et al. (20) studied the relative probability of 6-month recovery from an index course of major depression in subjects with and without MRI-confirmed vascular lesions. The only trends observed in this study were that subjects with lesions and later onset of depression tended toward poorer recovery.

In a subsequent study of 41 patients treated with ECT, Steffens et al. (40) examined the association between outcome of an acute course of ECT treatment and lesion ratings (dichotomized as Fazekas rating 0–1 versus 2–3). Patients with lower SCGMH ratings had significantly greater improvement on CGI-severity scores ($D = -3.2$) compared with patients with higher ratings. The number of treatments did not differ between groups (9.6 versus 10.3). For DWMH, there were no significant differences in clinical improvement or number of ECT treatments. These preliminary data offer support for the association between MRI lesion severity in subcortical gray matter and treatment resistance.

All these studies utilized relatively small samples, were naturalistic in design, and were limited in terms of image acquisition and inability to fully control for factors such as standardization of treatment. Recently, Salloway et al. (41) analyzed data from a 12-week randomized trial of sertraline versus placebo in geriatric major depression. A subset of 59 patients had received MRI scans as part of a substudy to examine MRI correlates of treatment response. In this subset, MRI hyperintensities were not found to be predictive of acute treatment response to sertraline or placebo.

Given the high frequency of MRI-defined T2H in elderly depressed patients, particularly those with late-onset depression, a systematic, large-scale study that examines whether MRI-defined T2H predicts treatment response to a standardized trial with a widely used antidepressant medication is clearly warranted. The importance of studying T2H in depression is suggested by a number of reports that show poorer outcomes and poorer antidepressant response, suggesting that the presence of these lesions may represent a more severe and chronic illness; however, not all studies are in agreement.

CONCLUSIONS

Based on these studies, Steffens et al. (42) have proposed criteria to chracterize vascular depression as follows: major depression occurring in the context of clinical and/or neuroimaging evidence of cerebrovascular disease or neuropsychological impairment. Clinical evidence would include history of stroke or transient ischemic attacks or focal neurological signs or symptoms. Neuroimaging evidence would include gray or white matter hyperintensities in keeping with the 1988 criteria of Fazekas et al., confluent white matter lesions, or cortical or subcortical infarcts. Neuropsychological impairment would be manifest by disturbance of executive function, memory, or speed of information processing. The diagnosis would be supported by older age, absence of a family history of depression, depression onset after age 50 or after a vascular event, psychomotor retardation, apathy, anhedonia, and impairment in activities of daily living.

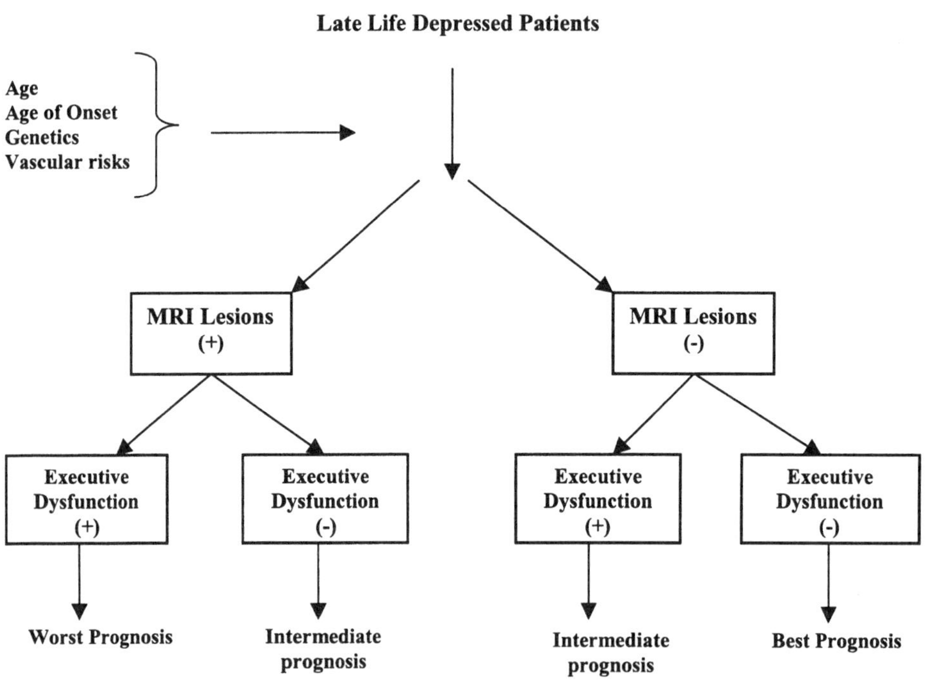

FIGURE 3 A hypothetical model for the effect of both MRI-determined T2H and frontal executive dysfunction (ED) is outlined above. We hypothesize that patients who have severe T2H lesions, greater ED, or both will have lower remission rates to treatment, greater relapse rates, and poor long-term outcomes.

Conceptually, a depression that responds to revascularization would also meet the criteria for "vascular depression."

Of the studies that examined the association between T2H lesion severity and response to antidepressant treatment, two studies found an association with poor treatment response (15,38). In addition, several studies have found that in addition to overall lesion severity, lesion location—in deep frontal white matter and basal ganglia—was importantly associated with depression. This is in accordance with neuropsychological findings, in patients with vascular depression, of impairment in frontal lobe function, in particular executive dysfunction and psychomotor slowing. Few prior studies have obtained neuropsychological data simultaneously with MRI data on T2H and only one study (28) has reported on the use of both MRI lesion severity and neuropsychological data as predictors in treatment response.

Extrapolating the available findings, we have developed a hypothetical model (Fig. 3) of the potential interactions between MRI lesions and executive dysfunction as well as how these may interact to influence treatment outcomes. Duke and Washington Universities have begun a prospective treatment trial to test this hypothesis. If such a hypothesis were to be confirmed, then treatments aimed at correcting the vascular deficits (e.g., vasodilators, antiplatelet agents) or those that target specific frontal neurotransmitter systems (e.g., dopamine agonists) may be worth investigating.

REFERENCES

1. Post F. The Significance of Affective Symptoms in Old Age. Maudsley Monographs 10. London: Oxford University Press, 1962.
2. Robinson RG, Starkstein SE. Mood disorders following stroke: new findings and future directions. J Geriatr Psychiatry 1989; 22:1–15.
3. Fazekas F, Kleinert R, Offenbacher H, Payer F, Schmidt R, Kleinert G, Radner H, Lechner H. The morphologic correlate of incidental punctate white matter hyperintensities on MR images. AJNR 1991; 12:915–921.
4. Mirsen TR, Lee DH, Wong CJ, Diaz JF, Fox AJ, Hachinski VC, Merskey H. Clinical correlates of white-matter changes on magnetic resonance imaging scans of the brain. Arch Neurol 1991; 48:1015–1021.
5. Krishnan KR, Goli V, Ellinwood EH, France RD, Blazer DG, Nemeroff CB. Leukoencephalopathy in patients diagnosed as major depressive. Biol Psychiatry 1988; 23:519–522.
6. Coffey CE, Figiel GS, Djang WT, Saunders WB, Weiner RD. White matter hyperintensity on magnetic resonance imaging: clinical and neuroanatomic correlates in the depressed elderly. J Neuropsychiatry Clin Neurosci 1989; 1:135–144.
7. Coffey CE, Wilkinson WE, Weiner RD. Quantitative cerebral anatomy in depression. A controlled magnetic resonance imaging study. Arch Gen Psychiatry 1993; 50:7–16.
8. Soares JC and Mann JJ. The anatomy of mood disorders–review of structural neuroimaging studies. Biol Psychiatry 1997; 41:86–106.

9. Coffey CE, Figiel GS, Djang WT, Weiner RD. Subcortical hyperintensity on magnetic imaging: a comparison of normal and depressed elderly subjects. Am J Psychiatry 1990; 147:187–189.
10. Zubenko GS, Sullivan P, Nelson JP, Belle SH, Wolf G. Brain imaging abnormalities in mental disorders of late life. Arch Neurol 1990; 47:1107–1111.
11. Lesser IM, Miller BL, Boone KB, Hill-Gutierrez E, Mehringer CM, Wong K, Mena I. Brain injury and cognitive function in late-onset psychotic depression. J Neuropsychiatry Clin Neurosci 1991; 3:33–40.
12. Rabins PV, Pearlson GD, Aylward E, Kumar AJ, Dowell K. Cortical magnetic resonance imaging changes in elderly inpatients with major depression. Am J Psychiatry 1991; 148:617–620.
13. Howard RJ, Beats B, Forstl H, Graves P, Bingham J, Levy R. White matter changes in late onset depression: a magnetic resonance imaging study. Int J Geriatr Psychiatry 1993; 8:183–185.
14. Krishnan KR, McDonald WM, Doraiswamy PM. Neuroanatomical substrates of depression in the elderly. Eur Arch Psychiatry Clin Neurosci 1993; 243:41–46.
15. Hickie I, Scott E, Mitchell P, Wilhelm K, Austin MB, Bennett B. Subcortical hyperintensities on magnetic resonance imaging: clinical correlates and prognostic significance in patients with severe depression. Biol Psychiatry 1995; 37:151–160.
16. Guze BH, Szuba MP. Leukoencephalopathy and major depression: A preliminary report. Psychiatry Res 1992; 45:169–175.
17. Dupont RM, Jernigan TL, Heindel W, Butters N, Shafer K, Wilson T, Hesselink J, Gillin JC. Magnetic resonance imaging and mood disorders: localization of white matter and other subcortical abnormalities. Arch Gen Psychiatry 1995; 52:747–755.
18. Steffens DC, Helms MJ, Krishnan KRR, Burke GL. Cerebrovascular disease and depression symptoms in the Cardiovascular Health Study. Stroke 1999; 30:2159–2166.
19. Doraiswamy PM, MacFall J, Krishnan KR, O'Connor C, Wan X, Benaur M, Lewandowski M, Fortner M. Magnetic resonance assessment of cerebral perfusion in depressed cardiac patients: preliminary findings. Am J Psychiatry 1999; 156(10):1641–1643.
20. Krishnan KR, Hayes J, George L, Blazer D. Six-month outcomes for MRI-related vascular depression. Depression Anxiety 1998; 8:142–146.
21. Fujikawa T, Yamawaki S, and Touhouda Y. Incidence of silent cerebral infarction in patients with major depression. Stroke 1993; 24:1631–1634.
22. Fujikawa T, Yamawaki S, Touhouda Y. Background factors and clinical symptoms of major depression with silent cerebral infarction. Stroke 1994; 25:798–801.
23. Figiel GS, Krishnan KRR, Doraiswamy PM, Rao VP, Nemeroff CB, Boyko OB. Subcortical hyperintensities on brain magnetic resonance imaging: a comparison between late age onset and early onset elderly depressed subjects. Neurobiol Aging 1991; 26:245–247.
24. Krishnan K, Hays J, and Blazer D. MRI-defined vascular depression. Am J Psychiatry 1997; 154(4):497–501.
25. George AE, de Leon MJ, Kalnin A, Rosner L, Goodgold A, Chase N. Leukoencephalopathy in normal and pathologic aging: 2. MRI of brain lucencies. AJNR 1986; 7:567–570.
26. Roman GC. Senile dementia of the Binswanger type: a vascular form of dementia in the elderly. JAMA 1987; 258:1782–1788.

27. Jung HH, Bassetti C, Tournier-Lasserve E, Vahedi K, Arnaboldi M, Arifi VB, and Burgunder JM. Cerebral autosomal dominant arteriopathy with subcortical infarcts and leukoencephalopathy: a clinicopathological and genetic study of a Swiss family. J Neurol Neurosurg Psychiatry 1995; 59:138–143.
28. Simpson S, Jackson A, Baldwin RC, Burns A. Subcortical hyperintensities in late-life depression: acute response to treatment and neuropsychological impairment. Int Psychogeriatr 1997; 9(3):257–275.
29. Dahabra S, Ashton CH, Bahrainian M, et al. Structural and functional abnormalities in elderly patients clinically recovered from early- and late-onset depression. Biol Psychiatry 1998; 44:34–46.
30. Junque C, Pujol J, Vendrell P, Bruna O, Jodar M, Ribas JC, Vinas J, Capdevila A, Marti-Vilalta JL. Leuko-araiosis on magnetic resonance imaging and speed of mental processing. Arch Neurol 1990; 47:151–156.
31. Gupta SR, Naheedy MH, Young JC, Ghobrial M, Rubino FA, Hindo W. Periventricular white matter changes and dementia. Clinical, neuropsychological, radiological, and pathological correlation. Arch Neurol 1988; 45:637–641.
32. Van Swieten JC, Staal S, Kappelle LJ, Derix MM, van Gijn J. Are white matter lesions directly associated with cognitive impairment in patients with lacunar infarcts? J Neurol 1996; 243:196–200.
33. Kalayam B, Alexopoulos GS. Prefrontal dysfunction and treatment response in geriatric depression. Arch Gen Psychiatry 1999; 56(8):713–718.
34. Alexopoulos GS, Meyers BS, Young RC, Kalayam B, Kakuma T, Gabrielle M, Sirey JA, Hull J. Executive dysfunction and long-term outcomes of geriatric depression. Arch Gen Psychiatry 2000; 57(3):285–290.
35. Alexopoulos GS, Kiosses DN, Klimstra S, Kalayam B, Bruce ML. Clinical presentation of the "depression-executive dysfunction syndrome" of late life. Am J Geriatr Psychiatry 2002; 10(1):98–106.
36. Alexopoulos GS, Meyers BS, Young RC, Campbell S, Silbersweig D, Charlson M. "Vascular depression" hypothesis. Arch Gen Psychiatry 1997; 54(10):915–922.
37. Steffens DC, MacFall JR, Payne ME, Welsh-Bohmer KA, Krishnan, KR. Grey-matter lesions and dementia. Lancet 2000; 356:1686–1687.
38. Simpson S, Baldwin RC, Jackson A, Burns AS. Is subcortical disease associated with a poor response to antidepressants? Neurological, neuropsychological and neuroradiological findings in late-life depression. Psychol Med 1998; 28:1015–1026.
39. O'Brien J, Ames D, Chiu E, Schweitzer I, Desmond P, Tress B. Severe deep white matter lesions and outcome in elderly patients with major depressive disorder: follow up study. Br Med J 1998; 317:982–984.
40. Steffens DC, Conway CR, Dombeck CB, Wagner HR, Tupler LA, Weiner RD. Severity of subcortical gray matter hyperintensity predicts ECT response in geriatric depression. J ECT 2001; 17(1):45–49.
41. Salloway S, Boyle PA, Correia S, Malloy PF, Cahn-Weiner DA, Schneider L, Krishnan KR, Nakra R. Am J Geriatr Psychiatry 2002; 10(1):107–111.
42. Steffens DC, Krishnan KR. Structural neuroimaging and mood disorders: recent findings, implications for classification, and future directions. Biol Psychiatry 1998; 43(10):705–712.

8

Caregiver Depression

Fred Silverstone
McLean Hospital, Belmont, Massachusetts, U.S.A.

Nava Vogel
Belmont Council on Aging, Belmont, Massachusetts, U.S.A.

INTRODUCTION

For multiple reasons, we have begun to witness a dramatic increase in the need for family members to become involved in the care of their aging relatives. By the year 2030, an estimated 20% of the U.S. population will be 65 years of age or older (Koizumi, 1998). While the elderly population continues to increase, a growing burden has been placed on family caregivers by cutbacks in health care funding and in insurance coverage that have reduced the accessibility of outpatient and home-based care services, by abbreviated medical and psychiatric hospital stays, and by deinstitutionalization of psychiatric patients. Between 1988 and 1996, the number of caregiving households in the United States tripled to approximately 22 million. By 2003, an estimated one-fifth of U.S. households will provide care (Koizumi, 1998).

Beyond direct financial impact, an indirect cost to society is imposed by the decreased productivity of caregivers. Already, more than 14 million part- or full-time employees care for relatives while remaining employed. U.S. businesses bear an estimated $11 to $29 billion annual loss due to absences alone, and the total estimated annual cost of decreased productivity among caregivers is estimated to exceed $196 billion (Koizumi, 1998). A recent Canadian study estimated that 15% of the adult population of Ontario was providing care to family members (Barnet, 1999). In Britian, approximately 7 million informal caregivers spend anywhere between 20 and 100 hr per week performing caregiving responsibilities (Thomas, 1993). This chapter reviews the definition of *caregiver burden* and explores its impact, with particular attention to how caregiving increases the caregivers' risk for depressive disorders.

OBJECTIVE VERSUS SUBJECTIVE CAREGIVER BURDEN

Caregiver burden refers to "the physical, psychological or emotional, social and financial problems that can be experienced by family members or friends caring for impaired older adults" (Llindick, 1986). Caregivers provide assistance to elderly patients with physical health problems such as cancer, diabetes, Parkinson's disease, heart disease, arthritis, macular degeneration, stroke, hip replacements, and many other problems. Psychiatric illnesses that may require caregiving include the dementias, depression, anxiety, panic disorders, bipolar illness, and psychotic disorders such as schizophrenia.

The now extensive literature on caregiver burden and the mentally ill first began to surface during the 1960s. Toward the end of the 1970s, Hatfield (1978) differentiated objective burden from subjective burden. Objective burden comprised financial costs and other verifiable, observable allocation of resources. Subjective burden considered the emotional and psychosocial impacts of caregiving (Thompson, 1982). Caregivers of depressed older adults experience objective burden through providing transportation, performing housework, preparing meals, giving personal hygiene care, and offering financial help. They experience additional subjective burden through the need to assure safety, address behavioral disturbances, cope with excessive dependency, and weather disruptions in sleep, social routines, personal relationships, and the usual activities of daily living and work (Baronet, 1999).

CAREGIVING CAN BE HAZARDOUS TO YOUR HEALTH

As caregiving by nonprofessionals has increased, the need for caregivers themselves to receive care has become a major concern. Family members forced to provide care in order to compensate for diminishing hospital stays and limited home services too easily become "hidden patients" themselves (Andolsek 1988). Such caregivers then are at increased risk for health complications. A study by Schulz and Beach (1999) involving 400 older adult caregivers and 400 controls living with their spouses showed that caregiving is an independent risk factor for mortality. They found that caregivers who reported high levels of burden when caring for their spouses were 63% more likely to die within a subsequent 4-year period than noncaregiving controls. Caregivers had significantly higher rates of depression, anxiety, and poorer physical health, often due to inadequate time for self-care. Estimated rates of depression among caregivers range between 18 and 47% (Livingston, 1996), and 17.5% of caregivers have been found to have anxiety disorders (Livingston, 1996). Usage of psychotropic drugs by caregivers is increased, although no significant differences in alcohol consumption have been found (Cochrane, 1997).

At a physiological level, intriguing studies have even suggested that caregivers' immune status is compromised. Viral illnesses, for example, have been shown to last longer in caregivers than in noncaregiving controls (Kiccolt-Glaser, 1991). Comparisons of caregivers to controls given influenza vaccine found decreased antibody response among the caregivers. This was attributed to their increased levels of emotional distress and decreased activation of the hypothalamic-pituitary-adrenal axis, consistent with the observation that caregivers show increased levels of salivary cortisol concentrations (Vedhara, 1999).

DEPRESSION IN CAREGIVERS OF DEMENTIA PATIENTS

Several authors have attempted to identify the risk factors that predict depression in caregivers of Alzheimer's disease patients. Disease severity appears an important factor, since depression was more common among caregivers of patients whose Mini-Mental State Exam (MMSE) scores were below 17 (Howard, 1998). Similarly, the presence of behavioral disturbances—such as withdrawal, agitation, and verbal or behavioral disinhibition—correlated with increased caregiver depression (Howard, 1998). Impaired activities of daily living and depression in the Alzheimer's disease patients themselves, but not age or gender, have been associated with caregiver depression (Shua-Haim, 2001). Caregiving spouses became increasingly at risk for depression, too, when faced with the patients' increasing emotional and social withdrawal and the diminished capacity for intimacy that increased as the disease progressed (Bauer, 2001). Emotional and social withdrawal may also characterize patients with severe depression, suggesting similar concerns in the caretakers of these patients. There is a need for studies to determine how factors such as disease severity, degree of assistance required to perform activities of daily living, and extent of relationship impairment affect the caregivers of depressed patients.

OUTCOMES OF PROVIDING ASSISTANCE TO CAREGIVERS

Most of what we know about assisting caregivers is drawn from studies of those who care for older adults with Alzheimer's disease. The Health Care Financing

Administration has studied outcomes associated with providing assistance to these caregivers utilizing a case management and community care program for dementia patients and their caregivers. As part of the Omnibus Budget Reconciliation Act, known as the Medicare Alzheimer's Disease Demonstration Evaluation (MADDE), caregivers received education and training about Alzheimer's disease, individualized case management services, and attended caregiver support groups. In addition, community long-term-care reimbursement was provided ($299–$699 per client per month for the payment of formal care services). Expected results included decreased rates of depression and anxiety, improved physical health, and improved quality of life in caregivers as well as increased satisfaction with care received by patients.

The actual findings of the MADDE, however, demonstrated little improvement in caregiver burden or rates of depression. One interpretation of these findings was that the intensity of intervention and amount of reimbursement was too low for benefits to be detected. A need for more intensive assistance available more hours per day and days per week during periods of crisis might have made more of a difference. Also, more extensive training and education for caregivers, support group involvement, and peer counseling might have improved outcomes (Newcomer, 1999). The more intensive support provided in another study, one that examined the effectiveness of using home health nurses to decrease burden and depression of elderly caregivers, did indeed demonstrate a decrease in caregiver burden and depression (Mignon, 2000).

Beneficial effects to Alzheimer's disease family caregivers have also been shown using focused interventions based on cognitive-behavioral therapy approaches. In a British study, a combination of education, stress management, and coping skills training was provided for caregivers in 14 sessions over a 28-week period. An important outcome was the demonstration of fewer behavioral disturbances among the caregivers' care recipients (Marriott, 2000). In an American study implemented by the National Institute of Mental Health (NIMH) and the National Institute on Aging (NIA) and designated Project Assist (Rose 1990), both cognitive-behavioral therapy (CBT) and psychodynamic psychotherapies provided to older caregiving spouses were shown to be beneficial.

FAMILY IMPACT

The family care of patients with Alzheimer's disease and probably that of many other infirm elderly adults falls disproportionately on the shoulders of the family's women. Men almost always want their wives to be their primary providers of care, for example, while women are far less likely to want their husbands to be their primary caregivers. Women are able to provide both task-focused and emotional support to their husbands, but they often find it preferable to get help for themselves from other women, primarily their daughters, siblings, relatives, and friends. When an elder patient lives alone, he or she is likely to get help from adult children or other relatives.

A family's characteristic values, communication style, and approach to conflict resolution all impact on caregiving and caregiver burden. Characteristically hostile families with limited affilation and impaired communication do poorly with caregiving. Families composed of highly autonomous members rely more on formal supports. Collectivist families who engage in positive conflict resolution strategies provide significantly more help and emotional support (Lieberman, 1999).

Families able to use "cognitive empathy," which involves interest and understanding while maintaining an objective, more or less matter-of-fact approach, experience less stress as a result of caregiving. In cognitive empathy, feelings are contained while the distressed individual is given undivided, wholehearted but thoughtful and reflective attention. Lee and colleagues (2001) compared caregivers who showed cognitive empathy with caregivers who showed a less objective "emotional empathy" in a study of 140 informal caregivers of older adults. Those with emotional empathy responded to the emotional experiences of the care recipient in a way that was easily overwhelming. Those with a more cognitive style of empathizing were better able to maintain perspective. They showed a greater intellectual understanding of the care recipient's experience and were less depressed and less stressed. Their greater ability to engage and detach seemed to improve their quality of life. Even caregivers who have not learned to make use of cognitive empathy during their developmental adult years can learn to use this approach (Lee, 2001).

Other characteristics of well-functioning families coping effectively while providing care for a mentally ill relative include acceptance of the illness, cohesion among family members, flexibility and tolerance, patience, willingness to accept and seek outside support from friends, community organizations and professionals, solution-oriented problem-solving skills, and an absence of violence and of alcohol and substance abuse (Marsh, 1998). Such families draw upon their greater resilience in bearing the stress of caregiving and rebounding from adversity.

CAREGIVERS OF DEPRESSED ELDERS: VIGNETTES AND CLINICAL RECOMMENDATIONS

Caregivers of patients with Alzheimer's disease, AIDS, cancer, and other diseases have received greater attention recently, but there is very little public awareness of the burden borne by those who care for elders suffering from depression. While the limitations and needs of demented patients may be readily understood by the public and by professionals, it is often more difficult for caregivers to accept the depressed elder's needs, which can require similar levels of support and time.

Adult children who become caregivers to their aging parents often struggle with the difficult process of redefining their relationship to their parents. The adult child needs to achieve "filial maturity," the ability to renounce his or her own needs and desires for parenting from the elder care recipient (Bleckner, 1965) in order to accept the role of providing care. The provision of care to a parent can thus be laden with conflict and stress when the care provider's needs are not fully relinquished. Some adult children may continue to long for parental approval that was never previously received, seeking fruitlessly for this reward by agreeing to provide care.

The case of Ms. G. illustrates this point. At age 50, she had still never experienced a sense of being sufficiently valued by her mother, yet when her mother became frail she leaped at the opportunity to care for her. After a year, she was referred for treatment because she became sad and depressed. She reported to the clinician that she had hoped that her mother could finally appreciate her, because it was now so obvious how much she was doing for her. Instead, she was met with the devaluation and coldness that characterized their lifelong relationship. After several months of psychotherapy, she came to accept the likelihood that her wish for acceptance would never be granted. As a result, she was able to place her mother in a supported nursing facility, which eased her own emotional stress while more effectively meeting her mother's complicated physical and emotional needs.

The process of attaining filial maturity involves a role change rather than a role reversal, contrary to the expectations of many caregivers, who expect that providing care will reverse the direction of the parent-child relationship (APA, 1996). Even while the elder appears to require that the child perform activities similar to the parenting of a child, the basic, child-parent relationship remains. Elaine Brody's explorations (1985) into the psychodynamics of the child-parent relationship at the latter end of the life cycle reveal that the nature of the emotional stress experienced by the caregiver can often be linked to unrealistic expectations. The adult child somehow feels that he or she should be able to reciprocate the kind of care that the parent once gave. The care of an elder, however, does not result in increased independence and a lessening of the caregiver's burden. The attempt to provide the equivalent of what one received during childhood, therefore, can easily lead to frustration, disappointment, depression, and fatigue.

Caregiving requires acknowledging changes in the recipient's autonomy. Caregivers who are looking after their aging parents for example, may need to mourn the loss of being able to turn to those parents for the emotional and practical resources they came to depend on in their youth. As with most significant losses, failure to successfully acknowledge and mourn this change can set the stage for a state of depression.

In many cases, the actual provider of care to an elderly family member is not the one whose relationship with the care recipient was most resilient and successful. Rather, convenience may play an important role. Studies show that it is typically the child who is unemployed or underemployed, unmarried, childless, or geographically closest to the parent who becomes the primary care provider (Ikels, 1985). Some of these factors increase the psychological vulnerability of the care provider. In addition, the financial demands of caregiving may be impossible to meet. On the other hand, a caregiver who obtains some economic compensation from this role may develop an uneasy sense of dependency. Psychological regression can develop, leading to conflict, depression, and—in extreme circumstances—even abuse of the elder.

The case of Sandra, the 77-year-old caregiver to her 102-year-old mother, illustrates some of these dynamics. Sandra, a freelance writer, was the one daughter among three who found herself with only limited financial resources at the time and age when her mother needed care. She moved into the family home at age 60, but as the years progressed, the burden of care increased while she herself was aging. As she gradually become overwhelmed, the house became cluttered and uncared for to such a degree that it posed a health and safety hazard. The daughter caregiver also showed signs of extreme hostility that required the intervention of a social worker trained in abuse cases.

In addition to some of the dynamics already described, caregivers who must provide help to a spouse face an additional stress when the care recipient's illness results in diminished intimacy and a reduced capacity for usual activities. The alteration of roles that may result is often difficult for husbands whose wives formerly shouldered greater responsibility for relationship maintenance or for household duties. The stress of the husband may be further aggravated by feelings of isolation and the sense that it is not socially acceptable to be in the caregiving role.

ETHNIC AND SOCIAL CLASS VARIATIONS IN THE CAREGIVING RELATIONSHIP

The effects of ethnic and social class factors on the caregiving relationship are important for family members and involved clinicians to understand. As a general matter, families of white, middle-class Americans provide fewer hours of direct caregiving than those of nonwhites, families of lower socioeconomic levels, or immigrants to this country. African Americans provide an average of 10 hr of care per week more than their white counterparts. First-generation Asians and Hispanics provide more hours than whites and also tend to be younger when their caregiving careers begin (Abraham, 1992). With increasing levels of social mobility and assimilation into American culture, more of the care is provided by nonfamily caregivers. If the caregiver has a large and supportive extended family, there may be less stress. However, if the caregiver is isolated from the larger family and cultural group, levels of stress may be high and the caregiver may be at risk for depression.

The case of Sonia, a midde-aged woman of Syrian descent and a gifted ceramic artist who was caring for her frail mother of 80, demonstrates this vulnerability. Sonia did not have any of her family in the United States, yet she was adamant that her mother never be institutionalized or be left alone with a care provider in the home, as this would be unacceptable and disrespectful to an elder in her country of origin. The demands of the mother's care increased, however, until Sonia became a prisoner in her own home. Her isolation and conflict led to depression and a need for intervention.

A CAREGIVER SUPPORT GROUP

Caregivers who lack social support and experience caregiving as increasing a sense of isolation are more vulnerable to developing depression. This association has been demonstrated in a number of studies (Yates, 1999; Israel and Heaney, 1997). Caregiver support groups, now proliferating in many communities, provide one promising means of reducing caregivers' isolation and need for support.

At our institution, a caregiver support group that has been meeting regularly during the past year has been able to offer various kinds of support for its members at different stages in its development. It took several months for the group to grow to a size of 4–8 members. Meetings occur weekly and last for 1 hr. Salient themes for these caregivers include conflicts with siblings around care of the elder, negotiating difficult decisions with the elder—such as moves to assisted living, and the emotional challenges of watching a loved one decline physically, mentally, or both. Over the year, a noticeable change occurred in the interchanges among these group members. Participants who initially appeared to require much feedback from the facilitators came to look increasingly to other members for feedback and support. The somber and reserved initial tone of the group's meetings developed into a more widely varying, sometimes humorous interaction. Although the group included caregivers of elders with a variety of physical and mental conditions, a few of the care recipients were depressed elders. One middle-aged caregiver whose mother has been diagnosed with depression reported how difficult it was to stand helplessly by, listening to her mother's expression of unrelenting despair and her litany of exaggerated complaints. Her attempts to persuade her mother to view the circumstances of her life differently were consistently met with rejection, and the daughter's valiant efforts to provide her with constant companionship and uplifting activities had limited results. Over the course of 6 months, while participating in the group, she reported changes in responses to her mother. As she increasingly accepted and acknowledged her mother's pessimistic appraisals of life, her sense of burnout diminished. The daughter attributed her changed caregiving approach to the feedback she received from many others who guided her in this direction.

Another initially depressed caregiver in the group reported how frustrated she was in caring for her difficult and frail 93-year-old mother. Given the mother's reported symptoms, the group's facilitator began to question whether the mother herself was experiencing a depression, masked by behavioral symptoms. Once the mother's depression was indeed diagnosed by a physician and the group was able to provide some psychoeducation on handling someone with depression, the caregiver expressed less frustration. When the caregiving group members developed depression, this group helped to mobilize their attention to their own needs and encouraged their efforts to cope in different, more effective ways with the stresses of caregiving.

CAREGIVER BURDEN POSTDEATH

While the pain of bereavement is well recognized, one aspect of bereavement that is often overlooked involves the continuation of caregiver stress even beyond the deceased's departure. Studies of depression among caregivers after the death of a loved one reveal caregiver depression to be a persistent condition. Although we might have assumed that the death of an elder with cognitive impairment or terminal cancer would bring relief from caregiving responsibilities, in fact several researchers have found that the subjective burden continues for as long as 3–4 years after the recipient's death. Even after objective burdens such as the financial and physical tolls of caring subside, a subjective burden persists in the form of emotional issues such as adjustment to the loss of the bereaved, loneliness, isolation, and loss of caregiving role. In one study, the occurrence of frequent and intrusive ruminative thoughts and the quality and quantity of social supports prior to the care recipient's death were shown to be the strongest predictors of postcaregiving depression (Robinson-Whelan, 2001).

PSYCHODYNAMIC ISSUES

Providing care for an elderly depressed loved one evokes a kaleidoscope of feelings and emotions, including hopelessness, bewilderment, surprise, compassion, frustration, disappointment, anger, resentment, denial, sadness, guilt, impatience, resignation, and at other times a sense of hopefulness, gratification, and even fulfillment. Most caregivers go through periods of adjustment, including fluctuations of attachment and separation, codependency, and autonomy in the course of providing care. The care of a recipient whose illnesses remit and relapse can be difficult emotionally because of the uncertainty associated with a shifting prognosis. A depressed individual may have been decompensating but then respond to therapy, having a period of remission with renewed energy and a return of independence, autonomy, and greater interest in intimacy. The caregiver—who may have become detached due to anger, frustration, or strategies for self-preservation—may now attempt to reestablish feelings of mutuality in the relationship, which had been temporarily lost. The partner who had not been able to share in family decisions and responsibilities or actively engage in a loving relationship may now be capable and motivated to reciprocate. Major upheavals often occur due to financial stresses if the caregivers must reduce the time during which they are employed. Other sacrifices of time may take a caregiver away from community and family commitments and personal leisure outlets, leading to neglect of the caregivers' own physical and mental health needs. Emotional distancing but cognitive connecting may be helpful, along with other personal strategies including setting limits on the amount of caregiving. Creating time to learn coping skills and receive support, to engage in personally satisfying and stress reducing activities and interests both social and solitary in nature, and acknowledging positive aspects of the relationship also help.

CAREGIVER SUPPORTS

Just as the caregiver needs to be flexible, so does the system of supports established with adequate levels of intervention available at necessary times. Most communities offer caregiver support groups at either a local hospital, Council on Aging, or religious institution. Several organizations dedicated to helping caregivers maintain websites, for example the National Family Caregivers Association (NFCA) (*www.nfcacares.org*). These organizations offer practical advice for caregivers. Common tips include encouragement for caregivers to seek support and guidance from professionals, get education about the particular disease afflicting their loved one, and not to give up on leisure and socialization. These sites also point out that caregivers commonly neglect their own physical and mental health.

The NFCA commissioned a study on the value of caregivers recognizing themselves as a specific cohort. They found that caregivers who identified themselves fulfilling this role spoke more often with health care professionals, seeking resources, and increased willingness to preserve their health. Another outcome of caregiver self-recognition was increased unity in fighting for legislative action. Unfortunately, despite changed attitudes, the health of many respondents had suffered as a result of reduced exercise, poor diet, limited leisure time, and neglect of their own medical needs.

MEASURING CAREGIVER BURDEN AND CAREGIVER DEPRESSION

Numerous instruments have been developed to measure caregiver burden. Several are specifically targeted to assess caregivers of dementia patients while most other screens assessed caregivers of cancer patients. The Caregiver Strain Index (CSI) is a 13-question yes/no response tool used to measure objective strain in caregivers of hip replacement or arteriosclerotic heart disease in patients aged 65 or older. A positive response to 7 or more items indicates increased stress. The CSI measures employment, financial, physical, social and time impacts (Robinson, 1983). There are many other instruments—including the Screen for Caregiving Burden (Vitaliano, 1991) and the Burden Interview (Zarit, 1980). Assessments for depression, described in greater detail in Chapter 3 of this book, include the Geriatric Depression Scale, Short Form (Sheikh, 1986), Hamilton Depression Rating Scale (Hamilton, 1967), and Beck Depression Inventory (Beck et al., 1961).

CARING FOR CAREGIVERS: CASES FROM A GERIATRIC PARTIAL HOSPITAL PROGRAM (GPHP)

Partial hospital services, in some outpatient settings, offer a multifaceted and intensive approach to treating depression, anxiety, and other psychiatric problems of the elderly. Such programs often service depressed caregivers during their periods of more acute distress. Partial hospital programs typically meet weekdays, have emergency on-call staff for evenings and weekends, and provide several hours of treatment including psychoeducational, psychotherapeutic, and pharmacotherapeutic groups as well as individual interventions. In addition, family members, usually the primary caregivers, are encouraged to become involved in educational and therapeutic meetings. Groups help the patients develop skills in stress management, assertiveness training, building relationships, coping with family issues, defining and achieving goals, illness management, activity therapy, independent activities of daily living, and effective use of medications. Patients learn to monitor intrusive thoughts, practice stress reduction, develop goals, learn good health practices, cultivate leisure skills, receive practical help to resume independent functioning, and have daily opportunities to talk openly about personal issues and feelings.

CASE EXAMPLES

Depression After the Death of a Spouse

Karen

Karen, an 83-year-old retired real estate agent, was referred to the Geriatric Partial Hospital Program (GPHP), by her inpatient treatment team following hospitalization for depression with psychotic features. Her husband had recently passed away after a long decline from Alzheimer's disease. He had been a professional photographer. Karen and her husband married in their forties and were childless. They reportedly had a happy marriage with several interests in common.

Karen had cared for her husband at their home for several years while his dementia progressed and eventually had to place him in a local nursing home, where she visited him daily. Throughout his illness and decline, Karen relied solely upon herself to provide care. Her sister lived at the opposite end of the country, she had no children, and only one relative lived in a nearby area. Fiercely independent and previously very private about her emotional reactions, Karen was not the type to seek out professional help or services.

Shortly after her husband's death, Karen was admitted by her internist to a community hospital, from which she was transferred to our hospital's inpatient geriatric psychiatry service. She was severely depressed, with severe paranoid ideation and abnormalities of concentration, cognition, energy, appetite, and ability to perform the usual activities of daily living. She had not been locking her doors or windows and often wandered about town. There was evidence of excessive alcohol usage. Despite her severe depression, she was medically quite healthy, suffering only from mild hypertension and a nonessential tremor.

The local board of health had condemned Karen's home after visits by a social worker from the Council on Aging, who had been called by concerned neighbors. The Board of Health found large amounts of rotten food in her refrigerator and strewn about her kitchen. The filth had created insect infestations. Her bathroom and other rooms were piled with debris. In addition, she had failed to pay several bills and there were outstanding unpaid traffic violations, including a summons to appear in court for drunken driving. The plumbing and heating systems were in disrepair.

During her inpatient hospitalization, Karen was treated with medications including sertraline, olanzapine, and zolpidem. Neuropsychological testing revealed mild difficulties on tasks of executive functioning and in retrieval of new information. She was otherwise cognitively intact. Results were consistent with either a psychotic depression or the beginning stages of progressive dementia with frontal lobe dysfunction. Karen also received psychotherapy, psychoeducation, case management, and individual therapy to help her cope with bereavement and begin the recovery process.

Eventually, as she stabilized and symptoms subsided, she was discharged temporarily to the rest home where her mother resided. She chose this option in order to be with her mother, receive personal care, and continue to determine whether she would be able to return to her own home and live independently in the community. Her mother was remarkably cognitively and physically intact and she and Karen had always had a close, supportive relationship. Karen was also referred to the Geriatric Partial Hospital, where she continued to receive bereavement counseling, group therapy, individual psychotherapy, case management and psychopharmacological treatments. Gradually, her cognition, memory, sleep, appetite, energy, interest in activities, social contacts, and personal hygiene improved. She began taking daily walks, reading, and engaging with others. She was able to make visits to her home and eventually agreed to hire professionals to clean and rehabilitate her home rather than sell it and move to an assisted living facility. She agreed to stop driving and to hire a case manager and attorney to help with medication management, paying bills, and getting a cleaning service. She attended follow-up outpatient visits with a psychopharmacologist and was retested by neuropsychology 6 months after her hospitalization. Her executive functioning improved, as did her retrieval of new information, leading to the conclusion that her prior difficulties were due to her psychotic depression. Approximately 1 year after her hospitalization, she was able to return to her newly renovated home. She was able to accompany her 103-year-old mother on trips to Oregon, Michigan, and Tennessee to visit relatives. To this day, she has continued to socialize with friends and neighbors, take walks, read, and attend activities at her local senior center. A cousin who lives nearby visits often and has become a very involved helper.

Karen's recovery can be attributed to good medical interventions and her acceptance of intensive support services. Could her perilous state of mental health have been recognized at an earlier point, and would she have accepted help? Should the nursing home caring for her husband have been more vigilant in reaching out and urging participation in a caregiver group? Perhaps such outreach would have prevented her eventual development of a psychotic depression.

Husbands Caring for Depressed Wives: A Comparison of Three Couples' Coping Styles

The three vignettes that follow illustrate differences in coping styles among three male spouse primary caregivers.

Mr. and Mrs. H.

Mrs. H was referred to the Geriatric Partial Hospital by her psychiatrist after unsuccessful outpatient treatment of her persistent depression and anxiety. Her troubles began a decade earlier, after she was laid off from her job as a design engineer while she was in her early sixties. A few years later, she was diagnosed with Parkinson's disease. Mrs. H. and her husband were both Jewish engineers who left Russia in the 1970s in response to antisemitism and limited career opportunities. Mrs. H. reported a traumatic childhood, having endured the German invasion of Russia when she was a preteen. She survived winters with no heat and very little to eat. She and her family escaped by crossing a frozen lake during the night behind enemy lines. Mrs. H. had one son who is married with children and lives in a nearby community.

Efforts to treat her depression and anxiety with a variety of medications were made by her outpatient team, and the patient began a trial of L-dopa/carbidopa to control her Parkinson's. She also was diagnosed wtih gastric reflux disease and hypertension. Her cognition, concentration, interests, self-care, motivation, energy, and ability to perform activities of daily living gradually declined. She gave up playing the piano, reading, walking her dog, and socializing with friends. She also began experiencing daily panic attacks. At these moments, her blood pressure and pulse increased, her face became flushed with a mask-like affect, her voice was inaudible, and she complained of being unable to breathe. The frequency of these episodes increased, with Mrs. H. becoming more and more agoraphobic. She also became increasingly fearful of being alone, and eventually Mr. H. had to retire from his job as an engineer, creating additional financial hardships, frustration, and despair. Unable to leave his wife unattended, he became resentful of her dependency needs and the marriage steadily declined. As Mrs. H. became increasingly dependent, Mr. H. was deeply conflicted by his feelings of resentment, loss, selfishness and selflessness, hope and hopelessness. Initially a devoted and optimistic advocate, he was gradually worn down by his inability to attend to his wife's needs in the way he felt he should.

When Mrs. H. first came to the Partial Hospital, she began to show improvements in her mood and motivation, responding to the combination of treatments provided and the daily structure of getting out of the house; plans were made to continue this out-of-home structure. She was referred to a local social day program, which she attended three times weekly; however, she relapsed with the decrease in therapy, and her high blood pressure continued to unsettle staff at the social day program. Mrs. H. was rehospitalized at her primary medical facility, stabilized, and referred once more to the Geriatric Partial Hospital, where she had a consultation for electroconvulsive therapy (ECT). After she began a trial of outpatient ECT, her treatment team felt that inpatient monitoring during ECT would be safer, and she was admitted to the geriatric inpatient unit. Unfortunately, despite optimism in the outcome of ECT, staff continued to be concerned about the patient's high blood pressure, so she was transferred to a general hospital for continuation of ECT. The medical hospital team decided that the risks of ECT outweighed the benefits and her treatment was stopped; however, she did have neurology consultations and three different physicians ruled out Parkinson's disease! Mrs. H. was discharged to her home and returned to the Geriatric Partial Hospital. Her antiparkinsonian medication was discontinued and she began to show improvements in cognition, energy, mood, and motivation. She tried playing the piano for the first time in years and started to take walks with her husband and their dog.

These improvements, unfortunately, were fleeting. She soon decompensated once again, with a return of her previous symptoms. Her neurologist ultimately rediagnosed her with Parkinson's disease but started a different medication, pramipexole, in hopes of avoiding the anxiety apparently associated with the L-dopa treatment. Mr. H. found his hopes rekindled and then shattered again and again. He resisted engaging in the psychotherapy that was recommended to help him cope better, claiming it would be a waste of time and that he'd rather face his difficulties on his own. He had few friends or family members to turn to for nonprofessional support.

Over time, Mr. H became increasingly depressed and eventually required independent assessment and treatment. His financial stresses, loss of professional role identity, and social isolation were unbearable. He complained that the quality of his marriage had completely disintegrated and that he was now a parent taking care of a chronically disabled child. He had lost his loving partner and companion. He had been forced to becomes the shopper, cook, housecleaner, bill payer, nurse, and safety monitor for his wife but felt little gratification with these roles. He did not take opportunities for relaxation and very little respite was available from family, friends, or social services. He was grieving over his lost former life and had lost hope for the future. In fact, he envisioned becoming even more destitute and isolated, and he often worried about his own health in addition to his wife's. Mr. H.'s insurance, a managed health care plan, appeared to obstruct the provision of services to his wife, and Mr. H.'s response was often a pessimistic and despairing acceptance. Over time and despite his own treatment, he appeared increasingly depressed and angry about his apparently insoluble predicament.

Mr. and Mrs. E.

Mrs. E., a married, retired professional health care worker and mother of three, was referred to the Geriatric Partial Hospital after an episode of inpatient care for depression and anxiety characterized by a marked decline in her ability to care for herself, perform daily routines, and tolerate being alone. In addition, she was engaging in self-injurious activities, such as biting and scratching and calling out "Help me!" in public places. Mrs. E. often expressed ambivalence about her relationship with Mr. E. Mrs. E.'s other major medical problems included mild cerebral palsy. Mrs. E. often worried about the long-term impact of this disease and feared she would have to live in a nursing home, separated from her spouse. Upon discharge from the inpatient psychiatric unit, she went temporarily to an assisted living facility. Her spouse made several visits weekly to see her and consistently urged her to return home as soon as possible.

Mrs. E. had attended college in New York City, after which she had a successful career as a social worker. She married and raised three children. Although depressed at various times and often in treatment as an outpatient, she was able to function as a mother and wife and to work with disturbed children. In addition, she managed to maintain her home, enjoyed cooking, and participated in several community activities including temple functions, volunteer groups, and taking adult-learner classes. Summer vacations were spent at Cape Cod and she and her spouse managed rental property.

Mrs. E. continued to receive support from a couples therapist, a case manager/therapist, a psychiatrist, and an outpatient support group. She was eventually able to leave the assisted living facility, return home, and start a social day program. She also enrolled in classes at her senior center and a local college. Her husband accompanied her to art class and remained close by in the event that she had an anxiety attack or developed the need to call for help. She took adult continuing education at a local college with her husband and the two enjoyed studying together. As her mental status improved, she took on more responsibilities at home, resumed cooking, and hired a home companion/helper to assist with the shopping and cleaning. She was able to remain at home alone for increasingly longer intervals without panic and gradually reduced her frequent therapy sessions and emergency calls for help. Eventually, she took a vacation trip to Florida for the first time in years!

Mr. E.'s life continued to be fulfilling and, although often interrupted, he was patient and accepting. Throughout his wife's illness, Mr. E. continued to live an active life, playing tennis, volunteering in the community, managing rental properties, and interacting with his children and grandchildren. Mr. E. also attended couples therapy on a weekly basis and drove his wife to several medical appointments and groups. While he waited for her at these times, he would read or take a nap. Despite medical problems of his own, he maintained a hopeful attitude and enjoyed many aspects of his life. He was able to afford to pay a homemaker and case manager out of pocket, expenses that amounted to far less than would the cost of care in an assisted living facility. Mr. E. showed a loving yet detached attitude toward his wife and did not easily become overwhelmed by her disability. He was often caring, extremely patient, and accepting, maintaining his hopes about her potential to return to health. He often pushed her to the limit to maintain interaction as a couple despite her apathy, ambivalence, and sometimes resistance. The net result, however, was to maximize his wife's ongoing ability to remain an involved spouse to the extent that this was possible for her. He conveyed encouragement and appreciation for whatever companionship she could offer, for example, when preparing diner, he would have his wife cook with him, gently offering her a choice of tasks but insisting on her company. He became talented in using behavioral strategies and enjoyed brainstorming with professional staff.

Mr. and Mrs. L.

Ms. L. met her husband after leaving war-torn Europe and being sent to England. Both she and her spouse were from families with the foresight and means to get them to relative safety. After the war, the couple relocated to the United States and raised a family. Both were professionals who developed accomplished careers. Ms. L.'s recurrent episodes of depression disrupted her family life and her career, but these episodes were never prolonged and she was repeatedly able to resume her normal routines. During the year prior to her referral to the Geriatric Partial Hospital, she became severely depressed and began a series of antidepressant trials. Unfortunately, she achieved minimal improvement with either medications or ECT.

Eventually, she was hospitalized, given additional ineffective medication trials, and then referred to the Geriatric Partial Hospital. There, she continued with medication trials, and also participated in group and individual therapy services. During this time, her husband decided to go on his annual winter vacation to ski with wartime friends in the Alps. Ms. L. had always previously accompanied her husband on these reunion vacations but was in no shape to do so on this occasion. Mr. L. made arrangements to have family and professional home companion services available 24 hr a day and traveled to the reunion alone.

Throughout his wife's illness, Mr. L continued to work, socialize, and participate in his normal community activities. He hired home companions to stay with his wife when he was not home and arranged for his children to stay with her while he took his vacation. He was determined to both care for his wife and care for himself, maintaining professional and other commitments. He was able to set clear boundaries and to advocate strongly for professional services. Ms. L. continuously rejected attempts by Mr. L. to provide reassurance and hope for a better future. She often told staff and her husband that there was nothing any one could do for her to improve her mental state. Mr. L. had financial and professional resources, skills in advocating, knowledge, and the ability to care for himself while caring for his spouse. Although angered and hurt by what she perceived to be neglect, the patient also accepted her husband's decisions and plans. Mr. L. was a survivor and had been challenged his whole life to be self-reliant and adaptive to circumstances beyond his control. In fact, his acceptance of his wife's uncertain recovery provided justification for his own course of action.

In contrasting these three couples' coping styles, we can learn about the perils of caregiving and gather insights about providing support to caregivers. While Mr. H. became immobilized by his own depression in the course of caring for his depressed wife, both Mr. E. and Mr. L. managed to cope, thrive, and continue relatively more normal routines. All three husbands had to contend with major changes in their relationships with their wives; in particular, they coped with feelings of active rejection, abandonment, and diminished intimacy as well as the need for becoming advocates for their wives' care and providers of transportation and other types of concrete assistance. Lives that had been joined in partnership became, as described by the husbands, more "one-sided." Each husband assumed, with minimal assistance, the management of household responsibilities. Each expressed guilt over the wish for his wife to resume a more active role, and each struggled with the loss of mutuality, companionship, and sexual intimacy. Each complained of feeling unloved. In one case, sexual relations became a complicated bartering item, an expected reward for all of the spousal sacrifice. Mr. L.'s coping, which relied on a stance of cognitive empathy and the maintainence of an active and hopeful relationship to his wife and her depression, appeared quite resilient.

Mr. R.

Mr. R., an 85-year-old married, retired, and financially successful businessman, was referred for partial hospital services due to depression and anxiety. The chief precipitants of his depression were the placement of his wife in an assisted living facility due to advancing Alzheimer's disease and a hip fracture necessitating use of a walker. Mr. R. presented initially with mood lability and frequently burst uncontrollably into tears. He had not seen his wife for the several weeks since he had been hospitalized for his hip fracture and her move out of their home overlapped with his hospitalization. In addition, Mr. R. had suffered the loss of his siblings over recent years.

The patient had initially tried to convince his daughter to take his wife into her home rather than place her in an assisted living facility. The daughter, although having a close and loving relationship with her mother, had her own family to care for as well as a career and felt that her mother would be better cared for at a facility specializing in the care of elders with dementia. When the daughter refused to care for her mother at her home, the patient refused to speak to her and took legal action to remove her from his will. In therapy, he dwelt on his feelings of betrayal. He shared his views of having spoiled his children and their obligation to care for their elderly parents as he saw fit. In therapy, Mr. R. was attention-seeking and focused on his own dependency needs but willing to recognize and attempt to modify his behaviors. With the support of the partial program as well as a community-based caregiver support group and counseling, he was able to accept the reality of his wife's illness, finally start visiting her, and start to work through his anger and disappointment with his daughter. He became invested in striving to be self-reliant and independent with daily living routines. He also started to plan more fulfilling ways to spend time—for example, by reactivating his volunteer status at a local college library.

RECOMMENDATIONS

Given the often severe consequences of depression on the older adult and the caregiver, ameliorative and preventive measures must be sought and provided. Awareness of the issues by a variety of groups capable of effecting solutions is the first step towards achieving those solutions. For health care professionals, increased use of screening examinations for depression among elderly patients is recommended. The primary care physician is often the most appropriate professional in the health care system who can identify and diagnose depression among older patients (Brusch 2002). However, both lay and professional individuals who come into contact with the elderly should be aware of the signs, symptoms and consequences of depression. Health care professionals should also be attuned to recognizing the problems of caregivers and to be prepared to provide supports and special care to them as well.

For clinicians, the best approach for addressing the emotional needs of caregivers is to provide psychoeducational help. Training can be provided via a psychoeducational course or from skills taught and incorporated into individual supportive work with a counselor. Training caregivers to adopt the attitude of cognitive empathy rather than emotional empathy can improve their well-being and more effectively avoid emotional exhaustion. Assisting the caregiver to understand and identify with the role is also important, as role identification is a prerequisite for learning how to meet one's own needs as a caregiver. A caregiver support group can be particularly beneficial in developing healthy coping strategies. In addition, caregivers need practical, resource-oriented information to local supports and ancillary services in the community. These supports include respite, home health care, and legal and financial assistance as well as senior housing options (see list of informational resources at the end of this chapter).

Public awareness is vital for advancing the cause of identifying caregiver needs of the depressed elderly. Community agencies serving the elderly—such as councils on aging, public and private home-care agancies—are but some of the venues where general information about services to this population should be provided.

Finally, the mental health needs of both caregiver and patient require advocacy on many levels. Political lobbying for extended mental health coverage for the caregivers and adequate psychiatric care for the elderly among managed health care plans and other private health insurance plans may be necessary to adequately address the problem. Advocacy for increased governmental support of respite care and public health insurance coverage of the mental health needs of caregiver and depressed elders alike is required as well. Research should be financed and supported for rigorous evaluation of programs designed to treat depressed elderly patients and their caregiver families so that quality control and meaningful improvement of treatment outcomes can be substantiated.

CONCLUSION

As family caregiving becomes increasingly common in our society, we can expect to see increasing numbers of depressed caregivers. As the clinical case vignettes provided here demonstrate, many of these caregivers are themselves caring for a depressed spouse or parent. While caregivers of medically ill relatives experience many burdens, the stresses of those who attend to the needs of a depressed relative may include some unique feature, such as the waxing and waning course of the disability, the associated withdrawal from interaction and intimacy, the social stigmatization of depression, and the difficulty for some caregivers to comprehend the degree of dysfunction that can be associated with a disease that produces no obvious physical disability.

Whatever the care recipient's primary illness, it may be possible to lighten the caregiver's burden to some degree by encouraging development of cognitive empathy, emphasizing the need to avoid neglecting his or her own emotional and physical health needs, providing psychoeducational opportunities and supports such as the caregivers' group described here, promoting awareness of supportive resources, and advocating for further public assistance to the medically or mentally ill and further research into the needs of these individuals and of their caregivers. Additional research on caregiver depression should address, among other questions, whether caregivers of depressed relatives are themselves especially vulnerable to developing caregiver depression.

REFERENCES

Abraham LK. Mama Might Be Better Off Dead: The Failure of Health Care in Urban America. Chicago: University of Chicago Press, 1992, p. 151.

Andolsek KM. Clapp-Chang NE, Gehlbach SH, Morre I. Prevalance of caregiving. Family practice. Arch Inter Med 1988; 148:2177–2180.

APA HelpCenter. "Elder care more than 'Parenting a Parent': family and relationships—get the facts. American Psychological Association 1996. www.helping.apa.org/family/elderly.html.

Barnet A-M. Factors associated with caregiver burden in mental illness. Clin Psych Rev 1999; 19:819–841.

Baronet A. Effects associated with caregiver burden in mental illness. Clin Psych Rev 1999; 19(7):819–841.

Bauer M, Maddox M, Kirk L, Burns T, Kuskowski M. Progressive dementia: personal and relational impacts on caregiving wives. Am J Alzheimer Dis Other Dementias 2001; 16(6):329–334.

Beck AT, Ward CH, Mendelson M, Mock J, Erbaugh J. Arch Gen Psychiatry 1961; 4: 561–571.

Bleckner M. Social work and family relationships in later life with some thoughts on filial maturity. In: Strauss E, Streib GF, eds. Social Structure and the Family: Generational Relations. Englewood Cliffs, NJ: Prentice-Hall, 1965.

Brody E. Parent-care as a normative life stressor. Gerontologist 1986; 25:19–29.
Brown LJ, Potter JF, Foster BG. Caregiver burden should be evaluated during geriatric assessment. J Am Geriatr Soc 1990; 38:455–460.
Brusch JL. Depression in the elderly. paper delivered at the Cambridge Health Alliance, Cambridge, MA, June 4, 2002.
Burns A, Lawlor B, Craig S. Assessment Scales in Old Age Psychiatry. London: Dunitz, 2001.
Cochrane J, Goering PN, Rogers JM. The mental health of informal caregivers in Ontario: an epidemiological survey. Am J Public Health 1997; 87:2002–2007.
Hamilton M. Development of a rating scale for primary depressive illness. Br J Soc Clin Psychol 1967; 6:278–296.
Hatfield AB. Psychological cost of schizophrenia and the family. Social Work 1978; 24: 335–359.
Heaney CA, Istael BA. Social networks and social support. In Lanz K, Lewis FM, Rimer BK, eds. Health Behavior and Health Education. San Francisco: Jossey-Bass, 1997, chap. 9.
Howard DG et al. Depressive symptomatology in first degree family caregivers of Alzheimer disease patients: a cross-ethnic comparison Am J Alzheimer Dis Assoc Disord 1998; 4:340–346.
Ikels C. The process of care-taker selection. In: Hess BB, Markson EW. eds. Growing Old in America, 3rd ed. New Brunswick, NJ: Transaction, 1985, pp 136–150.
Kiccolt-Glaser JK, Dura JR, Spercher CE, Trask OJ, Glaser R. Spousal caregivers of dementia victims: longitudinal changes in immunity and health. Psychosom Med 1991; 53:345–362.
Koizumi LS et al., eds. The Public Health: 1998 Healthcare—Almanac and Yearbook. New York: Faulkner & Gray, 1998, p 263.
Lee H, Brennan P, Daly B. Relationship of empathy to appraisal, depression, and life satisfaction and physical health in informal caregivers of older adults. Res Nursing Health 2001; 24:44–56.
Lieberman M, Fischer L. The effects of family conflict resolution and decision-making on the provision of help for an elder with Alzheimer's disease. Gerontologist 1999, 39(2):159–166.
Livingston G, Manla M, Kalua C. Depression and other psychiatric morbidity in care of elderly people living at home. Br Med J 1996; 312:153–156.
Llindick G, Gwyther L. Caregiver well being: a multidimensional examination of family caregivers of demented adults. Gerontologist 1986; 26(3):253.
Marriott A et al. Effectiveness of cognitive behavioral family intervention reducing the burden of care in carers of patients with Alzheimer's disease. Br J Psychiatry 2000; 176:557-561.
Marsh DT. Serious Mental Illness and the Family. New York: Wiley, 1998.
Mignon D. Effectiveness of use of home health nurses to decrease burden of depression of elderly caregivers. J Psychosoc Nurs 2000; 38(7):34–41.
Newcomer R. Effects of the Medicare Alzheimer's Disease Demonstration on Caregiver Burden and Depression. Health Services Research, 34(3):691–714, 1999.
Roach MJ. Caregiver and family burden measures. Center to Improve Care of the Dying. www.gwu.edu.

Robinson BC. Validation of a caregiver strain index. J. Gerontol 1983; 38:344–348.
Robinson-Whelan S et al. Long-term caregiving: what happens when it ends? J Abnorm Psychol 2001; 110(4):573–584.
Rose J. and DelMaestro S. Separation and individuation conflict as a model for understanding distressed caregivers: psychodynamic and cognitive case studies. Gerontologist 1990; 30(5):6693–6697.
Schulz R. Beach SR. Caregiving as a risk factor for mortality. The caregiver health effects study. JAMA 1999; 282:2215–2219.
Sheikh JI, Yesavage JA: Geriatric Depression Scale (GDS): Recent evidence and development of a shorter version. In: Brink TL, ed. Clinical Gerontology: Guide to Assessment and Intervention. Binghamton, NY: Haworth Press, 1986, pp 165–173.
Shua-Haim J, Haim T, Shi Y, Kuo Y, Smith J: Depression among Alzheimer caregivers: identifying risk factors. Am J Alzheimer Dis Other Dementias. 2001; 16(6):353–359.
Thomas L. The personal cost of caring. Elder Care 1993; 5(4):5.
Thompson EH, Doll W. The burden of families coping with the mentally ill: an invisible crisis. Fam Rel 1982; 31:379–388.
Vedhara K et al. Chronic stress in elderly carers of dementia patients and antibody response to influenza vaccination. Lancet 1999; 353:9153.
Vitaliano P, Russo J, Young H, Becker J, Maiuro R. The screen for caregiver burden. Gerontologist, 1991; 31(1):76–83.
Yates ME, Tennstedt S, Chang B. Contributors to and mediators of psychological well-being for informal caregivers. J Gerontol Ser B-Psychol Sci Soc Sci 1999; 546(1): 12–22.
Zarit SH, Reever KE, Bach-Peterson J. Relatives of the impaired elderly: correlates of feelings of burden. Gerontologist 1989; 20:649–655.

General Resources for Family Caregivers

Information and Referral

Alzheimer's Association National Office
919 North Michigan Avenue, Suite 1000
Chicago, IL 60611-1676
Phone: 312-335-8700
Fax: 312-335-8700
Toll-free: 1-800-272-3900
www.alz.org

Children of Aging Parents (CAPS)
1609 Woodburn Road, Suite 302-A
Woodbourn Office Campus
Levittown, PA 19057
Phone: 215-945-6900

Fax: 215-945-8720
Toll-free:1-800-227-7294
Website: www.careguide.net

Eldercare America, Inc.
1141 Loxford Terrace
Silver Spring, MD 20901
Phone: 301-593-1621
Fax: 301-593-1621

National Alliance for Caregiving (NAC)
4720 Montgomery Lane, Suite 642
Bethesda, MD 20814
Phone: 301-718-8444
Fax: 301-652-7711

National Family Caregivers Association (NFCA)
10605 Concord Street, Suite 501
Kensington, MD 20895-2504
Phone: 301-942-2302
Toll-free: 1-800-896-3650
Website: www.nfcacares.org

National Quality Caregiving Coalition (NQCC)
Rosalynn Carter Institute for Human Development
Georgia Southwestern State University
800 Wheatley Street
Americus, GA 31709-4693
Phone: 912-928-1234
Fax: 912-931-2663
Website: rci.gsw.edu

Well Spouse Foundation
30 East 40th Street
New York, NY 10018
Phone: 212-685-8815
Fax: 212-685-8815
Fax: 212-685-8676
Toll-free: 1-800-838-0879
Website: www.wellspouse.org

Caregiver Self-Help and Literature

Lebow G, Kane B. Coping With Your Difficult Older Parent: A Guide for Stressed Out Children. New York: Quill–HarperCollins, 1999.
Mace NL, Rabin PV. The 36 Hour Day: A Family Guide to Caring for Persons with Alzheimer's Disease, Related Dementing Illness and Memory Loss in Later Life. Baltimore: Johns Hopkins University Press, 2001.

Understanding Depression

Contact the Manic-Depressive Disease Association at:
Phone: 617-855-2795
Website: www.mddaboston.org

HomeCare/Respite
Information is available through you local Visiting Nurses Association.

Assisted Living/N.H. Care or Adult Day Health
Information is available through your state office of elder affairs.

Legal/Financial Assistance

Information is available through the elder law section of your state's bar association and your local department of public welfare.

Local Community Services

For transportation, nutrition, home-delivered meals, social services, volunteer opportunities, government entitlement programs, senior center activities, and other local resources, contact your city or town council on aging, sometimes referred to as the town office of elder services.

Resources

National Information Center of the U.S. Administration on Aging
Telephone: 202-619-7501

American Association of Retired Persons: a free caregiver resource kit (No. D15267)
Telephone: 202-479-3410

Children of Aging Parents
Telephone: 800-227-7294
Web address: http://www.careguide.cgi/caps/capshome.htm

National Family Caregivers Association
Telephone: 800-896-3650
Web address: http://www.nfcacares.org

The Well Spouse Foundation
Telephone: 800-838-0879
Web address: http://www.wellspouse.org

Caregiverzone.com
Web address: http://www.caregiverzone.com

9

Pharmacotherapy of Late-Life Depression
Review and Recommendations

James M. Ellison
McLean Hospital, Belmont, and Harvard Medical School, Boston, Massachusetts, U.S.A.

E. Yusuf Sivrioglu*
Uludag University Medical School, Bursa, Turkey, and McLean Hospital, Belmont, Massachusetts, U.S.A.

Sumer Verma
McLean Hospital, Belmont, Harvard Medical School, Boston, and Boston University School of Medicine, Boston, Massachusetts, U.S.A.

Noah M. Meyers†
University of Pittsburgh School of Medicine, Pittsburgh, Pennsylvania, U.S.A.

INTRODUCTION

Antidepressant medications are the most thoroughly researched and most frequently employed modality for treating late-life depression. Though their bene-

*Supported by the Scientific and Technical Research Council of Turkey (TUBITAK) NATO Science Fellowship grant.
†*Current affiliation*: Cornell University, Ithaca, New York, U.S.A.

fits have repeatedly been shown superior to those of placebo in treating depressed elderly research subjects, many questions about their use in clinical populations remain unresolved. Which of the many available antidepressants should be chosen initially? Are there strong differences between classes or between agents within a class? How should treatment approaches be modified in the care of special populations of depressed elderly such as those with "vascular depression," dementia, a history of CVA, or treatment resistance? How long should a treatment trial be extended? Under what circumstances and for how long should maintenance treatment be prescribed? And, finally, what gaps are there in our knowledge to guide the design and implementation of more informative future studies? This chapter will briefly review antidepressants currently available in the United States, then address the issues relevant to the special needs of elderly depressed patients by reviewing the available English-language evidence base for treatment decisions regarding the pharmacotherapy of late-life depression.

IDENTIFYING THE EVIDENCE BASE

Our approach to treating late-life depression has evolved from review of all available published, English-language randomized controlled trials (1–71) of pharmacotherapy of acute depression in elderly populations as well as four thoughtful meta-analyses on this topic (72–75) and a recent expert consensus guideline panel (76) on the treatment of depressive disorders in older patients. The 73 randomized controlled trials were identified by a Medline search and subsequent iterative review of all English-language citations within the identified studies until no further trials were discovered.

Heterocyclic antidepressants were the agents most frequently reported, and SSRIs the next most often encountered. Seven studies were identified for monoamine oxidase inhibitors. Three studies were identified for bupropion or bupropion SR, three for mirtazapine, one for venlafaxine, and none for nefazodone. An additional 29 trials were found for agents not currently available in the United States: moclobemide, mianserin, adinazolam, sulpiride, viloxazine, lofepramine, and nomifensine.

The most frequent type of trial was a comparison of two antidepressants. This paradigm accounted for 44 of the studies we identified. Fifteen of the published randomized controlled trials reported comparisons between an antidepressant and a placebo. Comparisons between two active agents and a placebo were reported in eleven studies. In three studies, three agents were compared to a placebo. A variety of rating scales were used to assess response, with the majority of studies relying upon the Hamilton Depression Rating Scale or the Montgomery Asberg Depression Rating Scale.

Seven of the reviewed studies were carried out in depressed, demented subjects. Three were carried out in depressed, poststroke subjects. Only three studies were carried out exclusively among residents in long-term care settings, while 26 drew upon outpatient populations, 14 obtained subjects solely from an inpatient population, and the remaining 17 mixed inpatients with outpatients. No recruitment site was reported in thirteen studies.

None of these studies reported a mean age less than 60. Minimum age among the studies we reviewed was 50, whereas the maximum reported age extended to 98. More than 80% of the trial cohorts contained more women than men, with a mean proportion of women among samples at 65%. Many of the studies excluded acutely suicidal or severely medically ill individuals. The durations of these trials varied from 3 to 26 weeks, with a mean of 7.4 weeks. The number of subjects receiving a specific agent varied greatly among studies, from 7 to 336, with a mean of 45. Fewer than half the studies (41.6%) exceeded 6 weeks in duration.

AN OVERVIEW OF ANTIDEPRESSANTS

An enormous literature now describes the clinical features of the available antidepressants, their mechanisms of action, their dosing, adverse effects, drug interactions, and appropriate duration of treatment. Several excellent textbooks (77–80) include thorough, useful descriptions of the use of antidepressants in treating elderly patients. Here, we will offer a brief review of antidepressants currently available in the United States, highlighting their mechanisms of action, dosing, adverse effects, and drug interactions. This will pave the way to an evidence-based discussion of antidepressant choice and optimal use among elderly patients.

According to a popular classification system (81), antidepressants currently available in the United States are hypothesized to exert their antidepressant effects by one of seven mechanisms. Each of these mechanisms enhances neurotransmission dependent on norepinephrine, serotonin, or dopamine. The heterocyclics and serotonin reuptake inhibitors accomplish this by inhibiting transport of neurotransmitters back into presynaptic cells following release into the synapse. Mirtazapine works through a different mechanism, antagonizing the inhibitory presynaptic noradrenergic autoreceptors and thereby augmenting norepinephrine release by presynaptic cells. Monoamine oxidase inhibitors increase the availability of norepinephrine and serotonin by inhibiting the enzymatic destruction of these neurotransmitters intracellularly and in the synapse.

Each class of antidepressants has—besides its characteristic mechanism of action—additional pharmacodynamic actions and pharmacokinetic properties that may contribute to adverse reactions. Antidepressant drugs within a specific class often differ from each other in their pharmacokinetics as well as in their pharmacodynamics. Although a thorough review of each antidepressant falls beyond the scope of this chapter, we will highlight the major distinctions between antidepressant classes and among members of each class with respect to treatment of older adults.

The *serotonin reuptake inhibitors* (SRIs) have become the most commonly prescribed antidepressants in the United States, primarily as a result of their ease of use and generally well-tolerated side effect profile. The SRIs include a group of "selective" serotonin reuptake inhibitors (SSRIs) as well as two other agents, venlafaxine (Effexor and Effexor XR) and nefazodone (Serzone), which possess additional pharmacodynamic effects. Fluoxetine (Prozac, Prozac Weekly, and others), sertraline (Zoloft), paroxetine (Paxil and Paxil CR), fluvoxamine (Luvox), citalopram (Celexa), and escitalopram (Lexapro) comprise the SSRIs. These antidepressants possess distinctly different properties from the heterocyclics or monoamine oxidase inhibitors, which were more popular before the 1990's, although their efficacy in treating depression is considered comparable. Their selectivity confers a more specific neurotransmitter effect, so in general they lack additional pharmacodynamic effects that may produce adverse clinical responses. The SRIs lack the anti-adrenergic effect responsible for postural hypotension, the antihistaminic effect associated with sedation and increased appetite, and with the exception of paroxetine the SRIs lack anticholinergic effects associated with dry mouth, constipation, urinary hesitancy or retention, and erectile dysfunction. At therapeutic dosing levels, cardiac toxicity is inconsequential, and overdoses with SRIs are less dangerous than with heterocyclics or monoamine oxidase inhibitors.

In addition to serotonin reuptake inhibition, venlafaxine also blocks the reuptake of norepinephrine and dopamine. Nefazodone, in addition to inhibiting serotonin reuptake, also blocks the postsynaptic 5HT2 receptor, a characteristic thought to mitigate some SRI side effects such as anxiety and sexual dysfunction. These antidepressants, too, lack significant anti-adrenergic, antihistaminic, and anticholinergic effects. A weakly selective serotonergic drug, trazodone, is used by many geriatric psychiatrists as a hypnotic agent or as a treatment for agitation in demented patients (82). Because of its associated sedative and orthostatic effects, and because of the rare but serious complications of priapism, confusion, or memory disturbances it is less frequently used as an antidepressant monotherapy (83).

Though considered more tolerable than previous antidepressants by many clinicians, SRIs are not completely without adverse effects. Furthermore, the frequency of their adverse effects among elderly subjects in particular is similar to that seen with heterocyclic antidepressants (72,74). Their most frequent adverse effects include nausea, anxiety, anorexia, diarrhea, dizziness, nervousness, headache, and insomnia. Not infrequently, they reduce libido or impair sexual performance. They appear capable of inducing mania in bipolar individuals. Hyponatremia, a rare SRI adverse effect in general, is more frequently seen among elderly patients. Extrapyramidal side effects such as akathisia are occasionally observed. Weight loss, an early concern with fluoxetine, is thought to be associated with pretreatment high body mass index (84). Paroxetine's anticholinergic properties and association with discontinuation symptoms have been considered relative disadvantages in comparison to the other SRIs. Paroxetine CR, if associated with a longer duration of action, may be less likely to produce discontinuation symptoms and therefore advantageous in patients sensitive to that adverse effect. Venlafaxine's tendency at higher dose levels to increase supine diastolic blood pressure is regarded by some clinicians as a relative drawback when treating the elderly, many of whom already have elevated blood pressure.

SRI studies in the elderly have most frequently been carried out in medically healthy, relatively young elderly populations. Our literature search identified 38 placebo-controlled trials or comparison trials in which an SRI was administered to acutely depressed elderly subjects. Fluoxetine was the studied drug in 14 trials, paroxetine in 11, sertraline in 9, citalopram in 4, fluvoxamine in 3, and venlafaxine in one. In an additional six trials, trazodone was administered, and in one trial, trazodone CR (not available in the United States) was the studied drug.

Several generalizations can be made about the SRI studies among elderly depressed subjects. First, nearly all comparisons of SRIs to placebo show the SRI to be more efficacious. Second, the comparisons of SRIs to heterocyclics or other antidepressants show similar efficacy. Finally, a number of the comparisons of SRIs with heterocyclics conclude that the SRIs are better tolerated, with a lower incidence of side effects. Within the SRIs, however, a qualitative overview of studies does not readily suggest one to be superior to the others. Only three randomized controlled trials, in fact, compare one SRI to another. In a comparison of paroxetine to fluoxetine (63), a significantly lower HAM-D score was noted in favor of paroxetine at the third week, but this difference did not persist by the end of the study. However, at week 6, paroxetine-treated patients had significantly higher response rates compared with fluoxetine-treated patients. Sertraline, similarly, showed a trend toward greater decrease in HAM-D scores at the end of the second week, although this advantage was not sustained (52). In another study comparing sertraline with fluoxetine, Finkel (18) reports that the reduction of HAM-D scores was similar at the end of the study, but the number of responders was significantly greater among sertraline-treated patients.

Four meta-analyses have examined the pharmacotherapy trials for geriatric depression. Their conclusions are in agreement that SRIs treat geriatric depression with efficacy similar to that of the heterocyclics. The earliest meta-analysis (73) combined two comparison studies to conclude that fluoxetine showed less severe adverse effects than two tricyclic agents (amitriptyline or dothiepin), but the later meta-analyses show no significant difference or only a nonsignificant trend (75) toward reduced adverse effects with SRIs versus heterocyclics. A recently published consensus guideline, drawing upon the expertise of a panel of acknowledged experts in geriatric psychopharmacology (76), endorsed the first-line use of SRIs in geriatric depression on the basis of their proven efficacy and possibly greater tolerability. Among members of the SRI class, the consensus guideline rated citalopram and sertraline most highly as treatments of choice, while paroxetine and fluoxetine received lower ratings. Although fewer studies have examined citalopram than sertraline in geriatric populations, these antidepressants both possess minimal interactions with the cytochrome P450 enzymes, an elimination half-life sufficiently long to justify once daily dosing, and a side effect profile at least as tolerable as those of other SRIs. Escitalopram, one of two isomers contained in the racemic antidepressant citalopram, has recently become available for clinical use in the US. If the single isomer produces a more tolerable side effect profile, as claimed on the basis of early results, escitalopram may prove a useful medication for geriatric patients. No studies in elderly cohorts, however, are yet available.

In agreement with the consensus guideline, our recommendation for an initial citalopram dose is 10 to 20 mg/d; for an initial sertraline dose, we recommend 25 to 50 mg/d. Care must then be taken to increase dosing as tolerated, aiming for resolution of depressive symptoms. This result is most likely to be achieved, in our experience, at final dosing levels of 20 to 40 mg/d for citalopram and 50 to 150 mg/d for sertraline—levels higher than the expert consensus guideline's average target dosing range but within the limits of suggested maximal dosing. Venlafaxine XR may be an especially useful choice for patients who fail to respond to an initial SSRI regimen, provided blood pressure is appropriately monitored to detect venlafaxine-associated increases. Nefazodone may be useful in some anxious elderly patients who fail the initial SSRI trial, but because of its CYP3A4 inhibition—as well as recent reports (85,86) and an FDA warning (87) linking its use with several cases of liver failure—nefazodone is not considered among the first-line choices for elderly patients. Table 1 lists these antidepressants as well as the other antidepressants currently available in the United States, with suggested dose ranges in elderly patients whose health status does not require individualized lowering of doses.

The non-SRI antidepressants of newer availability include bupropion immediate release (IR), bupropion slow release (SR), and mirtazapine. These antidepressants are often used and have been investigated in elderly depressed subjects, but less is known about their relative advantages and disadvantages than about either the SRIs or heterocyclics. Bupropion is unique among available antidepressants in its nonserotonergic dopamine and norepinephrine reuptake blocking mechanism. Though unavailable for some years after its initial marketing because of concern about increased seizure risk, its seizure-inducing rate

TABLE 1 Antidepressants for Use in Late-Life Depression

Generic Name	Brand Name	Available Dosage Forms	Starting Dose Range (mg/d)	Usual Geriatric Dose Range (mg/d)	Notes
Tricyclic Antidepressants (TCAs)					
Nortriptyline	Pamelor, Aventyl, and others	10, 25, 50, 75 mg tablets; oral solution 10 mg/5 ml	10–25	25–100	TCA with least postural hypotension Follow plasma levels Therapeutic window 50–150 ng/ml (Response is likely to decrease beyond therapeutic range maximum)
Desipramine	Norpramin and others	10, 25, 50, 75, 100, 150 mg tablets	10–25	25–150	TCA with least anticholinergic effect Therapeutic blood range 75–150 ng/ml (Response is unlikely to improve above therapeutic range maximum)
Doxepin	Sinequan and others	10, 25, 50, 75, 100, 150 mg tablets; oral solution 10 mg/ml	NR	NR	Strong anticholinergic and sedative effect Plasma level:efficacy relation is not established Strong antihistaminic (H_2) effect

TABLE 1 *Continued*

Generic Name	Brand Name	Available Dosage Forms	Starting Dose Range (mg/d)	Usual Geriatric Dose Range (mg/d)	Notes
Protriptyline	Vivactyl	5, 10 mg tablets	NR	NR	One of the least sedating of heterocyclics Orthostatic hypotension, cardiovascular toxicity, and anticholinergic side effects Extremely long elimination half-life (140 hr)
Imipramine	Tofranil and others	10, 25, 50 mg tablets; injectable solution	NR	NR	Sedative and anticholinergic effects less severe then amitriptyline Frequently causes postural hypotension Therapeutic blood range 75–150 ng/ml (Response is unlikely to improve above therapeutic range maximum)
Amitriptyline	Elavil and others	10, 25, 50, 75, 100, 150 mg tablets; injectable solution	NR	NR	Strong sedative effect Frequent anticholinergic effects Low doses and monitoring of plasma levels can minimize anticholinergic side effects

Clomipramine	Anafranil	25, 50, 75 mg capsules	NR	NR	Strong sedative, anticholinergic, hypotensive, and cardiac side effects
Trimipramine	Surmontil	25, 50, 100 mg capsules	NR	NR	Strong anticholinergic and sedative effect Strong H_2 blocker
Selective Serotonin Reuptake Inhibitors (SSRIs)					
Fluoxetine	Prozac and others	10 mg tb.; 10, 20, 40 mg cap.; 20/5 ml oral concentrate	10	10–40	Oral solution available
	Prozac Weekly	90 mg enterically coated cap	90 once weekly		Initiate after establishment of daily regimen of 20 mg/d, waiting 1 week after last daily dose
Sertraline	Zoloft	25, 50, 100 mg tb.; 20 mg/ml oral concentrate	25	50–200	Oral solution available
Fluvoxamine	Luvox	25, 50, 100 mg tb.	25	50–200	
Paroxetine	Paxil	10, 20, 30, 40 mg tb.; 10 mg/5 ml oral solution	10	10–40	Possesses mild anticholinergic effects
Paroxetine CR	Paxil CR	12.5, 25 mg CR tb.	12.5	12.5–25	
Citalopram	Celexa	10, 20, 40 mg tb.; 10 mg/5 ml oral concentrate	10	10–40	
Escitalopram	Lexapro	10, 20 mg tb.	5	10–20	No RCT in geriatric

TABLE 1 *Continued*

Generic Name	Brand Name	Available Dosage Forms	Starting Dose Range (mg/d)	Usual Geriatric Dose Range (mg/d)	Notes
Serotonin Antagonist and Reuptake Inhibitors (SARIs)					
Nefazodone	Serzone	50, 100, 150, 200, 250 mg tb.	50 bid	100–500	Sedating for many patients
Trazodone	Desyrel and others	50, 100, 150 mg tb.	25–50	25–200	Dose range applies to trazodone's common use, as a hypnotic agent often combined with another antidepressant
Serotonin Norepinephrine Reuptake Inhibitor (SNRI)					
Venlafaxine	Effexor	25, 37.5, 50, 75, 100 mg tb.	25	50–225	Blood pressure elevation associated with higher dose range
	Effexor XR	37.5, 75, 150 mg capsule	37.5	50–300	
Norepinephrine Dopamine Reuptake Inhibitor (NDRI)					
Bupropion	Wellbutrin and others Wellbutrin SR	75, 100 mg tb. 100, 150, 200 mg SR tb.	75 100	100–300 100–450	Contraindicated with eating disorders, caution with seizure disorders

Noradrenergic and Specific Serotonergic Antidepressant (NaSSA)					
Mirtazapine	Remeron	15, 30, 45 mg tb.;	15	15–45	
	Remerson Soltab	15, 30, 45 mg orally disintegrating tablet			
Monoamine Oxidase Inhibitors (MAOIs)					
Phenelzine	Nardil	15 mg tb.	15	15–45	Requires restrictions of diet and coadministered medications
Tranylcypromine	Parnate	10 mg tb.	10	10–40	
Isocarboxazid	Marplan	10 mg tb.	10	10–40	
Stimulants					
Methylphenidate	Ritalin	5, 10, 20 mg tb.	2.5	10 bid	
	Ritalin SR and others	20 mg tb.		20 (may be substituted once dose of methylphenidate is established)	Several new preparations of extended release methylphenidate are also available
Dextroamphetamine	Dexedrine, Dexedrine Spansules, and others	5, 10 mg tablets; 5, 10, 15 mg extended-release capsules	2.5	10 bid	

Source: Antidepressant classification system is from Stahl SM. Essential Psychopharmacology, ed 2. New York: Cambridge University Press, 2001.

Chart is modified from Refs. 78 and 118.

among patients with no history of seizures, coadministered seizure-facilitating drugs, or other risk factors is considered acceptably low. The SR preparation (bupropion SR) is associated with a lower risk of seizures than the IR form. Seizure risk is further decreased by administering the IR form of bupropion on a three-times-daily regimen or the SR form on a twice-daily regimen—with no greater than 450 mg/d total IR dose or 400 mg/d total SR dose and with no single dose exceeding 200 mg. Seizure risk should be included in the potential adverse effects discussed with the patient considering a bupropion trial. The elderly are predisposed to accumulate bupropion and its metabolites (88) and these may contribute to bupropion's side effects, the most frequent of which are headache, somnolence, insomnia, agitation, dizziness, diarrhea, dry mouth, or nausea. An unusual side effect reported in several elderly patients on bupropion was the tendency to fall backwards (89). Bupropion is in general regarded as an inferior treatment in patients with a concurrent anxiety disorder, but a comparison of bupropion SR to paroxetine in elderly depressed subjects showed similar rates of agitation with both drugs and no greater increase in anxiety symptoms during treatment with either (70). In addition, preliminary findings in a small sample of younger adults suggested bupropion to be safer than other antidepressants when treating depression in bipolar patients (90). As noted in Table 1, bupropion IR can be initiated at 75 mg per day and bupropion SR at 100 mg/d. Dose increases spaced at least a week apart will allow equilibration of blood levels to each new steady state.

Mirtazapine, another agent with a unique mechanism of action, joins antagonism of presynaptic noradrenergic α_2 presynaptic autoreceptors and heteroreceptors with antagonism of H_1, 5-HT_2, and 5-HT_3 receptors. The resulting clinical effect is a depression-reducing increase in synaptic norepinephrine and serotonin levels accompanied by sedation, appetite enhancement, and minimal nausea. This combination of effects might be anticipated to help anxious, insomniac, anorexic elderly depressives. The three available controlled trials in elderly depressed subjects provide some support for mirtazapine's use and showed it to be as effective and well tolerated as amitriptyline, trazodone, or paroxetine (27,28,62). Clinicians are advised to resist the temptation to begin mirtazapine therapy at doses below 15 mg/d, since excessively low dosing is associated with a predominantly sedating, antihistaminic effect that may deter the patient from proceeding further with the course of treatment. Patients may question the notion, though it appears to be supported by clinical observations, that higher doses of this antidepressant are less sedating than lower doses.

Heterocyclic antidepressant studies in the elderly, similarly to studies of SRIs, are most frequently reported in medically healthy, relatively young elderly populations. Our literature search identified 50 placebo-controlled trials or comparison trials in which a heterocyclic was administered to acutely depressed elderly subjects. Amitriptyline and imipramine were the most frequently studied, with 14 trials each. There were 10 nortriptyline trials, 5 doxepin trials, 3 trials each for dothiepin and maprotiline, and 1 for desipramine. No randomized controlled trials were identified for clomipramine, protriptyline, or trimipramine.

The heterocyclics comprise the tricyclic antidepressants and the essentially similar single tetracyclic agent, maprotiline. Among the tricyclic antidepressants, available agents are characterized as tertiary or secondary amines. The tertiary amines amitriptyline, imipramine, trimipramine, doxepin, clomipramine, and amoxapine are more lipid soluble and thus produce higher levels of central nervous system anticholinergic effects, postural hypotension, and sedation. In elderly patients, these effects are of great importance if they increase the likelihood of severe constipation with impaction, urinary retention in men with preexisting prostatic hypertrophy, or a hip-fracturing fall. Meaningful standards have been established to guide dosing of the tricyclics based on serum level measurements, particularly for nortriptyline, imipramine, and desipramine. Measurement of plasma levels is particularly useful in treating elderly patients because the therapeutic index of the medications is lower with older individuals. The use of levels can avoid either overly cautious, inadequate dosing or excessively high doses that may increase the risk of medical complications.

The many extraneous pharmacodynamic effects of tertiary amine tricyclics have earned for amitriptyline, at least, the designation of "polypharmacy in a pill" and the recommendation of some authorities to avoid prescribing this antidepressant to elderly patients (91). Clomipramine, though known for its less tolerable side effect profile, is considered an excellent treatment for younger adults with obsessive compulsive disorder, which may be present concurrently with depression. In the one available controlled study of its use in the elderly (25), a comparison with paroxetine, it was shown to be similarly efficacious but with more severe adverse effects. Amoxapine, finally, is unique among available antidepressants for possessing both norepinephrine and serotonin presynaptic reuptake blocking effects as well as postsynaptic dopamine-blocking activity. Although it was initially hoped to provide a superior option for treating psychotic depressions, its potential toxicity is considerable and no controlled trials describe its use in treating late-life depression.

The secondary amines—nortriptyline, desipramine and protriptyline—are, by contrast, regarded as effective and safe agents for treating elderly depressed patients. Nortriptyline—which is associated with less severe anticholinergic and orthostatic effects than the tertiary amine tricyclics—is the tricyclic most recommended for use in elderly patients. When its use is optimized by monitoring serum levels, nortriptyline is as well tolerated as SRIs and as effective. Roose and Suthers (92) caution that nortriptyline treatment is associated with significant anticholinergic effects, an increase in heart rate, and less improvement of quality of life than was associated with sertraline in one comparison study. On the other hand, nortriptyline has demonstrated its efficacy in a nursing home cohort (36), a population in which it is particularly difficult to show antidepressant effects exceeding placebo. Furthermore, two studies show nortriptyline to be well tolerated and efficacious in the less often studied "old old" population, adults greater than 70 years of age.

Beyond nortriptyline and desipramine, which is the subject of one randomized controlled trial in older subjects, the other heterocyclic antidepressants are less frequently recommended for use in the elderly.

Maprotiline, a tetracyclic relative of the tricyclics created by the addition of an ethylene bridge across the tricyclic's middle ring, is considered as effective as any tricyclic but shares a similar range of side effects. Maprotiline's major disadvantages are its long half-life (which means a slow development of a steady-state serum level and longer illness following overdose) and its increased association with seizures, especially with excessively rapid upward titration of dosage. In addition, it occasionally causes a skin rash, which clears after discontinuation of the drug.

Many clinicians consider the side effect profile of heterocyclics problematic for older patients. Use of heterocyclic antidepressants can be accompanied by side effects including sedation, confusion, urinary retention, exacerbation of glaucoma, blurred vision, increase in heart rate, delayed ventricular conduction, dry mouth, constipation, fatigue, dizziness, atrial fibrillation, orthostatic hypotension, falls, and gait disturbance. Compared to the serotonergic agents, heterocyclic antidepressants are more dangerous in overdose.

The cardiovascular side effects of heterocyclics have attracted particular attention and require special mention. Heterocyclic antidepressants possess a quinidine-like property of slowing cardiac conduction that renders them undesirable for treatment of patients with bundle branch disease. Orthostatic hypotension, which may endanger elderly individuals with unstable gait or marginal perfusion of heart or brain, appears to be less pronounced with nortriptyline than other members of the class (95). These properties do not contraindicate the use of heterocyclics in older patients but do emphasize the value of attentive monitoring of adverse effects and use of serum levels as appropriate to achieve adequate treatment levels while minimizing administration of excessively large, potentially toxic doses. Monitoring of nortriptyline or desipramine levels by reducing excessive dosing also helps to reduce accumulation of cardiotoxic hydroxy-metabolites that may endanger older patients, particularly those with renal impairment (78). The four meta-analyses find heterocyclics to be as effective as other agents for the treatment of geriatric depression, with possible nonsignificant trends toward both more severe adverse effects and greater efficacy among those who tolerate the medication. The expert consensus guideline group, however, reserves first-line use of heterocyclics only for "severe depression," in which nortriptyline is designated a highly ranking alternate to SSRIs. Studies in which nortriptyline's use was accompanied by monitoring of plasma levels have shown particularly good outcomes, with best responses to nortriptyline when plasma levels are measured between 60 and 260 ng/ml. The consensus guideline recommends starting at 10 to 30 mg/d and aiming for target plasma levels between 50 and 150 ng/ml, usually achieved at doses between 40 and 100 mg/d. Dosing recommendations for other heterocyclics are listed in Table 1.

Monoamine oxidase inhibitors (MAOIs), used less frequently these days because of their potential for toxic drug–drug or drug–food interactions, are nonetheless as effective as other antidepressants in treating unipolar depression, and they may be even more effective in treating atypical depression, especially with concomitant panic attacks. This class of antidepressants works by competitively binding the monoamine oxidase (MAO) enzyme, a protein responsible for destroying catecholamines and indoleamines in presynaptic neurons and in the synapses. MAO located in the intestines also destroys ingested neurotransmitter-like chemicals, protecting the central nervous system against their potential effects. When MAO is inhibited, the body loses its defenses against such "false neurotransmitters," rendering it vulnerable to the "hypertensive crisis" reaction, which is the most serious MAOI adverse effect. Researchers have now delineated fairly clearly which foods or medications must be avoided by a patient taking an MAOI, so this adverse effect is preventable (see Table 2). It is worth emphasizing that these substances should be avoided several days before starting an MAOI and 7 to 14 days after stopping an MAOI. Recent case reports have also emphasized the danger of switching too rapidly between MAOIs, or between MAOIs and other antidepressants. After a trial of fluoxetine, for example, a full 5 weeks must elapse before the initial dose of an MAOI.

Additional MAOI side effects include increased appetite and weight gain, induction of mania or hypomania, orthostatic hypotension, sexual dysfunction including inhibition of orgasm, swelling of the ankles or feet, increased sweating, skin rash, constipation, drowsiness, dry mouth, insomnia, nightmares, or fatigue. Because MAOIs can produce transaminase elevations, periodic measurements of liver enzymes are useful.

Among the eight randomized controlled geriatric depression trials we identified for monoamine oxidase inhibitors, the treatment in six was moclobemide, a reversible inhibitor of MAO-A not available in this country. One trial investigated another unavailable MAOI, brofaromine, while only one trial addressed the use of phenelzine and none studied tranylcypromine or isocarboxazid. Thus, use of the three MAOIs available in the United States (see Table 1) occupies a secondary role in the treatment of late-life depression.

Stimulants such as amphetamines or methylphenidate, despite the frequency of their use, are supported as antidepressant agents in the elderly only by very limited controlled data (96). Methylphenidate's use as a monotherapy for late-life depression is advocated on the basis of one controlled trial among medically ill depressed geriatric subjects (97) and other uncontrolled clinical

TABLE 2 Foods and Medications Interacting with Monoamine Oxidase Inhibitors

Foods Containing Tyramine	
Avocados	Particularly if overripe.
Bananas	Reactions can occur if eaten in large amounts; tyramine levels high in peel.
Bean curd	Fermented bean curd, fermented soya bean, soya bean pastes, soy sauces, and miso soup, prepared from fermented bean curd: all contain tyramine in large amounts; miso soup has caused reactions.
Beer and ale	Major domestic brands do not contain appreciable amounts; some imported brands have had high levels; nonalcoholic beer may contain tyramine and should be avoided.
Caviar	Safe if vacuum-packed and eaten fresh or refrigerated only briefly.
Cheese	Reactions possible with most, except unfermented varieties such as cottage cheese; in others, tyramine concentration is higher near rind and close to fermentation holes.
Figs	Particularly if overripe.
Fish	Safe if fresh, but dried products should not be eaten; caution required in restaurants; vacuum-packed products are safe if eaten promptly or refrigerated only briefly.
Liver	Safe if very fresh, but rapidly accumulates tyramine; caution required in restaurants.
Milk products	Milk and yogurt appear to be safe.
Protein extracts	See also Soups; avoid liquid and powdered protein dietary supplements.
Meat	Safe if known to be fresh; caution required in restaurants.
Sausage	Fermented varieties such as bologna, pepperoni, and salami have a high tyramine content.
Shrimp paste	Contains large amounts of tyramine.
Soups	May contain protein extracts and should be avoided.

TABLE 2 *Continued*

Soy sauce	Contains large amounts of tyramine; reactions have occurred with teriyaki.
Wines	Generally do not contain tyramine, but many reactions have been reported with Chianti, champagne, and other wines.
Yeast extracts	Dietary supplements (e.g., Marmite) contain large amounts; yeast in baked goods, however, is safe.
Food Not Containing Tyramine	
Caffeine	A weak pressor agent; large amounts may cause reactions.
Chocolate	Contains phenylethylamine, a pressor agent that can cause reactions in large amounts.
Fava beans (broad beans, "Italian" green beans)	Contain dopamine, a pressor amine, particularly when overripe.
Ginseng	Some preparations have caused headache, tremulousness, and maniclike symptoms.
Liqueurs	Reactions reported with some (e.g., Chartreuse and Drambuie); cause unknown.
New Zealand prickly spinach	Single case report; patient ate large amounts.
Whiskey	Reactions have occurred; cause unknown.
Medications to Avoid	
Decongestants or cough suppressant	Sympathomimetics contained in OTC medications for respiratory symptoms or for dietary aids (e.g., phenylpropanolamine, pseudoephedrine), or the cough suppressant dextromethorphan.
Pain relievers*	Meperidine is VERY dangerous.
CNS depressants	Local and general anesthetics.*
Stimulants*	Amphetamine, cocaine, methylphenidate.
Monoamines or related compounds	L-dopa*, L-tryptophan, L-tyrosine, phenylalanine
Antihypertensives* (including β-blockers and thiazide diuretics)	Exaggerated hypotensive effect may occur
Other antidepressants*	Especially SRIs
Some herbal preparations	Containing ginseng or ma huang

*May be usable with precautions and careful monitoring.

Source: Modified from (1) Food interacting with MAO inhibitors. Med Lett Drugs Ther 31(785):11–12, 1989. (2) Ellison JM. Medications for mental disorders: a brief history and an overview of current uses. In: Ellison JM, ed. The Psychotherapist's Guide to Pharmacotherapy. Chicago: Year Book Medical Publishers, 1989, pp 119–143.

series that indicate significant response rates and limited adverse reactions. Stimulants are not recommended for first-line treatment by the expert consensus panel, but factors that may justify a stimulant trial for the treatment of depression typically include apathy or psychomotor retardation, concurrent medical illness, intolerance of standard antidepressants, and the need for a rapid response.

SHORTCOMINGS OF THE CURRENT EVIDENCE BASE FOR TREATMENT OF LATE-LIFE DEPRESSION

In our attempt to determine an optimal treatment approach for late-life depression, we have explored ways of pooling or meta-analyzing data from the available evidence base. The obstacles we have encountered are the same ones earlier faced by the authors of the meta-analyses already published on the pharmacotherapy of geriatric depression (72,73,74,75). To circumvent the obstacles created by comparing or pooling data from trials that vary so greatly, several of the meta-analytic reports rely upon drastically pared-down subsamples of published studies in reaching their conclusions. This approach, though it sacrifices much useful information, has been considered necessary because the published treatment studies differ so greatly in statistical methods, thoroughness of reporting, treatment parameters, and sample definition. Some of the key methodological issues will be described here for the purpose of illustrating ways in which future studies can be made more comparable.

To begin with, the studies that have served to demonstrate antidepressants' superiority to placebo are not as well-suited to determining whether one antidepressant is superior to another antidepressant of similar efficacy. A comparison between two effective antidepressants, as Thase (98) has pointed out, may require detection of a mean endpoint difference of as little as 2 HAMD points. Such a small difference is unreliably detected by studies enrolling fewer than 120 subjects per treatment group, accounting in part for the large number of negative trials in small treatment groups. The differences between active agents are presumably even smaller and more difficult to demonstrate (98).

Even when treatment differences between groups might be more conspicuous, an appropriate outcome measure must be chosen to detect them. As noted in Chapter 3, no current diagnostic instrument is ideal. The HAM-D, which is most frequently chosen, was not designed for elderly patients and may be excessively influenced by the presence of nonspecific somatic symptoms. Though typically used as an outcome measure for early antidepressant trials in demented, depressed subjects, the HAM-D is now often supplemented or replaced by newer scales, such as the Cornell Scale for Depression in Dementia (CSDD), that rely on behavioral observations and collateral reports, recognizing the impaired history-giving abilities of the patients. More recent studies of antidepressant trials have also more frequently supplemented the measurement of a change in depressive symptoms by a measurement of quality of life, recognizing that symptomatic change provides only a partial picture of effectiveness.

The design and quality of individual RCTs exploring antidepressant treatment of late-life depression vary greatly from study to study. We noted particularly a great deal of variation in thoroughness of reporting, dosing levels, and trial durations. In addition to employing small samples, some studies fail to report information necessary to a metanalysis, such as standard error of the mean changes in depression measurements over the course of the treatment trial. Antidepressant dosage magnitude, too, varies across a wide range. Mittman, in her meta-analysis (75), converted antidepressant doses to a standardized defined daily dose (DDD), defined as the average dose of the drug per day for adults, when it is prescribed for its main indication and showed a range of 0.33 to 3.0 for tricyclic antidepressants, and of 0.33 to 4 for SSRIs, where 1.0 represented an appropriate daily dose. Duration of trials, too, has varied dramatically. Mittman calculated average trial durations for trials with tricyclics (5.3 ± 1.2 weeks), SSRIs (5.7 ± 1.0 weeks), and placebo (5.3 ± 1.3 weeks). Our own analysis (which included additional studies) found an average trial duration of 7.35 ± 3.56 weeks. These durations are alarmingly short when we consider the finding by Dew (99) that 19% of eventual responders among elderly subjects in an antidepressant trial failed to respond by week 10 but did so subsequently.

As a final methodological comment, we reiterate the well-known observation that pharmacotherapy studies among older subjects have not adequately addressed the inherent diversity of the elderly population. Perhaps three decades of life are represented among such cohorts. There may be important differences between the drug response pattern and optimal dosing strategy, the pharmacokinetics, and the drug interactions for a 65-year-old compared to a 90-year-old. Beyond the changes associated with normal aging, many elderly depressed individuals are also affected by one or more chronic illnesses that may influence antidepressant choice or drug response. Elders affected by such neurological processes as Alzheimer's disease, other dementias, stroke, or cerebrovascular disease may respond differently than healthy elders to a specific antidepressant. The syndrome of depression with executive dysfunction, for example, may represent a specific variant depressive syndrome that is dependent on the presence of small vessel cerebrovascular disease, different in its manifestations, and different in its therapeutic response pattern. The presence of cardiovascular disease, hepatic disease, renal disease, or endocrinopathies will further alter the pharmacokinetics and pharmacodynamics of a prescribed antidepressant, affecting the patterns of responsiveness and of adverse outcomes. The oldest patients, those with more severe medical illnesses, the demented, and those sequestered in long-term care facilities may be the most challenging to treat and also the least explicitly studied. We will include here, therefore, some recommendations tailored to treatment of specific geriatric depressive subgroups: those with psychotic depression, depression with dementia, depression with executive dysfunction, poststroke depression, depression in long-term care settings, and treatment resistant depression.

Depression with psychotic features or *psychotic depression* is more prevalent among older than younger individuals with major depression (100). The standard of treatment for delusional depression has been to combine an antidepressant with an antipsychotic agent, though elderly patients often show difficulty with the side effects produced by a sufficiently high level of antipsychotic medication. ECT, a nonpharmacologic approach covered in Chapter 11, is often considered as the treatment for delusional depression in older patients because of its proven efficacy and tolerability, which may exceed that of combination pharmacotherapy. Controlled studies of olanzapine and the other atypical antipsychotics may in time justify their preferred use in treating late-life delusional depression, since olanzapine has already been shown effective in younger delusionally depressed subjects (101,102). Antipsychotic agents for use in geriatric mood disorders are summarized in Table 3.

Among demented patients, perhaps half will undergo significant depression. *Depression comorbid with dementia*, however, may too often be overlooked by clinicians. Apathy, passivity, decreased initiative, and poor concentration are associated with both depression and dementia and are therefore diagnostically nonspecific. Several placebo-controlled antidepressant trials (103) have shown antidepressant treatment to be beneficial in groups of depressed demented subjects. The expert consensus guideline on depressive disorders in older adults emphasizes the importance of concurrent psychosocial intervention and recommends as preferred antidepressants citalopram, sertraline, and venlafaxine XR (76). Streim and colleagues (104) noted a preferential response to low-dose nortriptyline rather than standard dose treatment in a cognitively impaired subgroup of depressed, frail nursing home subjects.

The syndrome of *depression with executive dysfunction*, a syndrome that overlaps that of *vascular depression*, was first defined by Alexopoulos as occurring first at or after age 65 and associated with "clinical and/or laboratory evidence of vascular disease or vascular risk factors" (105). The clinical and pathophysiological features of this syndrome are described in detail in Chapter 7 of this book, and a few additional comments here will address treatment approach. Although any recommendations must be regarded as tentative for this newly characterized subgroup of depressed individuals, optimization of vascular health should be considered through use of such agents as antioxidants, thrombolytics, calcium and sodium channel antagonists, NMDA receptor antagonists, GABA antagonists, antiapoptotic agents, and others (105). Dopaminergic antidepressants or augmentors (106) may find a role as well, and carefully designed trials will be needed to explore this important frontier in pharmacotherapy.

Poststroke depression has been estimated to occur in 20–40% of stroke

TABLE 3 Selected Antipsychotic Agents for Use in Late-Life Mood Disorders

Generic Name	Trade Name	Starting Dose Range (mg/d)	Treatment Dose Range (mg/d)	Notes
Typical Antipsychotic Agents (high potency)				
Haloperidol	Haldol and others	0.5	2–10	Available as oral solution, IM injection, IV injection
	Haldol decanoate and others	12.5 IM q 14–28 days	50–200 IM q 28 days	Depot injectable preparation
Perphenazine	Trilafon and others	2	4–32	Available as oral solution
Fluphenazine	Prolixin and others	0.5	2–10	Available as oral solution or IM injection
	Prolixin decanoate Prolixin enanthate	12.5 IM q 7–14 days	12.5–50 IM q 14–21 days	Available as depot injectable preparation
Atypical Antipsychotic Agents				
Risperidone	Risperdal	0.25	0.5–6	Available also as oral solution
Olanzapine	Zyprexa	2.5	2.5–15	Available also as orally disintegrating tablet
Quetiapine	Seroquel	25	50–500	Sedative, low in EPS
Clozapine	Clozaril and others	6.25	25–200	Anticholinergic, low in EPS
Ziprasidone	Geodon	20	20 bid–60 bid	Monitoring of QTc suggested Available for IM injection
Aripiprazole	Abilify	7.5–15	15–30	Awaiting data in geriatric populations

Source: Adapted from Kennedy GJ. Geriatric Mental Health Care. New York: Guilford Press, 2000.

victims (107). Although DSM-IV lists stroke as one of the rare conditions causing depression, the increase in the elderly population has already meant 600,000 new cases of stroke each year. Improvements in medical care and increased survival after CVA will account for a substantial number of poststroke depressions in the near future. Our evidence base search identified three (42,59,71) English-language, randomized placebo controlled trials of pharmacotherapy of depression in elderly poststroke subjects. One of the three studies compared fluoxetine to placebo (42), one study compared fluoxetine to nortriptyline or placebo (59), and one study compared nortriptyline to placebo (71). Variations in diagnostic criteria, study duration, duration since last stroke, and length of treatment make it difficult to combine data from these studies. Two, however, found nortriptyline to be superior to placebo (42,59). Furthermore, one of the comparisons found nortriptyline to be superior to fluoxetine in subjects with poststroke depression (59). Stimulants, which some clinicians consider an effective treatment for poststroke depression, have not been studied in this role under controlled conditions (108), but methylphenidate has reduced apathy and fatigue and improved quality of life in an open trial (108,109).

Five percent of the elderly population of the United States resides in *long-term care facilities* (LTCF), and estimates suggest that up to half of these individuals suffer from clinically significant depressive symptoms. A recent study, however, suggested that only 55% of the depressed LTCF residents received antidepressants and 32% of these were treated with subtherapeutic dosing (110). We have identified four RCTs for pharmacotherapy of major depression in which subjects were recruited solely from LTCFs. Of these, one compared nortriptyline to placebo (36), one compared sertraline to placebo (44), one compared amitriptyline to nomifensine (24), and one compared two different doses of nortriptyline (104). Study durations were 7, 8, 4 and 10 weeks, respectively. Nortriptyline was found to be superior to placebo, but authors noted that only 2 in 3 subjects could complete the trial and emphasized the need for close monitoring of side effects (36). Streim et al. reported a relationship between plasma levels of nortriptyline and clinical improvement defining a therapeutic window. Cognitively intact elderly responded to regular doses of drug while cognitively impaired elderly responded better to low doses (104). In one study, sertraline showed no significant benefits over placebo in treating depressed subjects with late-stage Alzheimer's disease (44). In the remaining study (24), nomifensine was better for reactive depression and amitriptyline for endogenous depression. The most significant conclusion to draw from these studies is that more investigations are needed in long-term care settings.

With *treatment-resistant depression*, which is nonresponsive to appropriately implemented standard interventions, several interventions have been proposed for elderly patients. In partial responders, an augmentation strategy may be more practical. Lithium augmentation, the most credibly documented option, can be successful at blood levels between 0.4 and 0.8 mmol/l (111). Bupropion has safely been used in medically frail elderly subjects as an augmenter to serotonergic agents (112). In postmenopausal depressed elderly women, Schneider and colleagues (113) demonstrated an augmenting effect when estrogen replacement therapy (ERT) was added to fluoxetine 20 mg/d. In one report, a brief pulse of dexamethasone aided treatment of two elderly patients with resistant depression (114). When no partial response has occurred, a switch to a different antidepressant—often one with a different mechanism of action—is preferred by many clinicians. Treatment trials to support one or another of these approaches or to compare their results remain to be done.

PARAMETERS OF TREATMENT CONTINUATION

Data from antidepressant trials of longer duration support the claim that, compared with younger adults, older subjects require longer intervals of treatment in order to achieve full antidepressant effectiveness. Georgotas and colleagues (115), for example, reported results from a comparison of phenelzine and nortriptyline among geriatric depressives and emphasized that most symptoms did not show significant improvement before the fourth week of treatment. In a study of nortriptyline treatment (99) mentioned earlier in this chapter, Dew and colleagues found that a significant subgroup of drug-responsive elderly subjects did not meet criteria for recovery until the tenth week. A more modest trial duration is recommended by the expert consensus guideline (76), which endorses waiting a minimum of 2 to 3 weeks and as long as 7.5 weeks before considering an antidepressant trial adequate.

MAINTENANCE THERAPY

Current issues regarding maintenance therapy are addressed in Chapter 14 of this book. There is as yet no clear consensus about the optimal criteria for or duration of maintenance pharmacotherapy in the elderly, but consensus exists for more liberal and lengthy maintenance treatments than those used in younger depressives. Repeatedly, undertreatment has been shown to be a factor in poor outcome and early relapse. Maintenance treatment, on the other hand, has been shown to be effective in older patients and should be pursued actively. Factors such as the number and severity of depressive episodes, response to treatment, concomitant anxiety symptoms (76), and delayed response to treatment during the first episode (116) may be important factors to consider in planning the duration of maintenance treatment. The recent expert consensus guideline recommends that treatment extend for 1 year or longer after a severe first episode, and for three or more years following a third or subsequent episode (76). Additional research is needed to guide and assess the effectiveness of maintenance antidepressant treatment in the medically ill, very old, or cognitively impaired elderly.

CONCLUSION

The ideal antidepressant for treating late-life depression remains to be identified. Experience with available agents, however, has identified some desirable characteristics for superior results with older patients. These are indicated in Table 4, adapting DeVane's approach (117).

As this chapter has made clear, none of the currently available agents matches this list of ideal characteristics. With growing numbers of depressed elderly patients experiencing depression and seeking treatment, it will be increasingly important to determine and promote optimal pharmacotherapy practices for specialists and primary care clinicians. Identifying superior agents and establishing meaningful comparison data among them will require more standardized and more powerful approaches than we observe in many of the studies

TABLE 4 Characteristics of an Ideal Antidepressant for Late-Life Depression

Efficacy characteristics
Alleviates symptoms, producing response or remission
Produces therapeutic benefits rapidly
Achieves effectiveness with all or most patients
Maintains effectiveness in continuation and maintenance phases of treatment
Safety and tolerability characteristics
Remains affordable even when not covered by insurance
Produces only infrequent or mild adverse effects
Induces minimal toxicity in overdose
Improves or does not impair cognition
Enhances quality of life and functionality
Pharmacokinetic characteristics
Possesses minimal anticholinergic, antidopaminergic, antiadrenergic, antihistaminic, or cardiotoxic effects
Yields predictable dose:effect relationship
Follows consistent and predictable pattern of disposition
Has a wide therapeutic index
Is inactivated/eliminated by multiple pathways
Has an elimination half-life suitable for once-daily dosing
Participates rarely in pharmacokinetic (including CYP450) drug–drug interactions

Source: Adapted from 117.

we reviewed. Currently available studies only partially answer our questions, largely because they lack statistical power, comparable design, or sufficiently thorough reporting. Underpowered studies make it difficult to assume that "not significantly different from" is synonymous with "equal to" (98). Furthermore, our identification of only five studies in which an investigated drug led to unfavorable overall results (lack of therapeutic benefits in four studies [51,55,59,61] and side effect problems in the other [36]) suggests a systematic bias against availability of negative studies, the so-called "file drawer effect" by which positive studies find their way more easily into publication. We would hope to see in future studies a design that includes sufficient statistical power to detect reliably the possible differences among compared drugs; use of standardized measures for efficacy and side effects; inclusion and subgroup analysis of patients with special characteristics (men vs. women, "old old," demented, poststroke, executive dysfunction); standard format for reporting so that statistical techniques are described in detail and data such as F- and t-statistics, standard deviations and standard errors are included; and reporting of negative as well as positive trials. In this way, our effectiveness in treating late-life depression can be improved, resulting in better acute and longer term outcomes, increased survival, and enhanced quality of life for our patients.

REFERENCES

1. Altamura A, Mauri M, Rudas N, et al. Clinical activity and tolerability of trazodone, mianserin, and amitriptyline in elderly subjects with major depression: a controlled multicenter trial. Clin Neuropharm 12(suppl 1):525–533; 534–537, 1989.
2. Altamura A, Percudani M, Guercetti G, Invernizzi G. Efficacy and tolerability of fluoxetine in the elderly: a double-blind study versus amitriptyline. Int Clin Psychopharm 4:(suppl 1):103–106, 1989.
3. Ather S, Ankier S, Middleton R. A double-blind evaluation of trazadone in the treatment of depression in the elderly. Br J Clin Prac 39:192–199, 1985.
4. Bayer A, Pathy M, Cameron A, et al. A comparative study of conventional and controlled-release formulations of trazodone in elderly depressed patients. Clin Neuropharm 12(suppl 1):S50–S55, 1989.
5. Bondareff W, Alpert M, Friedhoff A, et al. Comparison of sertraline and nortriptyline in the treatment of major depressive disorder in late life. Am J Psychiatry 157(7):729–736, 2000.
6. Branconnier R, Cole J, Ghazvinian S, et al. Clinical pharmacology of bupropion and imipramine in elderly depressives. J Clin Psychiatry 44(5):130–133, 1983.
7. Cohn C, Shrivastava R, Mendels J, et al. Double-blind, multicenter comparison of sertraline and amitriptyline in elderly depressed patients. J Clin Psychiatry 51(12 suppl B):B28–B33, 1990.
8. Cohn J, Varga L, Lyford A. A two-center double-blind study of nomifensine,

imipramine, and placebo in depressed geriatric outpatients. J Clin Psychiatry 44: 68–72, 1984.
9. De Vanna M, Kummer J, Agnoli A, et al. Moclobemide compared with second-generation antidepressants in elderly people. Acta Psychiatr Scand 360:64–66, 1990.
10. Dorman T. Sleep and paroxetine: a comparison with mianserin in elderly depressed patients. Int Clin Psychopharm 6(suppl 4):53–58, 1992.
11. Dunner D, Cohn J, Walshe T III, et al. Two combined, multicenter double-blind studies of paroxetine and doxepin in geriatric patients. J Clin Psychiatry 53(suppl 2): 57–60, 1992.
12. Eklund K, Dunbar G, Pinder R, Steffensen K. Mianserin and imipramine in the treatment of elderly depressed patients. Acta Psychiatr Scand 320:55–59, 1985.
13. Evans M, Hammond M, Wilson K, et al. Placebo-controlled treatment trial of depression in elderly physically ill patients. Int J Geriatr Psychiatry 12:817–824, 1997.
14. Fairweather JS, Kerr DB, Harrison D. A double-blind comparison of the effects of fluoxetine and amitriptyline on cognitive functioning in elderly depressed patients. Hum Psychopharm 8:41–47, 1993.
15. Falk W, Rosenbaum J, Otto M, et al. Fluoxetine versus trazodone in depressed patients. J Geriatr Psychiatry Neurol 2:208–214, 1989.
16. Feighner J, Boyer W, Hendrickson G, et al. A controlled trial of adinazolam versus desipramine in geriatric depression. Int Clin Psychopharm 5:227–232, 1990.
17. Feighner J, Cohn J. Double-blind comparative trials of fluoxetine and doxepin in geriatric patients with major depressive disorder. J Clin Psychiatry 46(3):20–25, 1985.
18. Finkel S, Richter E, Clary C, Batzar E. Comparative efficacy of sertraline versus fluoxetine in patients age 70 or over with major depression. Am J Geriatr Psychiatry 7(3):221–227, 1999.
19. Forlenza O, Almeida O, Stoppe A, et al. Antidepressant efficacy and safety of low-dose sertraline and standard-dose imipramine for the treatment of depression in older adults: results from a double-blind, randomized, controlled clinical trial. Int Psychogeriatr 13(1):75–84, 2001.
20. Forlenza O, Stoppe A Jr, Hirata E, Ferreira R. Antidepressant efficacy of sertraline and imipramine for the treatment of major depression in elderly outpatients. Sao Paulo Med J 118(4):99–104, 2000.
21. Georgotas A, McCue R, Hapworth W, et al. Comparative efficacy and safety of MAOIs versus TCAs in treating depression in the elderly. Biol Psychiatry 21: 1155–1166, 1986.
22. Geretsegger C, Stuppaeck C, Mair M, et al. Multicenter double blind study of paroxetine and amitriptyline in elderly depressed patients. Psychopharmacol 119: 227–281, 1995.
23 Gerner R, Estabrook W, Steuer J, Jarvik L. Treatment of geriatric depression with trazodone, imipramine, and placebo: a double-blind study. J Clin Psychiatry 41(6): 216–219, 1980.
24. Goldstein S, Birnbom F, Laliberte R. Nomifesine in the treatment of depressed geriatric patients. J Clin Psychiatry 43:7, 1982.
25. Guilibert E, Pelicier Y, Archambault J, et al. A double-blind, multicentre study of

paroxetine versus clomipramine in depressed elderly patients. Acta Psychiatr Scand 80:350(suppl):132–134, 1989.
26. Gwirtsman H, Ahles S, Halaris A, et al. Therapeutic superiority of maprotiline versus doxepin in geriatric depression. J Clin Psychiatry 44:449–453, 1983.
27. Halikas J. Org 3770 (mirtazapine) versus trazodone: a placebo controlled trial in depressed elderly patients. Hum Psychopharm 10:S125–S133, 1995.
28. Hoyberg O, Maragakis B, Mullin J, et al. A double-blind multicentre comparison of mirtazapine and amitriptyline in elderly depressed patients. Acta Psychiatr Scand 93:184–190, 1996.
29. Hutchinson D, Tong S, Moon C, et al. Paroxetine in the treatment of elderly depressed patients in general practice: a double-blind comparison with amitriptyline. Int Clin Psychopharmacol 6(suppl 4):43–51, 1992.
30. Jansen W, Siegfried K. Nomifensine in geriatric inpatients: a placebo-controlled study. J Clin Psychiatry 45(4):63–67, 1984.
31. Jarvik L, Mintz J, Steuer J, Gerner R. Treating geriatric depression: a 26-week interim analysis. J Am Geriatr Soc 30(11): 713–717, 1982.
32. Kane J, Cole K, Sarantkos S, et al. Safety and efficacy of bupropion in elderly patients: preliminary observations. J Clin Psychiatry 44(5):134–136, 1983.
33. Karlsson I, Godderis J, Lima C, et al. A randomized, double-blind comparison of the efficacy and safety of citalopram compared to mianserin in elderly, depressed patients with or without mild to moderate dementia. Int J Geriatr Psychiatry 15: 295–305, 2000.
34. Katona C, Bercoff E, Chiu E, et al. Reboxetine versus imipramine in the treatment of elderly patients with depressive disorder: a double-blind randomised trial. J Affect Disord 55:203–213, 1999.
35. Katona C, Hunter B, Bray J. A double-blind comparison of the efficacy and safety of paroxetine and imipramine in the treatment of depression with dementia. Int J Geriatr Psychiatry 13:100–108, 1998.
36. Katz I, Simpson G, Curlik S, et al. Pharmacologic treatment of major depression for elderly patients in residential care settings. J Clin Psychiatry 51(suppl 7):41–47, 1990.
37. Kivela S, Lehtomaki E, Kivekas J. Sulpride and placebo in depressed elderly outpatients: a double-blind study. Int J Geriatr Psychiatry 2:255–260, 1987.
38. Kretschmar J. Mianserin and amitriptyline in elderly hospitalized patients with depressive illness: a double-blind trial. Curr Med Ther Opin 6(suppl 7):144–151, 1980.
39. Kyle C, Peterson H, Overo K. Comparison of the tolerability and efficacy of citalopram and amitriptyline in elderly depressed patients treated in general practice. Dep and Anxiety 8:147–153, 1998.
40. La Pia S, Giorgio D, Ciriello R. Evaluation of the efficacy, tolerability, and therapeutic profile of fluoxetine versus mianserin in the treatment of depressive disorders in the elderly. Curr Ther Res 52(6):847–858, 1992.
41. Lakshmanan M, Mion L, Frengly D. Effective low dose tricyclic antidepressant treatment for depressed geriatric rehabilitation patients. J Am Geriatr Soc 34:421–426, 1986.
42. Lipsey J, Robinson R, Pearlson G, et al. Nortriptyline treatment of post-stroke depression: a double-blind study. Lancet 1(8372):297–300, 1984.

43. Lyketsos C, Sheppard J, Steele C, et al. Randomized, placebo-controlled, double-blind clinical trial of sertraline in the treatment of depression complicating Alzheimer's disease: initial results from the depression in Alzheimer's disease study. Am J Psychiatry 157(10):1686–1689, 2000.
44. Magai C, Kennedy G, Cohen C, Gomberg D. A controlled clinical trial of sertraline in the treatment of depression in nursing home patients with late-stage Alzheimer's disease. Am J Geriatr Psychiatry 8(1):66–74, 2000.
45. Mahapatra S, Hackett D. A randomized, double-blind, parallel-group comparison of venlafaxine and dothiepin in geriatric patients with major depression. Int J Clin Prac 51(4):209–213, 1997.
46. Merideth C, Feighner J, Hendrickson G. A double-blind comparative evaluation of the efficacy and safety of nomifensine, imipramine and placebo in depressed geriatric outpatients. J Clin Psychiatry 45(4):73–77, 1984.
47. Moller H, Volz H. Brofaromine in elderly major depressed patients—a comparative trial versus imipramine. Eur Neuropsychpharm 3:501–510, 1993.
48. Mulsant B, Pollock B, Nebes R, et al. A twelve-week, double-blind, randomized comparison of nortriptyline and paroxetine in older depressed inpatients and outpatients. Am J Geriatr Psychiatry 9:406–414, 2001.
49. Mulsant B, Sweet R, Rosen J, et al. A double-blind randomized comparison of nortriptyline plus perphenazine versus nortriptyline plus placebo in the treatment of psychotic depression in late life. J Clin Psychiatry 62:597–604, 2001.
50. Nair N, Amin M, Holm P, et al. Moclobemide and nortriptyline in elderly depressed patients: a randomized, multicentre trial against placebo. J Affect Disord 33:1–9, 1995.
51. Navarro V, Gasto C, Torres X, et al. Citalopram versus nortriptyline in late-life depression: a 12-week randomized single-blind study. Acta Psychiatr Scand 103: 435–440, 2001.
52. Newhouse P, Krishnan K, Doraiswamy P, et al. A double-blind comparison of sertraline and fluoxetine in depressed elderly outpatients. J Clin Psychiatry 61: 559–568, 2000.
53. Nyth A, Gottfires C, Lyby K, et al. A controlled multicenter clinical study of citalopram and placebo in elderly depressed patients with and without concomitant dementia. Acta Psychiatr Scand 86:138–145, 1992.
54. Pancheri P, Delle CR, Donnini M, et al. Effects of moclobemide on depressive symptoms and cognitive performance in a geriatric population: a controlled comparative study versus imipramine. Clin Neuropharm 17(suppl 1):S58–S73, 1994.
55. Petracca G, Chemerinski E, Starkstein S. A double-blind, placebo-controlled study of fluoxetine in depressed patients with Alzheimer's disease. Int Psychogeriatr 13(2):233–240, 2001.
56. Phanjoo A, Wonnacott S, Hodgson A. A double-blind comparative multicentre study of fluvoxamine and mianserin in the treatment of major depressive episode in elderly people. Acta Psychiatr Scand 83:476–479, 1991.
57. Rahman M, Akhtar M, Savla N, et al. A double-blind, randomised comparison of fluvoxamine with dothiepin in the treatment of depression in elderly patients. Br J Clin Prac 45(4):255–258, 1991.
58. Reynolds CF III, Miller M, Pasternak R, et al. Treatment of bereavement-related

major depressive episodes in later life: a controlled study of acute and continuation treatment with nortriptyline and interpersonal psychotherapy. Am J Psychiatry 156(2):202–208, 1999.
59. Robinson R, Schultz S, Castillo C, et al. Nortriptyline versus fluoxetine in the treatment of depression and in short-term recovery after stroke: a placebo controlled, double-blind study. Am J Psychiatry 157:351–359, 2000.
60. Roth M, Mountjoy C, Amrein R. Moclobemide in elderly patients with cognitive decline and depression: an international double-blind, placebo-controlled trial. Br J Psychiatry 168:149–157, 1996.
61. Salloway S, Boyle P, Correia S, et al. The relationship of MRI subcortal hyperintensities to treatment response in a trial of sertraline in geriatric depressed outpatients. Am J Geriatr Psychiatry 10:107–111, 2002.
62. Schatzberg AF, Kremer C, Rodrigues HE, Murphy GM, et al. Double-blind, randomized comparison of mirtazapine and paroxetine in elderly depressed patients. Am J Geriatr Psychiatry 10:541–550, 2002.
63. Schone W, Ludwig M. A double-blind study of paroxetine compared with fluoxetine in geriatric patients with major depression. J Clin Psychopharm 13(6 suppl 2):34S–39S, 1993.
64. Seigfried K, O'Connolly M. Cognitive and psychomotor effects of different antidepressants in the treatment of old age depression. Int Clin Psychopharm 1:231–243, 1986.
65. Taragano F, Lyketsos C, Mangone C, et al. A double-blind, randomised, fixed-dose trial of fluoxetine vs. amitriptyline in the treatment of major depression complicating Alzheimer's disease. Psychosomatics 38:246–252, 1997.
66. Tiller J, Maguire K, Davies B. A sequential double-blind controlled study of moclobemide and mianserin in elderly patients. Int J Geriatr Psychiatry 5:199–204, 1990.
67. Tollefson G, Bosomworth J, Heiligenstein J, et al. A double-blind, placebo-controlled clinical trial of fluoxetine in geriatric patients with major depression. Int Psychogeriatr 7(1):89–104, 1995.
68. Waite J, Grundy E, Arie T. A controlled trial of antidepressant medication in elderly inpatients. Int Clin Psychopharm 1:113–126, 1986.
69. Wakelin J. Fluvoxamine in the treatment of the older depressed patient: double-blind, placebo-controlled data. Int Clin Psychopharm 1:221–230, 1986.
70. Weihs K, Settle E Jr, Batey S, et al. Bupropion sustained release versus paroxetine for the treatment of depression in the elderly. J Clin Psychiatry 61:196–202, 2000.
71. Wiart L, Petit H, Joseph P, et al. Fluoxetine in early poststroke depression: a double-blind placebo-controlled study. Stroke 31(8):1829–1832, 2000.
72. Gerson S, Belin T, Kaufman A, Mintz J, Jarvik L. Pharmacological and psychological treatments for depressed older patients: a meta-analysis and overview of recent findings. Harvard Rev Psychiatry 7:1–28, 1999.
73. Klawansky S. Meta-analysis on the treatment of depression in late life. In: Schneider LS, Reynolds CF III, Lebowitz BD, Friedhoff AJ, eds. A Friedhoff, ed. Diagnosis and Treatment of Depression in Late Life: Results of the NIH Consensus Development Conference. Washington, DC: American Psychiatric Press, 1994.
74. Wilson K, Mottram P, Sivanranthan A, Nightingale A. Antidepressants versus

placebo for the depressed elderly. Cochrane Database Syst Rev 2:CD000561, 2001.
75. Mittmann N, Herrmann N, Einarson T, et al. The efficacy, safety and tolerability of antidepressants in late life depression: a meta-analysis. Journal of Affective Disorders 46:191–217, 1997.
76. Alexopoulos G, Katz I, Reynolds CI, Carpenter D, Docherty J. The expert consensus guide line series pharmacotherapy of depressive disorders in older patients. Postgraduate Medicine Special Report (Oct):1–86, 2001.
77. Katona C. Depression in Old Age. Chichester, UK: John Wiley & Sons, 1994.
78. Salzman C, ed. Clinical Geriatric Psychopharmacology, ed 3, Baltimore, MD: Williams & Wilkins, 2001.
79. Nelson J, ed. Geriatric Psychopharmacology. New York: Marcel Dekker, Inc., 1998.
80. Jacobson S, Pies R, Greenblatt D. Handbook of Geriatric Psychopharmacology. Washington, DC: American Psychiatric Press, 2002.
81. Stahl S, Muntner N. Essential Psychopharmacology: Neuroscientific Basis and Practical Applications. Cambridge, UK: Cambridge University Press, 2000.
82. Sultzer D, Gray K, Gunay I, et al. A double-blind comparison of trazodone and haloperidol for treatment of agitation in patients with dementia. Am J Geriatr Psychiatry 5:60–69, 1997.
83. Rothschild A. The diagnosis and treatment of late-life depression. J Clin Psychiatry 57(suppl 5):5–11, 1996.
84. Goldstein D, Hamilton S, Masica D, et al. Fluoxetine in medically stable, depressed geriatric patients: effects on weight. J Clin Psychopharmacol 17:365–369, 1997.
85. Aranda-Michel J et al. Nefazodone-induced acute liver failure: report of three cases. Ann Intern Med 130:285–288, 1999.
86. Schirren CA, Baretton G. Nefazodone-induced acute liver failure. Am J Gastroenterol 95:1596–1597, 2000.
87. Schwetz BA. From the Food and Drug Administration. JAMA 287:1103, 2002.
88. Sweet R, Pollock B, Kirshner M, et al. Pharmacokinetics of single- and multiple-dose bupropion in elderly patients with depression. J Clin Pharmacol 35:876–884, 1995.
89. Szuba M, Leuchter A. Falling backward in two elderly patients taking bupropion. J Clin Psychiatry 53:157–159, 1992.
90. Sachs G, Lafter B, Stoll A, et al. A double-blind trial of bupropion versus desipramine for bipolar depression. J Clin Psychiatry 55:391–393, 1994.
91. Beers M. Explicit criteria for determining potentially inappropriate medication use by the elderly: an update. Arch Intern Med 157:1531–1536, 1997.
92. Roose S, Suthers K. Antidepressant response in late-life depression. J Clin Psychiatry 59(suppl 10):4–8, 1998.
93. Finkel SI, Richter EM, Clary CM. Comparative efficacy and safety of sertraline versus nortriptyline in major depression in patients 70 and older. Int Psychogeriatr 11:85–99, 1999.
94. Oslin D, Streim J, Katz I, et al. Heuristic comparison of sertraline with nortriptyline for the treatment of depression in frail elderly patients. Am J Geriatr Psychiatry 8:141–149, 2000.

95. Roose S, Glassman A, Siris S, et al. Comparison of imipramine and nortriptyline induced orthostatic hypotension: a meaningful difference. J Clin Psychopharm 1(5):316–319, 1981.
96. Satel S, Nelson J. Stimulants in the treatment of depression: a critical overview. J Clin Psychiatry 50:241–249, 1989.
97. Wallace A, Kofoed L, West A. Double-blind, placebo-controlled trial of methylphenidate in older, depressed, medically ill patients. Am J Psychiatry 152:929–931, 1995.
98. Thase M. Comparing the methods used to compare antidepressants. Psychopharm Bull 36(suppl 1):4–18, 2002.
99. Dew M et al. Temporal profiles of the course of depression during the treatment: predictors of pathways toward recovery in the elderly. Arch Gen Psychiatry 54: 1016–1024, 1997.
100. Meyers B, Greenberg R. Late-life delusional depression. J Affect Disord 11:133–137, 1986.
101. Konig F, von Hippel C, Petersdorff T, et al. First experiences in combination therapy using olanzapine with ssris (citalopram, paroxetine) in delusional depression. Neuropsychobiology 43:170–174, 2001.
102. Rothschild A, Bates K, Boehringer K, Syed A. Olanzapine response in psychotic depression. J Clin Psychiatry 60:116–118, 1999.
103. Olin J, Katz I, Meyers B, Schneider L, Lebowitz B. Provisional diagnostic criteria for depression of Alzheimer disease: rationale and background. Am J Geriatr Psychiatry 10:129–141, 2002.
104. Streim J et al. Drug treatment of depression in frail elderly nursing home residents. Am J Geriatr Psychiatry 8:150–159, 2000.
105. Alexopoulos G et al. Vascular depression hypothesis. Arch Gen Psychiatry 54: 915–922, 1997.
106. Alexopoulos G. The depression-executive dysfunction syndrome of late life: a specific target for D_3 agonists? Am J Geriatr Psychiatry 9:22–29, 2001.
107. Robinson R. Treatment issues in poststroke depression. Dep and Anxiety 8(suppl 1):85–90, 1998.
108. Whyte EM, Mulsant BH. Post stroke depression: epidemiology, pathophysiology, and biological treatment. Biol Psychiatry 52:253–264, 2002.
109. Lazarus L et al. Efficacy and side effects of methylphenidate for poststroke depression. J Clin Psychiatry 53:447–449, 1992.
110. Brown M, Lapane K, Luisi A. The management of depression in older nursing home residents. J Am Geriatr Soc 50:69–76, 2002.
111. Katona C. The management of depression in old age. In Depression in Old Age. Chichester, UK: John Wiley & Sons, 1994, pp 93–121.
112. Spier S. Use of bupropion with SRIs and venlafaxine. Depress Anxiety 7:73–75, 1998.
113. Schneider L, Small G, Hamilton S, et al. Estrogen replacement and response to fluoxetine in a multicenter geriatric depression trial. Am J Geriatr Psychiatry 5: 97–106, 1997.
114. Bodani M, Sheehan B, Philpot M. The use of dexamethasone in elderly patients

with antidepressant-resistant depressive illness. J Psychopharmacol 13:196–197, 1999.
115. Georgotas A, McCue R, Friedman E, et al. Response of depressive symptoms to nortriptyline, phenelzine and placebo. Br J Psychiatry 151:102–106, 1987.
116. Flint A, Rifat S. The effect of treatment on the two-year course of late-life depression. Br J Psychiatry 170:268–272, 1997.
117. DeVane C. Pharmacological characteristics of ideal antidepressants in the 21st century. J Clin Psychiatry 61(suppl 11):4–8, 2000.
118. Ellison JM, Gottlieb G: Recognition and management of late life mood disorders. In: Sirven JI, Malamut BL, eds. Clinical Neurology of the Older Adult. Philadelphia: Lippincott Williams & Wilkins, 2002.

10

Barriers and Solutions to Medication Adherence

Rein Tideiksaar
ElderCare Companies, Inc., Philadelphia, Pennsylvania, U.S.A.

INTRODUCTION

Adherence, or the patient's accurate and consistent implementation of a care provider's therapeutic instructions, is essential to effective treatment. One of the factors that makes pharmacotherapy of depression in elderly patients particularly complex and challenging is the high rate of medication nonadherence among older patients. It is estimated that about one-third of older individuals always adhere, one-third never adhere, and one-third sometimes adhere with their medications (Lim and Woodward, 1999).

Nonadherence becomes an important clinical issue when the failure to follow prescribed medication regimes detracts from the effective treatment of a disease. The consequences of medication nonadherence can be both serious and costly. The worsening of a chronic condition resulting from not taking a medication may deceive the clinician into prescribing an even larger dose. This, in turn, can lead to serious adverse effects if the patient begins to take the medication as intended. When even more medications are added, in order to reduce adverse effects of the primary medication, the result may be an unreasonably complicated medication regimen. Any inappropriate or insufficient therapeutic response or adverse medication reactions resulting from nonadherence may require additional medical visits in order to render care, or emergency room and hospital visits if the patient's condition is severe. In turn, poor disease control can drastically change the health status of an older person and may pave the way for premature long-term nursing home placement.

Nonadherence with pharmacotherapy substantially impairs the treatment of depression among elderly patients. To the extent that health professionals can recognize and diminish this important barrier to treatment—and encourage better adherence to therapy—patients are likely to benefit from improved medical outcomes. Part of the health care provider's responsibility in ensuring good patient outcomes is to understand the various factors that either enhance or impede adherence with medications.

Early identification of the nonadherent patient, unfortunately, is sometimes difficult or even impossible. Good adherence with one medication regimen does not necessarily mean that a patient will adhere to instructions with another one. Furthermore, the absence of questions about how to take a medication does not always indicate that the patient fully understands the prescriber's instructions. In other words, adherence should not be assumed in any patient. However, elderly patients who are socially isolated (i.e., who lack involved and available caregivers), take multiple medications (e.g., usually more than four medications), have memory problems, financial difficulties, and/or sensory problems (e.g., vision and hearing impairment) are most likely not to adhere to a prescribed regimen.

Adherence to an antidepressant regimen is inherently problematic because of the nature of the disease. Even though antidepressants are relatively well-tolerated medications, depressed patients are three times as likely as nondepressed patients to be nonadherent with pharmacotherapy (DiMatteo et al., 2000). Although antidepressants are moderately effective in treating depression in later life, the pessimism or apathy associated with depression can produce nonadherence and undermine even the best treatment plan.

Providers often assume adherence to a medication regimen, but may be misled by hopelessness, therapeutic optimism, trust, or the limitations of knowledge that can be associated with infrequent follow-up visits. No matter how well providers think that they know a patient, their judgments about medication adherence are often inaccurate. Furthermore, when providers become aware that a patient is nonadherent, they may respond in a blaming manner or even with anger and rejection, as though nonadherence represents a patient's willful decision to be disobedient or contrary. This can exacerbate problems in the clinician's relationship with his or her patient. Rather, providers must learn that nonadherence often indicates that a patient's medication regimen is too complex, impractical, or intolerable for some reason and requires reconsideration and perhaps revision in order to meet the patient's needs. The reasons for nonadherence are varied and complex. This chapter reviews the common reasons for medication nonadherence and provides solutions to increase the likelihood of medication adherence in elderly patients.

REASONS FOR NONADHERENCE

Several factors are known to increase medication nonadherence in elderly patients. Some of the most important ones are outlined below.

Severity of the Disease or Disability

Diseases that produce severe symptoms or disability are generally associated with improved medication adherence. Conversely, a lack of overt symptoms and/or disability is associated with nonadherence. Similarly, the presence of multiple chronic diseases may encourage nonadherence, since elderly patients may be less able to distinguish the symptoms of a depressive disorder from symptoms associated with other comorbid illnesses.

Perceived Value of Treatment

Patients' perceptions about the seriousness or nature of their illnesses and the benefits of pharmacotherapy can often affect their willingness to adhere to a therapeutic regimen. If taking a medication is viewed by the patient as admitting to the presence of depression, failure to adhere to therapy may allow the patient to deny the presence of the illness. Because depression is accompanied by a degree of hopelessness, depressed patients may lack a positive attitude regarding the benefits and efficacy of treatment.

Duration of Treatment

The more extended a treatment, the greater the risk of nonadherence. Because late-life depression often requires long-term treatment, the risk of patient nonadherence with prescribed medications is great.

Understanding of the Disease and Its Treatment

A lack of acceptance of the diagnosis and treatment plan, a lack of concern about one's health in general, and, more specifically, thinking that depression does not pose a problem or threat to one's well-being can lead to nonadherence. Also, depression's symptoms can wax and wane, allowing patients to conclude that they are "better" and need not continue taking antidepressant medications. In addition, the beneficial effects of an antidepressant may be slow to appear, often requiring more than a month for full effect in an elderly patient. A patient who becomes discouraged by limited or delayed improvement may decide to discontinue the medication.

Relationship with Provider

A perception of the provider as warm, caring, friendly, and accessible encourages medication adherence. Poor communication between the patient and provider or a lack of apparent concern can lead to nonadherence.

Satisfaction with Provider Visits

Barriers to adherence often occur as early as the patient's initial visit with the provider. Patients who felt they were made to wait too long or that they were treated with insufficient concern or respect may be less likely to follow the instructions for taking medications. After an unsatisfying visit, a patient may leave the provider's office without a complete understanding of the rationale for therapy or the therapeutic regimen. Long waiting times to obtain an appointment may also contribute to nonadherence.

A STRATEGY FOR IMPROVING MEDICATION ADHERENCE

Common scenarios for nonadherence in elderly patients include failure to have a prescription filled, taking medications incorrectly, or stopping medications prematurely. Tables 1–3 suggest solutions specific to each of these scenarios.

Dementia and Fear of Falling: Two Additional Influences on Adherence

When depression is accompanied by cognitive impairment due to dementia, adherence can be seriously impaired. Fear of falling, by contrast, undermines adherence in both demented and cognitively intact depressed individuals. Each of these conditions is common among elderly depressed patients. They are discussed individually below.

Dementia

Elderly patients with dementia experience the same chronic medical conditions as other elderly patients, but their cognitive difficulties may seriously undermine their ability to take medications as prescribed. As dementia progresses, it becomes increasingly difficult for the patient to remember which pills to take and when, and it also becomes more difficult for the patient to report adverse effects. Many elders with mild dementia believe that they are successfully managing the cognitive demands of taking medications when in actuality they are taking too

TABLE 1 Failure to Obtain/Take Medication

Reason	Solution
Patient doesn't understand need for medication.	Educate patient about the treatment regimen and its rationale, giving clear explanation of the diagnosis, prognosis, and potential consequences of treatment and nontreatment. Provide written medication instructions. Enlist the help of significant others, family members, or other care providers when appropriate and feasible.
Inconvenience, limited mobility, or lack of transportation makes trip to pharmacy impractical	Explore mail order pharmacy options. Arrange for the pharmacy to deliver medications. Enlist help of family members, if available and willing.
High cost of medications deters patient from filling prescriptions	Use the lowest effective dose of medication. Consider less costly alternatives such as splitting of higher-dose tablets to provide a less costly low dose of medication, prescribing generic medications when available, or switching to alternative medications that are available in a generic form. Explore "patient assistance programs" that will supply low-income patients with low-cost medications.
Patient avoids obtaining medication by instead using medications that were prescribed to a friend or family member suffering from the same illness (i.e., depression).	Educate patient about the importance of matching specific medications to individual patient's needs including medications' differences in potential drug/drug interactions, effects on concurrent medical illnesses, and side effects.
Patient avoids obtaining medication by instead taking leftover medications from previous illness (i.e., depression).	Educate patient about medications' loss of potency over time and importance of discarding medications retained beyond expiration date.

TABLE 2 Taking Medications Improperly

Reason	Solution
Patient forgets to take some or all of prescribed medications.	When multiple medications are coprescribed, evaluate need for all medications involving other clinicians caring for patient and consider whether any can be given less frequently (e.g., once per day) or discontinued. Simplify medication regimen, when possible, by eliminating some medications or reducing the number of times medications are taken per day. Instruct patients to take medications at regularly scheduled time each day (i.e., when getting up in the morning, after dinner, at mealtime, etc.). Use memory aids (e.g., medication calendars, pillboxes), recognizing that effectiveness of such methods may require significant visual acuity and manual dexterity. Verify (e.g., with pill counts) that the appropriate amount of medication has been taken between assessments.
Patient doesn't understand medication instructions.	Provide written medication instructions in legible, bold, large print. Involve significant others or other care providers in medication administration when appropriate. Assess whether cognitive impairment or sensory impairment may be contributing to nonadherence and address these problems if present.
Patient takes too much or too little medications.	Assess patients' cognitive status to determine capacity to adhere to treatment regimen and assess whether additional supports are needed. Educate patient about the reasons for medication dosage and frequency. Explain that dosage increases or decreases should occur only after discussion with prescribing clinician.

TABLE 2 Continued

Reason	Solution
	Avoid "take as directed" instructions on pill bottles. This places burden of decision making on patients—a difficult task. Rather, be specific about medication directions.
Visual impairment interferes with adherence.	Color-code pill bottles (e.g., water pill in yellow container, antidepressant in blue container, etc.).
Pain, poor vision, and manual dexterity interfere with measuring liquids or breaking tablets prescribed in doses that require pill splitting.	Ascertain that patient's measuring spoon or device is properly marked in legible numerals. Ask pharmacist to prebreak scored tablets for patient. If patient has difficulty opening childproof tops or other packaging, ask pharmacist to dispense medications in easily opened, nonchildproof containers.

little or too much medication. They may mistakenly believe that they have taken their pills or may take extra doses of medications, having failed to remember that they already took them. Many elders with mild dementia can be helped with memory strategies involving external cues. Timing the administration of medications around meals and bedtime, using pillboxes that are organized daily or weekly, and involving family members or other caregivers are all measures that can increase adherence. Routine pill counts are a good idea in demented patients to assure that medications are being taken properly. Providers should consider assessing elderly patients for the presence of cognitive-impairment dementia if they repeatedly complain of problems in remembering to take their medications, report adverse effects attributable to using extra medications or omitting medications, and/or seem to show neither therapeutic effects nor side effects despite having been prescribed a suitable antidepressant regimen.

Fear of Falling

Approximately one-third of community-living elders fall each year, with the rate increasing to 40% for those over the age of 80 (Afken et al., 1994). It is estimated that about 50% of elders who have fallen report a fear of further falls (Yardley and Smith, 2002). In many ways, fear of falling among the elderly can

TABLE 3 Medications Are Discontinued Prematurely

Reason	Solution
Feeling better; lack of symptoms.	Educate patient about purpose and course of antidepressant therapy, including preventive benefits of continuation and maintenance therapy Generally, adherence with medications falls off as symptoms improve.
Not feeling better; patient believes medication will be ineffective.	Educate patient about what to expect from the medication, including potential side effects, delay before therapeutic benefits, and possible need to try more than one medication before arriving at an effective therapy.
Feeling worse; medication side effects are intolerable.	Evaluate current medication regimen; consider alternative medication dosing, timing, or medication.
	Evaluate for drug-drug and drug-food interactions that can result in adverse effects and nonadherence. Polypharmacy increases the risk of adverse interactions.
	Educate patient about proper medication administration regimen. Adverse effects can sometimes be alleviated by a change in timing of doses or by administering with food.

be as traumatic as a fall itself. Elderly patients with fear of falling often suffer from a loss of confidence in their ability to perform mobility tasks safely without falling. Even performing simple tasks such as reaching into a kitchen cabinet or stepping into a shower can create a great deal of anxiety and fear. As a result, many elderly patients start to restrict their everyday basic functional activities of daily living in order to prevent falls from occurring. This lack of activity can, in turn, lead to increasing weakness and frailty, which makes them more prone to falling. Eventually, fear of falling can lead to reduced quality of life and independence and hence an increased probability of being admitted to a long-term-care facility or nursing home for care.

Depression can be a preventable consequence of the fear of falling and its associated effects (e.g., lack of interest in pursuing activities, feelings of hopelessness). About 25% of elderly patients who are "very fearful" about falling show associated depression (Yardley and Smith, 2002). This group of elderly patients tends to be very dissatisfied with life, to restrict their physical or social activities, and to remain homebound for the most part. Treatment of depression with medication, unfortunately, can increase the risks of falls (Leipzig et al., 1999) and thereby exacerbate a patient's fears. Aside from the postural hypotension seen with some antidepressants, an additional reason for increased falling and increased fear is medication-induced gait abnormalities (Draganish et al., 2001). The fear of falling, however, should not preclude appropriate antidepressant treatment that can avert the morbidity of depressive illness. Elderly patients receiving antidepressants should be appropriately monitored and advised to stand and ambulate with care. In addition, the use of exercise and/or social activities as a treatment modality for depression should not proceed without first identifying and correcting the reasons for falls and attempting to increase the elderly patient's confidence in accomplishing mobility tasks.

SUMMARY

Nonadherence with antidepressant medication regimens is a significant problem in elderly patients. The basic steps to ensure patient adherence and optimize treatment benefits with medication regimens include the following:

Explaining to patients the nature of their illness and why medication is necessary and beneficial for the treatment of depression. If patients do not believe that medications are necessary and likely to not work, they will have little incentive to follow through.

Individualizing medication treatment (i.e., select a medication specific for the patient's symptoms of depression) and minimizing the treatment regimen. Use the smallest number of medications, at the lowest doses, administered as few times daily as possible. Complicated medication regimens hamper adherence, especially if multiple dosing of multiple medications is involved. Also, review the patient's current medications and consider the possibility of adverse interactions.

Explaining exactly what the patient should expect from their medication. Important items to cover include what the medication does, how it should be taken, what is the expected time course of response, what the major side effects are, and what the patient should do if side effects are experienced. Encourage the patient to ask questions. Telephone the patient 1 week after starting antidepressant medication, to check for early side effects and adherence, and to invite the patient to call if there are any problems. This can be very beneficial.

Minimizing inconvenience. Determine the patient's daily routine and try to fit the medication schedule into the patient's lifestyle (i.e., such as times of waking, evening meal, bedtime, etc.).

REFERENCES

Afken CL, Lach HW, Birge HW, Miller J. The prevalence and correlates of fear of falling in elderly persons living in the community. Am J Public Health 1994; 84: 565–570.

DiMatteo MR, Lepper HS, Croghan TW. Depression is a risk factor for noncompliance with medical treatment. Meta-analysis of the effects of anxiety and depression on patient adherence. Arch Intern Med 2000; 160:2101–2107.

Draganich LF, Zacny J, Klafta J, Karrison T. The effects of antidepressants on obstructed and unobstructed gait in healthy elderly people. J Gerontol 2001; 56A:M36–M41.

Lim WK, Woodward MC. Improving medication outcomes in older people. Aust J Hosp Pharm 1999; 29:103–107.

Leipzig R, Cumming R, Tinetti M. Drugs and falls in older people: a systemic review and meta-analysis: 1. Psychotropic drugs. J Am Geriatr Soc 1999; 47:30–39.

Yardley L, Smith H. A prospective study of the relationship between feared consequences of falling and avoidance of activity in community-living older people. Gerontologist 2002; 42:17–23.

11

Electroconvulsive Therapy for the Treatment of Late-Life Depression

Stephen Seiner and Michael E. Henry
McLean Hospital, Belmont, and Harvard Medical School, Boston, Massachusetts, U.S.A.

INTRODUCTION

Electroconvulsive therapy (ECT) is an underutilized treatment option for the treatment of severe mood disorders. Limitations of early ECT technique, adverse media portrayal, and a lack of education about the procedure have stigmatized ECT for decades, and significant advances in the procedure have not completely eliminated that stigma. Patients and family members are often surprised to find out that the procedure still exists and may be offended to have it offered to them as a treatment. This may be particularly true for geriatric patients who remember the early stigma of ECT.

Severe depression, however, is often debilitating and even life-threatening. Some cases of late-life depression respond poorly to standard psychotherapeutic and pharmacotherapeutic treatments. Even when treatment might otherwise succeed, elderly patients' compliance can present an obstacle to a successful outcome. The geriatric patient is also more sensitive to the side effects of medications, due to changes in drug metabolism, protein binding, and receptor sensitivity associated with aging. The result is that geriatric patients often require encouragement from their family members to get into and remain in treatment. Unfortunately, this may not occur until the patient has irretrievably lost many social supports and the family is desperate. It is often out of this desperation that these patients and their family members are finally referred for an ECT consultation. They are often afraid of the procedure but are usually reassured when provided with the facts about ECT's good safety record, impressive efficacy, and relatively mild side effects in most patients.

While ECT is often a very effective and appropriate choice for treating late-life depression, it must be administered with great care. The risks associated with ECT are higher in elderly patients with significant underlying medical disease. However, with thoughtful evaluation and planning, most patients, even those with significant medical disease, can undergo ECT with considerable safety.

INDICATIONS FOR ECT

Major Depression

Depression in the geriatric population is unique in several respects. The severity of geriatric depression can lead to increased medical morbidity and even mortality (Penninx et al., 1999; Schulz et al., 2000; Lee et al., 2001). These individuals often have diminished physical reserves with which to weather the poor nutrition and weight loss associated with depression, fewer social supports, and a decreased ability to rebuild their social network after isolating themselves during an episode of depression. They also have a higher rate of completed suicide (Lloyd et al., 1987; Milic, 2000). These factors combine to increase the urgency of treating their depression successfully. This urgency, together with the fact that geriatric depressed patients are less tolerant of pharmacological treatments than the general population (Peabody et al., 1986; Katz et al., 1990), suggests ECT should be routinely considered as a treatment for severely depressed older adults.

The efficacy data in geriatric patients strongly support the use of ECT. Several studies have suggested that the elderly may have higher response rates to ECT than the general population (Tew et al., 1999). In a large, prospective, multisite study of 268 patients, Tew and colleagues reported a response rate of 54% for patients under 60 years of age, 73% for patients aged 60 to 74, and 67% for those over age 75 (Tew et al., 1999). Other studies also support the use of ECT in the "old old" population (those over 75 years of age), finding ECT to be a relatively safe, well-tolerated, and effective treatment in this age group, with response rates reaching as high as 85% (Gormley, 1998; Manly et al., 2000). In a large, multisite, longitudinal study, the remission rates were reported for patients in different age groups receiving bilateral ECT for major depression. Patients over age 65 had a 90% remission rate, while those under age 45 showed a 70% response (O'Connor et al., 2001).

The efficacy of ECT for depression in patients with concurrent dementia remains inadequately explored. Rao and Lyketsos, however, did examine hospitalized patients receiving ECT who suffered from both dementia and depression (Rao et al., 2000) and found that ECT improved mood significantly by the time of discharge from the hospital. Although close to half of these patients developed delirium, there was a mild mean improvement in initial Mini-Mental State Exam (MMSE) scores of 1.62 by the time of discharge, suggesting that ECT may help relieve some of the cognitive impairment caused by depression. In case studies, ECT has also been reported to be effective in treating agitation and aggression in demented patients (Grant et al., 2001).

Psychotic Depression

ECT has consistently been shown to be an effective treatment for psychotic depression in the general population (Coryell, 1996; Coryell, 1998) and has been proposed by some as the first-line treatment for this condition when symptoms are severe or when patients are unable to take oral medications (Iwanami et al., 1999). A recent study by Petrides and colleagues demonstrated that psychotic depressed patients responded more quickly and robustly to ECT (bilateral) than did nonpsychotic depressed patients (Petrides et al., 2001), with response rates as high as 95%. Literature reviews and meta-analyses support ECT as being at least as effective in treating psychotic depression as "combination medication" treatment—a combination of antidepressant and antipsychotic medications. They further support ECT as being significantly more effective than either antidepressant or antipsychotic monotherapy (Parker et al., 1992). In a study of late-life psychotic depression, ECT was shown to be significantly *more* effective than combination medication treatment (Flint et al., 1998). It should be noted that the data on the newer pharmacological options for treating psychotic depression are limited; systematic studies that compare the efficacy of these and future agents to ECT are urgently needed.

Other Syndromes Associated with Late-Life Depression

Several syndromes, some of which are particularly present in the geriatric population and related to depression in late life, are responsive to ECT. Parkinson's disease has an extremely high rate of comorbid depression, reaching as high as 40% in some studies (Cummings et al., 1999). ECT, by virtue of its ability to increase central nervous system (CNS) dopamine turnover may be uniquely effective in treating the mood and the movement components of this condition (Glue et al., 1990; Fall et al., 1995; Moellentine et al., 1998). Maintenance ECT has also been reported to be helpful in case reports of patients with intractable or difficult-to-treat Parkinson's disease (Wengel et al., 1998; Fall et al., 1999).

Catatonia secondary to psychiatric conditions has also been shown to respond well to ECT, although ECT's effectiveness in treating catatonia due to medical or neurological conditions has not been as thoroughly studied (Rummans, 1993). Possible neurological and medical disorders underlying catatonia should be investigated thoroughly and treated as aggressively as possible (Rummans, 1993). A severe form of catatonia, known as malignant catatonia, has a high morbidity and even mortality associated with it and has been shown to respond well to ECT (Mann et al., 1990). Therefore, in patients with malignant catatonia, ECT should be strongly considered as an early treatment option. Neuroleptic malignant syndrome (NMS) may be related to malignant catatonia (Fink, 1996) and has been shown to be responsive to ECT in a review of the limited cases reported in the literature (Trollor et al., 1999).

Bipolar Disorder/Bipolar Depression

ECT has been shown to be effective for treatment of mania (Mukherjee et al., 1994), mixed affective states (Devanand et al., 2000), and bipolar depression (Ciapparelli et al., 2001) in mixed age populations. The severity of bipolar episodes and the frequency with which affected individuals cycle between manic and depressive episodes tend to increase as bipolar patients age (Satlin et al., 1998), making treatment more challenging and sometimes more urgent. Unfortunately, studies of ECT in geriatric bipolar patients are limited.

Mukherjee and colleagues reviewed 50 years of treatment of acute manic episodes with ECT and concluded that ECT is associated with remission or marked improvement in approximately 80% of mixed-age manic patients and can be helpful for manic patients who have not responded to pharmacological treatments (Mukherjee et al., 1994). The optimal placement of electrodes remains controversial, with some research supporting the preferential use of bilateral ECT for mania (Small et al., 1985), while other studies have found right unilateral treatment to be effective as well (Black et al., 1987).

Mixed bipolar mood states can be difficult to diagnose and particularly challenging to treat pharmacologically. Few studies have assessed ECT in mixed states, but the existing evidence appears to support its use in these patients. Devanand and colleagues found that 80% of patients with mixed affective states responded well to ECT, but they required longer hospital stays and a greater number of ECT treatments than bipolar depressed patients (Devanand et al., 2000). Ciapparelli, however, in a larger study, found that patients with mixed symptoms who were unresponsive to medication responded well to ECT and demonstrated a more rapid and robust response than bipolar depressed patients (Ciapparelli et al., 2001). The differences in the results of these two studies may reflect differences in electrode placement. All patients received bilateral ECT in the latter study; in the former, some received unilateral placement while others received bilateral placement or a combination.

In general adult populations, ECT has also been shown to be effective in bipolar depression (Devanand et al., 2000; Daly et al., 2001). There is some evidence that bipolar depression may show a more rapid response, requiring fewer treatments than unipolar depression (Daly et al., 2001). However, patients who appear to be responding early should be monitored closely for symptoms of emerging mania, as ECT like all other antidepressant treatments, can precipitate mania (Serby, 2001).

SPECIAL CONCERNS IN THE ELDERLY

The older patient presents some unique medical risks and psychological concerns that the treatment team must assess prior to initiating ECT. Complex medical conditions including cardiac risk factors combined with pulmonary and orthopedic difficulties are often the rule more than the exception. Dementia can certainly complicate the picture further and often imposes an increased burden on the family to help with treatment decisions. Special attention must be paid to the family dynamics when an elderly parent is being treated with ECT.

Medical Concerns

In the general population ECT is a very safe procedure, with reported mortality rates of approximately 4 deaths per 100,000 treatments (Abrams, 1997). There are no absolute contraindications to ECT, but there are several conditions that increase the risks associated with treatment. These risks, however, must be weighed against the risks of untreated depression, including increased cardiac risk (Avery et al., 1977), increased suicidal risk (Coppen, 2000; O'Connor et al., 2001), and increased overall medical morbidity and mortality (Penninx et al., 1999; Schulz et al., 2000; Lee et al., 2001). Without treatment, patients with unresponsive catatonia or severe psychotic depression often present a significant mortality and morbidity risk. In contrast, Philibert and colleagues reported that geriatric patients who received ECT had lower mortality rates at follow-up than those who had not received ECT (Philibert et al., 1995).

Cardiac Illness

Cardiovascular diseases, common among the elderly, are very relevant to the administration and safety of ECT. The rare deaths that occur during ECT are most often cardiac in nature (Abrams, 1997). With careful planning, informed consent, and appropriate medical backup, however, even patients with severe cardiac disease can be treated successfully with ECT. Zielinski and colleagues studied a series of depressed patients with serious cardiac disease who underwent ECT (Zielinski et al., 1993) and found a significantly increased rate of cardiac complications. Among 40 patients, they found eight "major" complications, including "persistent ECG changes lasting hours to days, accompanied by chest pain, asystole or persistent arrhythmias." Importantly though, they had no deaths, and 38 of the 40 patients were able to complete the study. In a retrospective study, Rice and colleagues examined 80 patients with cardiac risk factors who received ECT. They found the high-cardiac-risk group had more minor complications but no major complications (Rice et al., 1994).

Successful treatment of the depressed elderly patient with cardiac disease begins with a thorough history. ECT affects the heart through the autonomic nervous system via the vagus nerve, sympathetic tract, and circulating catecholamines sequentially (Welch et al., 1989). This results in predictable fluctuations in cardiac rhythm, pulse, and blood pressure during an average treatment.

Patients with major cardiac risk factors such as unstable or severe angina, recent myocardial infarction, significant arrhythmias, severe valvular disease, or decompensated congestive heart failure (Eagle et al., 1996) present the greatest safety concerns. These patients should have medical stabilization, cardiology consultation, evaluation of ischemia and left ventricular function, and correction of the underlying pathology if possible before ECT is performed (Applegate, 1997). The noninvasive evaluation can include an exercise tolerance test or a pharmacological stress test if the patient is unable to exercise and, if needed, an echocardiogram. A thallium study as part of the stress test can be particularly helpful in determining the amount of myocardial tissue at risk. In patients with an intermediate risk profile (Eagle et al., 1996)—such as mild angina, prior (not recent) myocardial infarction, compensated congestive heart failure, or diabetes mellitus—a determination of functional status should take place. If the patient has good functional status, ECT can take place along with appropriate medical treatment (Applegate, 1997). If functional status is poor, then a reassessment of the risk-to-benefit analysis is warranted. Cardiology consultation on these patients can help determine whether medical intervention to improve functional status should take place before ECT is attempted.

Immediately after myocardial infarction (MI), vulnerable myocardial tissue and increased irritability and risk of arrhythmia need to be considered. ECT can transiently increase cardiac output and demand, stressing vulnerable tissue; therefore, it is preferable to avoid ECT in the immediate post-MI period. What constitutes the immediate post-MI period is unclear. The American College of Cardiology National Database Library defines a recent MI one that occurred more than 7 days but less than 1 month earlier (Applegate, 1997). In general, the longer that one can allow the myocardial tissue to heal before ECT is initiated, the better. Given the high rate of post-MI depression and increased mortality associated with it (Frasure-Smith et al., 1993, 1995), however, ECT may have to be considered in extreme cases during the post-MI period. Consultation with a cardiologist and careful planning with anesthesiology can make ECT an option in a controlled general hospital setting.

Hypertension is one of the more common cardiovascular risk factors seen in geriatric ECT patients. Ideally, the patient's blood pressure should be optimized with daily medication before beginning ECT. For patients with a history of hypertension already controlled with blood pressure medication, it is usually best to continue the medication as scheduled throughout the ECT. Pretreatment with a beta blocker may help attenuate the hyperdynamic response to ECT (Castelli et al., 1995; Zvara et al., 1997), and can be considered in patients with excessively high blood pressures or tachycardia during ECT, especially in those with known cardiovascular disease (Dolinski et al., 1997). Such measures, however, should be employed with caution as overly aggressive treatment of hypertension or tachycardia can contribute to asystole, bradycardia, or hypotension during phases of the treatment when parasympathetic tone is prominent.

Another potential complicating cardiac factor is the presence of an internal pacemaker or automatic implantable cardioverter/defibrillator (AICD). In general, ECT does not significantly affect pacemakers, but a magnet must be immediately accessible to override any abnormal signals if necessary (Dolinski et al., 1997). Prior to a course of ECT, an AICD should be evaluated by a cardiac electrophysiologist to determine whether the defibrillator function should be turned off during treatments, although the pacemaker function should generally be left on (APA Task Force, 2001).

Atrial fibrillation can be a concern, as ECT may convert atrial fibrillation to normal sinus rhythm, at least transiently (Petrides et al., 1996). For this reason, anticoagulation is a reasonable prophylactic measure to prevent a mural thrombus from embolizing. Some elderly patients may not be able to tolerate anticoagulation due to risks of falling, gastrointestinal bleeding, or other hazards. In these cases and when the anticoagulation may not have been consistently therapeutic, a transesophogeal echocardiogram can be helpful to determine whether there is a mural thrombus or to better define the risk of embolic events.

In summary, the presence of significant cardiac disease should alert the clinician to the need for a careful assessment to minimize the risks of treatment with ECT. Consultation with a cardiologist and careful planning with the anesthesiologist usually lower the risk sufficiently to allow these patients to be treated successfully.

Pulmonary Illness

ECT involves the use of a muscle relaxant; therefore the patient must be ventilated during the procedure, usually with simple masked ventilation. Underlying lung pathology, however, can complicate this usually routine task. Any pulmonary complaint by elderly patients prior to or after treatment with ECT needs to be evaluated before further ECT should be attempted.

Chronic obstructive pulmonary disease (COPD), asthma, pneumonia, bronchitis, and other lung disease can increase the difficulty of maintaining adequate oxygen saturation, elevate the risk of bronchospasm, and put increased demands on the heart. Pretreatment with bronchodilators can be helpful in treating patients with COPD and asthma (Wingate et al., 1997). However, theophylline increases the risk of prolonged seizures and status epilepticus (Devanand et al., 1988; Rasmussen et al., 1993; Stewart, 1996) and should be discontinued unless absolutely necessary. The treatment team should make every effort to optimize pulmonary function. This could include the use of inhalers or nebulizers to improve air exchange for COPD or asthma, preoxygenation for low oxygen saturation, and proper antibiotic treatment for infectious lung disease.

Gastrointestinal Disease

Peptic ulcer disease, gastritis, gastric reflux disease, or swallowing difficulties secondary to stroke or other neurological disease can increase the risk of aspiration and/or laryngospasm in the elderly. Every effort should be made to limit aspiration risk as much as possible prior to the initiation of ECT. Examples include pretreatment with sodium citrate (antacid) to neutralize gastric contents, metoclopramide to increase gastric emptying, and H_2 blockers or proton pump inhibitors to decrease acid production (APA Task Force, 2001). Cricoid pressure is often used during the treatment to reduce the risk of aspiration, but the effectiveness of this is uncertain (Brimacombe et al., 1997). Pretreatment intubation can help to protect the airway during treatment of patients with more severe aspiration risk or with severe underlying lung disease, although this must be weighed against the risks of multiple intubations during a treatment course.

Musculoskeletal Disease

Since the adoption of muscle relaxants and anesthesia as routine elements of ECT, the risk of long bone fractures and other complications has dropped significantly. Because of the relative fragility of bones, joints, and especially vertebrae in the elderly, however, careful attention must be paid to the timing and degree of muscle relaxation. Prior to treatment, it is important to evaluate and compensate for active vertebral disk disease, recent fractures, or significant spinal stenosis. Consultation with a neurologist or orthopedist should be considered. In many of these patients, appropriate and adequate dosing of the muscle relaxant can decrease complications and limit the risk of ECT (APA Task Force, 2001).

Posttreatment falls are a potential side effect of ECT, possibly due to confusion, sedation, orthostasis due to pretreatment beta blockade, or memory loss. DeCarle and colleagues reported the number of ECT treatments and a diagnosis of Parkinson's disease were two independent risk factors for falls in the elderly receiving ECT (de Carle et al., 2000). Patients should be monitored closely prior to and during a course of ECT treatments for balance difficulties, confusion, orthostasis, sedation, and other signs that they may be at increased risk for falling.

Neurological Disease

ECT alters regional blood flow to the brain (Nobler et al., 2001) and brain metabolism (Henry et al., 2001), but it is unclear how these changes affect patients who have suffered a recent cerebrovascular accident (CVA). It is unknown how soon ECT can safely be performed after a CVA. Canine studies have suggested that it may take 9 weeks for the margins of the infarction to heal fully (Meyer, 1958); however, in clinical practice, patients have been successfully treated with ECT within 1 month of having a CVA (Murray et al., 1986; Welch, 1993). One case report of ECT as early as 7–14 days poststroke has been reported (Weintraub et al., 2000). A retrospective study of 19 geriatric poststroke patients who received ECT showed acute improvement in 95% (Currier et al., 1992). Although 5 patients developed ECT-related medical complications, none experienced exacerbation of pre-existing neurological deficits. In another study, ECT produced marked improvement in 12 of 14 patients with depression and a history of stroke; none showed worsening of their neurological status (Murray et al., 1986). There are case reports of neurological deficits arising during post-ECT recovery. These deficits, however, are rare and often transient (Miller et al., 1998).

Intracranial vascular masses such as aneurysm or vascular malformation, space-occupying lesions, or other causes of increased intracranial pressure should be considered to be associated with "substantially increased" risk, according to the APA task force on ECT (APA Task Force, 2001). The risks of herniation, intracranial bleed, or other neurological complications must be weighed carefully against potential benefits of treatment. In some cases, provision of ECT may be the most appropriate choice. A review by Salaris and colleagues, for example, found no adverse outcome among eight reported cases of ECT performed with patients with intracranial vascular masses (Salaris et al., 2000). Instances of successful ECT have also been reported in patients with brain tumors and elevated intracranial pressure (Patkar et al., 2000). Under such circumstances, ECT can sometimes be performed, but this requires an experienced anesthesiologist and consultation with a neurologist and neurosurgeon in order to lower risk as much as possible. Unfortunately, further study is needed to fully assess the risks that brain tumors pose for patients undergoing ECT. The psychiatrist, together with the patient and family, must carefully consider the risks and benefits of both treating and not treating with ECT, and other alternatives should also be considered.

In general, Parkinson's disease responds positively to ECT treatment, as described in greater detail above. Several studies have demonstrated that ECT can be helpful not only in treating the depression that is seen very commonly with Parkinson's disease, but also in relieving many of the neurological symptoms. The effects of ECT on progressive supranuclear palsy are not as clear. Other neurological illnesses—such as multiple sclerosis, polio, and paralysis—can present anesthesia risks; therefore, input from the anesthesiologist is crucial to defining the degree of risk. While challenging, patients with these neurological illnesses can often be treated effectively with ECT.

Malignancies

Depression is common in cancer patients, occurring in about one-quarter of these (Pirl et al., 1999); ECT has been used to treat depression successfully in patients with different forms of cancer (Beale et al., 1997; Blewett et al., 2000). One major concern that arises in using ECT in patients with systemic cancer is the risk of treating when cerebral metastases may affect safety. When there is evidence of current malignancy or even a history of cancers with a high likelihood of metastasis to the brain—especially lung cancer, breast cancer, and melanoma (Hochberg et al., 1991)—it is particularly prudent to consider neuroimaging of the brain. While special attention needs to be paid to tumors that have high rates of central nervous system metastasis, other systemic tumors may also raise clinicians' concern. As the treatment of systemic tumors continues to improve and patients survive longer, the incidence of central nervous system involvement can be expected to rise for most types of tumors (Hochberg et al., 1991). Neuroimaging, therefore, may be considered in patients with other types of systemic tumors as well. Any patient with a history of systemic cancer who also has focal neurological findings on exam should raise serious concern about central nervous system metastasis, warranting further neurological assessment, likely including neuroimaging. As depression can be a secondary neurological symptom of a brain tumor, it is reasonable to image the brain of any patient with a history of systemic cancer and new onset of depression.

ECT, as mentioned above, has been performed in patients with brain lesions; therefore the discovery of a brain metastasis does not necessarily prohibit ECT treatment. Of course, if a brain lesion is discovered in the pre-ECT workup, the potential prognosis and specific treatment of the lesion must be addressed, as well as the possibility that the lesion may be contributing to the mood symptoms that initially prompted the ECT consultation. The oncology team may feel that treatment of the tumor is a priority in increasing the overall chances of survival. Should the decision be made to proceed with ECT, knowledge of the existence of a brain metastasis can aid the treatment team in preparing adequately for ECT.

Memory Loss

Memory loss is perhaps the biggest concern of patients, regardless of age, and family members who are contemplating ECT. Typically, the memory loss is mild and usually resolves after the ECT has ended. In studies that have examined patients several months after ECT, no sustained cognitive disturbances were found (Weeks et al., 1980; Frith et al., 1983; Calev et al., 1991). A review of 39 papers addressing the long-term memory effects of ECT found that the majority of studies suggested that ECT does not normally cause long-term memory deficits, although a small number of studies did find subtle deficits months after ECT, particularly in personal autobiographical material (Taylor et al., 1982). While geriatric patients are thought to be at higher risk for memory loss during ECT due to a presumed decrease in cognitive reserve, studies have shown that elderly patients often tolerate the cognitive effects of ECT very well (Rubin et al., 1993; Brodaty et al, 2001). Sometimes cognition, initially impaired by severe depression, actually improves after ECT (Stoudemire et al, 1991, 1995).

The risk of memory loss becomes an even bigger concern when patients already have some memory loss or dementia at baseline. ECT can be performed when patients have dementia, but particular care has to be taken to monitor memory throughout the course of treatment. While there is not clear consensus on the best way to reduce memory loss in the elderly or in patients with dementia, the following basic guidelines should be considered:

1. Prescreen memory—This is important in documenting the level of baseline memory loss, if present. It allows for reasonable expectations as far as recovery of memory following ECT. Furthermore, it prevents pre-existing memory deficits from being attributed to ECT. The form of cognitive testing depends on the patient and can range from simple memory testing to formal neuropsychological testing.
2. Monitor memory throughout treatment—This can include formal testing, but observations of caregivers can be even more important. More frequent episodes of getting lost, forgetting things, or frank confusion are important to note. Helpful questions to ask the patient routinely include questions about recent events, daily activities, and orientation. These can easily be incorporated into the standard discussion about mood and overall improvement with the patient prior to each treatment.
3. Consider decreasing the frequency of treatments—When significant and disruptive memory loss is noted or if considerable memory loss was present prior to treatments, it is very reasonable to decrease the frequency of the treatments in the acute course from three times weekly to twice or even once a week. There is evidence that twice a week treatment can be as effective with less memory loss than thrice weekly treatment, although the response of treatment may not be as rapid (McAllister et al., 1987; Shapira et al, 1998). With increasing

pressure to decrease length of hospitalization, treatment teams are sometimes reluctant to do this, but it should be remembered that marked confusion can interrupt ECT and can result in longer hospitalization while waiting for patients to stabilize cognitively. Some patients can also be treated as outpatients if adequate supports can be arranged.

4. Favor unilateral over bilateral treatment when reasonable—Unilateral treatments are associated with less memory loss and confusion (Fromm-Auch, 1982; Rosenberg et al., 1984) and should be used preferentially if possible. Mixed or manic episodes or a history of nonresponse to unilateral treatments, however, may lead to preferential treatment with bilateral placement. In such cases, strong consideration should be given to a decreased frequency of treatment in dementia patients undergoing bilateral ECT.
5. Set expectations with patient and family—This is advisable in all cases but is particularly important in patients with dementia. Worsening memory loss and/or confusion is very upsetting to most patients and families, and education about this possibility ahead of time, as well as reassurance during the course of treatment, can be extremely helpful and is good clinical practice.

PSYCHOLOGICAL ISSUES

The following sections address psychological issues, including making the decision about ECT and family involvement in the ECT process.

Making the Decision

Suggesting ECT to a geriatric patient can present formidable challenges for a number of reasons. Geriatric patients have spent much of their adult lives during a time when the idea of "shock treatments" was even more stigmatized than it is now. In addition, geriatric depression may be hidden behind somatic symptoms, making it more difficult to diagnose. Perhaps the greatest obstacle arises when patients have somatic ruminations or delusions and refuse ECT because they feel that all of their difficulties are medical rather than psychiatric. Providing education, establishing an alliance between the patient and the treatment team, and involving the family can be helpful with delusional patients.

Patients, family, and physicians are often troubled with the decision regarding ECT when patients have suffered multiple losses. It is important to acknowledge losses, but when patients show symptoms of a complicated bereavement—such as severe depression, marked weight loss or dehydration, suicidal ideation, psychosis, or other symptoms of a major depressive episode—the diagnosis of major depression and appropriate treatment are also warranted. When ECT is performed in such patients, particular attention has to be paid to limit memory loss as much as possible, as patients worry about forgetting recent memories about their loved ones. If the loss is a very recent one, it may be worthwhile to delay ECT, if possible, to decrease the risk of jeopardizing these memories. Occasionally, patients will forget about the loss of their loved one immediately after an ECT treatment and then feel retraumatized as the memory soon returns. These issues need to be discussed carefully with the patient and family before proceeding with ECT.

Some patients may have had complications during ECT they received years ago, before the introduction of anesthesia and muscle relaxants. Others may have seen movies from decades ago, which portrayed ECT without anesthesia or as a punitive procedure. They will need education about the advances in ECT and anesthesia, as well as its clinical indications, in order to make an informed decision.

Family Involvement

Depressed patients frequently worry about being a "burden" to their families, and do not want their families to be concerned or involved. While it is important to respect patients' decisions about this, in general it is very important to have the family involved in the decision about ECT. Sometimes family members disagree about ECT—a situation better addressed early rather than ignored. A meeting that educates the family about ECT and addresses family concerns can be very helpful. Otherwise, family members may not realize they disagree until partway through the ECT course, when this disagreement may escalate and cause an interruption or cessation of the ECT. Patients may refuse ECT in order to pacify family disputes about the procedure, which can sometimes be avoided with simple family education.

Whenever there are conflicts between the wishes of the patient and those of the family, the patient's preference takes precedence as long as the patient has demonstrated competence to make this decision with true informed consent. When the patient is not competent to make such decisions, usually a health care proxy, guardian, or judge is involved in making this decision. Legal consultation around this issue usually defines the pertinent statutes and issues to be addressed prior to proceeding with treatment. In general, every effort should be made to bring the patient, treatment team, and family together with a unified plan.

MAINTENANCE TREATMENT

One of the challenges of ECT is determining how to keep the patient better once he or she has improved with the acute ECT course. Some patients may have a course of ECT and need no further pharmacological or ECT treatment, but they are the minority. Most patients referred for ECT have had multiple medication trials and often have long histories of relapsing depression. Therefore, relapse rates following ECT can be very high (Sackeim et al., 2001). For these patients some form of maintenance treatment is usually warranted, and this may include antidepressant pharmacological treatment, intensive psychotherapy, psychosocial intervention, maintenance ECT, or some combination of these.

Pharmacological Maintenance

Medications are the most typical form of maintenance treatment following ECT. Given that many ECT patients have already failed multiple medication trials, however, it can be difficult to choose an effective medication regimen. Relapse rates of patients receiving medication maintenance following ECT appears to be related to medication resistance prior to ECT (Sackeim et al., 1990; Wijkstra et al., 2000). If the pre-ECT regimen has been ineffective, it is usually advisable to switch or augment the regimen following ECT. Combination medication strategies, such as nortriptyline and lithium salts, have been studied with some success in reducing post-ECT relapse rates in medication resistant or psychotic depressed patients (Sackeim et al., 2001), decreasing relapse rates from 84–39% at 24 weeks post-ECT. Such combinations, however, can sometimes be difficult for elderly patients to tolerate. Because many patients have not had trials with monoamine oxidase inhibitors (MAOIs) and because of the demonstrated effectiveness of these medicines in helping treatment-resistant depression (Thase et al., 1992; Nolen et al., 1993), MAOIs are often an attractive choice for post-ECT maintenance pharmacological treatment. In addition, ECT can be used to treat the depression during the washout period needed to switch from another antidepressant to an MAOI. MAOIs can be difficult to tolerate due to their orthostatic effects, and great care needs to be taken in monitoring elderly patients initiated on this type of medication. This is especially true given the fairly complicated diet necessary when taking MAOIs and the potential memory loss post-ECT. Therefore, it is often advisable to have a family member helping to monitor the medication and diet at home—someone who can alert the physician if there are problems in managing these issues. Many geriatric patients, however, tolerate MAOIs without difficulty.

In general, psychotic depression has a higher relapse rate than nonpsychotic depression (Robinson et al., 1985; Parker et al., 1991), and this appears to hold true in the geriatric population as well (Flint et al., 1998). Therefore, aggressive treatment following ECT is appropriate. Some evidence suggests that early withdrawal of the antipsychotic medication post-ECT may result in higher relapse rates in these patients (Flint et al., 1998). Therefore, in patients with psychotic depression, antipsychotic treatment following ECT for a maintenance period of several months or even years in some cases is usually helpful; and when withdrawn, such treatment should be tapered slowly, with very close monitoring.

Maintenance or Continuation ECT

Some patients who have demonstrated medication resistance or intolerance of medication side effects choose to go on with ECT on a continuation or maintenance basis. The aim of continuation ECT is very much like tapering a medication after successful treatment. The rate of the taper should be tailored to each individual patient's needs but often consists of weekly treatments following the acute course for 2–4 weeks and then tapering that as tolerated. The goal of this may vary. For many patients, the aim is to prolong the ECT effect until an adequate maintenance medication regimen can be found. If the patient begins to show signs of relapse when the time between treatments is extended, it may represent the need for medication adjustment. The advantage of the continuation ECT in this example is that the ECT can be used to prevent relapse and rehospitalization while that medication adjustment is made. Once a patient appears stable on medication without relapse with monthly or greater intervals between ECT, the ECT is discontinued. Other patients are tired of multiple medication trials and side effects and are content to receive monthly maintenance treatments indefinitely. These patients and their outpatient treaters are instructed to report any early signs of relapse, as an adjustment of the treatment schedule to include a few closely spaced treatments can often prevent relapse (Fox, 2001).

Substantial evidence supports the efficacy of continuation or maintenance ECT treatment in preventing relapse (Petrides et al., 1994; Gagne et al., 2000; Fox, 2001). One recent study examined long-term follow-up of chronically depressed patients who had responded to an acute course of ECT. At 2 years, those who received continuation ECT with antidepressant treatment had a survival rate without relapse or recurrence of 93%, compared to 52% for those on antidepressant treatment alone (Gagne et al., 2000). Another study found that 1-year relapse rates for patients with psychotic depression dropped from 95–42% following the institution of continuation ECT for these patients at their facility (Petrides et al., 1994).

Psychosocial Maintenance

In examining data regarding the effectiveness of pharmacological or ECT maintenance treatment, it is easy to ignore the effect of psychosocial interventions. It is difficult to study the effect of treatment interventions such as individual psychotherapy, group therapy, social day programs, increased family involvement, or moving to a more suitable home environment, but those who work in geriatric psychiatry or medicine will testify to the importance of these interventions. It is therefore important, when treating elderly patients with ECT, to have the help of a geriatric clinician, social worker, or geriatric case manager to help the patient and family with supportive psychosocial measures.

SUMMARY

ECT is a powerful treatment that should be considered as an option in geriatric patients with mood disorders when other therapeutic options have failed or when the illness is so severe that delay in treatment can be life-threatening. As with any serious treatment, the risks and potential benefits need to be reviewed carefully with the patient and family. Elderly patients can present with medical or neurological problems that put them at somewhat higher risk with ECT, but in most patients these problems can be managed safely. Furthermore, because these patients are also at significant medical risk from the depression itself and may be more sensitive to the side effects of many antidepressants, the decision to *not* treat with ECT may in many cases present significant risk to the severely depressed geriatric patient.

REFERENCES

APA. The Practice of Electroconvulsive Therapy: Recommendations for Treatment, Training, and Privileging: A Task Force Report of the American Psychiatric Association, 2nd ed. Washington DC: American Psychiatric Association, 2001, pp 37–40.

Abrams R. The mortality rate with ECT. Convuls Ther 1997; 13(3):125–127.

Applegate RJ. Diagnosis and management of ischemic heart disease in the patient scheduled to undergo electroconvulsive therapy. Convuls Ther 1997; 13(3):128–144.

Avery D, Winokur G. The efficacy of electroconvulsive therapy and antidepressants in depression. Biol Psychiatry 1977; 12(4):507–523.

Beale MD, Kellner CH, Parsons PJ. ECT for the treatment of mood disorders in cancer patients. Convuls Ther 1997; 13(4):222–226.

Black DW, Winokur G, Nasrallah A. Treatment of mania: a naturalistic study of electroconvulsive therapy versus lithium in 438 patients. J Clin Psychiatry 1987; 48(4): 132–139.

Blewett AE, Kareem O. ECT in a patient with psychotic retarded depression, metastatic hepatic cancer, and esophageal varices. J ECT 2000; 16(3):291–294.

Brimacombe JR, Berry AM. Cricoid pressure. Can J Anaesth 1997; 44(4):414–425.

Brodaty H, Berle D, Hickie I, Mason C. "Side effects" of ECT are mainly depressive phenomena and are independent of age. J Affect Disord 2001; 66(2–3):237–245.

Calev A, Nigal D, Shapira B, Tubi N, Chazan S, Ben-Yehuda Y, Kugelmass S, Lerer B. Early and long-term effects of electroconvulsive therapy and depression on memory and other cognitive functions. J Nerv Ment Dis 1991; 179(9):526–533.

Castelli I, Steiner LA, Kaufmann MA, Alfille PH, Schouten R, Welch CA, Drop LJ. Comparative effects of esmolol and labetalol to attenuate hyperdynamic states after electroconvulsive therapy. Anesth Analg 1995; 80(3):557–561.

Ciapparelli A, Dell'Osso L, Tundo A, Pini S, Chiavacci MC, Di Sacco I, Cassano GB. Electroconvulsive therapy in medication-nonresponsive patients with mixed mania and bipolar depression. J Clin Psychiatry 2001; 62(7):552–555.

Coppen A. Lithium in unipolar depression and the prevention of suicide. J Clin Psychiatry 2000; 61(suppl 9):52–56.

Coryell W. Psychotic depression. J Clin Psychiatry 1996; 57(suppl 3):27–31; discussion, 49.

Coryell W. The treatment of psychotic depression. J Clin Psychiatry 1998; 59(suppl 1): 22–27; discussion, 28–29.

Cummings JL, Masterman DL. Depression in patients with Parkinson's disease. Int J Geriatr Psychiatry 1999; 14(9):711–718.

Currier MB, Murray GB, Welch CC. Electroconvulsive therapy for post-stroke depressed geriatric patients. J Neuropsychiatry Clin Neurosci 1992; 4(2):140–144.

Daly JJ, Prudic J, Devanand DP, Nobler MS, Lisanby SH, Peyser S, Roose SP, Sackeim HA. ECT in bipolar and unipolar depression: differences in speed of response. Bipolar Disord 2001; 3(2):95–104.

de Carle AJ, Kohn R. Electroconvulsive therapy and falls in the elderly. J ECT 2000; 16(3):252–257.

Devanand DP, Decina P, Sackeim HA, Prudic J. Status epilepticus following ECT in a patient receiving theophylline. J Clin Psychopharmacol 1988; 8(2):153.

Devanand DP, Polanco P, Cruz R, Shah S, Paykina N, Singh K, Majors L. The efficacy of ECT in mixed affective states. J ECT 2000; 16(1):32–37.

Dolinski S, Zvara D. Anesthetic considerations of cardiovascular risk during electroconvulsive therapy. Convuls Ther 1997; 13(3):157–164.

Eagle KA, Brundage BH, Chaitman BR, Ewy GA, Fleisher LA, Hertzer NR, Leppo JA, Ryan T, Schlant RC, Spencer WH III, Spittell JA Jr, Twiss RD, Ritchie JL, Cheitlin MD, Gardner TJ, Garson A Jr, Lewis RP, Gibbons RJ, O'Rourke RA, Ryan TJ. Guidelines for perioperative cardiovascular evaluation for noncardiac surgery. Report of the American College of Cardiology/American Heart Association Task Force on Practice Guidelines. Committee on Perioperative Cardiovascular Evaluation for Noncardiac Surgery. Circulation 1996; 93(6):1278–1317.

Fall PA, Ekman R, Granerus AK, Thorell LH, Walinder J. ECT in Parkinson's disease. Changes in motor symptoms, monoamine metabolites and neuropeptides. J Neural Transm Park Dis Dement Sect 1995; 10(2–3):129–140.

Fall PA, Granerus AK. Maintenance ECT in Parkinson's disease. J Neural Transm 1999; 106(7–8):737–741.

Fink M. Toxic serotonin syndrome or neuroleptic malignant syndrome? Pharmacopsychiatry 1996; 29(4):159–161.

Flint AJ, Rifat SL. The treatment of psychotic depression in later life: a comparison of pharmacotherapy and ECT. Int J Geriatr Psychiatry 1998; 13(1):23–28.

Flint AJ, Rifat SL. Two-year outcome of psychotic depression in late life. Am J Psychiatry 1998; 155(2):178–183.

Fox HA. Extended continuation and maintenance ECT for long-lasting episodes of major depression. J ECT 2001; 17(1):60–64.

Frasure-Smith N, Lesperance F, Talajic M. Depression following myocardial infarction. Impact on 6-month survival. JAMA 1993; 270(15):1819–1825.

Frasure-Smith N, Lesperance F, Talajic M. Depression and 18-month prognosis after myocardial infarction. Circulation 1995; 91(4):999–1005.
Frith CD, Stevens M, Johnstone EC, Deakin JF, Lawler P, Crow TJ. Effects of ECT and depression on various aspects of memory. Br J Psychiatry 1983; 142:610–617.
Fromm-Auch D. Comparison of unilateral and bilateral ECT: evidence for selective memory impairment. Br J Psychiatry 1982; 141:608–613.
Gagne GG, Jr., Furman MJ, Carpenter LL, Price LH. Efficacy of continuation ECT and antidepressant drugs compared to long-term antidepressants alone in depressed patients. Am J Psychiatry 2000; 157(12):1960–1965.
Glue P, Costello MJ, Pert A, Mele A, Nutt DJ. Regional neurotransmitter responses after acute and chronic electroconvulsive shock. Psychopharmacology 1990; 100(1): 60–65.
Gormley N. ECT should be treatment option in all cases of refractory depression. Br Med J 1998; 316(7126):233.
Grant JE, Mohan SN. Treatment of agitation and aggression in four demented patients using ECT. J ECT 2001; 17(3):205–209.
Henry ME, Schmidt ME, Matochik JA, Stoddard EP, Potter WZ. The effects of ECT on brain glucose: a pilot FDG PET study. J ECT 2001; 17(1):33–40.
Hochberg F, Pruitt A, Neoplastic diseases of the central nervous system. In: Wilson JD BE, Isselbacher KJ, Petersdorf RG, Martin JB, Fauci AS, Root RK, eds. Harrison's Principles of Internal Medicine. New York: McGraw-Hill, 1991, p 2014.
Iwanami A, Oyamada S, Shirayama Y, Kamijima K. Algorithms for the pharmacotherapy psychotic depression. Psychiatry Clin Neurosci 1999; 53(suppl):S45–S48.
Katz IR, Simpson GM, Curlik SM, Parmelee PA, Muhly C. Pharmacologic treatment of major depression for elderly patients in residential care settings. J Clin Psychiatry 1990; 51(suppl):41–47; discussion, 48.
Lee Y, Choi K, Lee YK. Association of comorbidity with depressive symptoms in community-dwelling older persons. Gerontology 2001; 47(5):254–262.
Lloyd L, Armour PK, Smith RJ. Suicide in Texas: a cohort analysis of trends in suicide rates, 1945–1980. Suicide Life Threat Behav 1987; 17(3):205–217.
Manly DT, Oakley SP Jr, Bloch RM. Electroconvulsive therapy in old-old patients. Am J Geriatr Psychiatry 2000; 8(3):232–236.
Mann S, Caroff S. Electroconvulsive therapy of the lethal catatonia syndrome: case report and review. Convuls Ther 1990; 6(3):239–247.
McAllister DA, Perri MG, Jordan RC, Rauscher FP, Sattin A. Effects of ECT given two vs three times weekly. Psychiatry Res 1987; 21(1):63–69.
Meyer J. Importance of ischemic damage to small vessels in experimental cerebral infarction. J Neuropathol Exp Neurol 1958; 17:571–585.
Milic CT. [Age as a suicide risk factor]. Vojnosanit Pregl 2000; 57(2):191–195.
Miller AR, Isenberg KE. Reversible ischemic neurologic deficit after ECT. J ECT 1998; 14(1):42–48.
Moellentine C, Rummans T, Ahlskog JE, Harmsen WS, Suman VJ, O'Connor MK, Black JL, Pileggi T. Effectiveness of ECT in patients with parkinsonism. J Neuropsychiatry Clin Neurosci 1998; 10(2):187–193.
Mukherjee S, Sackeim HA, Schnur DB. Electroconvulsive therapy of acute manic episodes: a review of 50 years' experience. Am J Psychiatry 1994; 151(2):169–176.

Murray GB, Shea V, Conn DK. Electroconvulsive therapy for poststroke depression. J Clin Psychiatry 1986; 47(5):258–260.

Nobler MS, Oquendo MA, Kegeles LS, Malone KM, Campbell CC, Sackeim HA, Mann JJ. Decreased regional brain metabolism after ect. Am J Psychiatry 2001; 158(2): 305–308.

Nolen WA, Haffmans PM, Bouvy PF, Duivenvoorden HJ. Monoamine oxidase inhibitors in resistant major depression. A double-blind comparison of brofaromine and tranylcypromine in patients resistant to tricyclic antidepressants. J Affect Disord 1993; 28(3):189–197.

O'Connor MK, Knapp R, Husain M, Rummans TA, Petrides G, Smith G, Mueller M, Snyder K, Bernstein H, Rush AJ, Fink M, Kellner C. The influence of age on the response of major depression to electroconvulsive therapy: a CORE Report. Am J Geriatr Psychiatry 2001; 9(4):382–390.

Parker G, Hadzi-Pavlovic D, Hickie I, Mitchell P, Wilhelm K, Brodaty H, Boyce P, Eyers K, Pedic F. Psychotic depression: a review and clinical experience. Aust N Z J Psychiatry 1991; 25(2):169–180.

Parker G, Roy K, Hadzi-Pavlovic D, Pedic F. Psychotic (delusional) depression: a meta-analysis of physical treatments. J Affect Disord 1992; 24(1):17–24.

Patkar AA, Hill KP, Weinstein SP, Schwartz SL. ECT in the presence of brain tumor and increased intracranial pressure: evaluation and reduction of risk. J ECT 2000; 16(2):189–197.

Peabody CA, Whiteford HA, Hollister LE. Antidepressants and the elderly. J Am Geriatr Soc 1986; 34(12):869–874.

Penninx BW, Geerlings SW, Deeg DJ, van Eijk JT, van Tilburg W, Beekman AT. Minor and major depression and the risk of death in older persons. Arch Gen Psychiatry 1999; 56(10):889–895.

Petrides G, Dhossche D, Fink M, Francis A. Continuation ECT: relapse prevention in affective disorders. Convuls Ther 1994; 10(3):189–194.

Petrides G, Fink M. Atrial fibrillation, anticoagulation, and electroconvulsive therapy. Convuls Ther 1996; 12(2):91–98.

Petrides G, Fink M, Husain MM, Knapp RG, Rush AJ, Mueller M, Rummans TA, O'Connor KM, Rasmussen KG Jr, Bernstein HJ, Biggs M, Bailine SH, Kellner CH. ECT remission rates in psychotic versus nonpsychotic depressed patients: a report from CORE. J ECT 2001; 17(4):244–253.

Philibert RA, Richards L, Lynch CF, Winokur G. Effect of ECT on mortality and clinical outcome in geriatric unipolar depression. J Clin Psychiatry 1995; 56(9):390–394.

Pirl WF, Roth AJ. Diagnosis and treatment of depression in cancer patients. Oncology (Huntingt) 1999; 13(9):1293–1301; discussion 1301–1292, 1305–1296.

Rao V, Lyketsos CG. The benefits and risks of ECT for patients with primary dementia who also suffer from depression. Int J Geriatr Psychiatry 2000; 15(8):729–735.

Rasmussen KG, Zorumski CF. Electroconvulsive therapy in patients taking theophylline. J Clin Psychiatry 1993; 54(11):427–431.

Rice EH, Sombrotto LB, Markowitz JC, Leon AC. Cardiovascular morbidity in high-risk patients during ECT. Am J Psychiatry 1994; 151(11):1627–1641.

Robinson DG, Spiker DG. Delusional depression. A one year follow-up. J Affect Disord 1985; 9(1):79–83.

Rosenberg J, Pettinati HM. Differential memory complaints after bilateral and unilateral ECT. Am J Psychiatry 1984; 141(9):1071–1074.

Rubin EH, Kinscherf DA, Figiel GS, Zorumski CF. The nature and time course of cognitive side effects during electroconvulsive therapy in the elderly. J Geriatr Psychiatry Neurol 1993; 6(2):78–83.

Rummans T. Medical indications for electroconvulsive therapy. Psychiatr Ann 1993; 23(1):27–32.

Sackeim HA, Haskett RF, Mulsant BH, Thase ME, Mann JJ, Pettinati HM, Greenberg RM, Crowe RR, Cooper TB, Prudic J. Continuation pharmacotherapy in the prevention of relapse following electroconvulsive therapy: a randomized controlled trial. JAMA 2001; 285(10):1299–1307.

Sackeim HA, Prudic J, Devanand DP, Decina P, Kerr B, Malitz S. The impact of medication resistance and continuation pharmacotherapy on relapse following response to electroconvulsive therapy in major depression. J Clin Psychopharmacol 1990; 10(2):96–104.

Salaris S, Szuba MP, Traber K. ECT and intracranial vascular masses. J ECT 2000; 16(2):198–203.

Satlin A, Liptzin B, Diagnosis and treatment of mania. In: Salzman C, ed. Clinical Geriatric Psychopharmacology. Baltimore: Williams & Wilkins, 1998, p 310.

Schulz R, Beach SR, Ives DG, Martire LM, Ariyo AA, Kop WJ. Association between depression and mortality in older adults: the Cardiovascular Health Study. Arch Intern Med 2000; 160(12):1761–1768.

Serby M. Manic reactions to ECT. Am J Geriatr Psychiatry 2001; 9(2):180.

Shapira B, Tubi N, Drexler H, Lidsky D, Calev A, Lerer B. Cost and benefit in the choice of ECT schedule. Twice versus three times weekly ECT. Br J Psychiatry 1998; 172:44–48.

Small JG, Small IF, Milstein V, Kellams JJ, Klapper MH. Manic symptoms: an indication for bilateral ECT. Biol Psychiatry 1985; 20(2):125–134.

Stewart JT. Prolongation of ECT-induced seizures with theophylline. J Am Geriatr Soc 1996; 44(4):475.

Stoudemire A, Hill CD, Morris R, Dalton ST. Improvement in depression-related cognitive dysfunction following ECT. J Neuropsychiatry Clin Neurosci 1995; 7(1): 31–34.

Stoudemire A, Hill CD, Morris R, Martino-Saltzman D, Markwalter H, Lewison B. Cognitive outcome following tricyclic and electroconvulsive treatment of major depression in the elderly. Am J Psychiatry 1991; 148(10):1336–1340.

Taylor JR, Tompkins R, Demers R, Anderson D. Electroconvulsive therapy and memory dysfunction: is there evidence for prolonged defects? Biol Psychiatry 1982; 17(10): 1169–1193.

Tew JD Jr, Mulsant BH, Haskett RF, Prudic J, Thase, ME, Crowe RR, Dolata D, Begley AE, Reynolds CF III, Sackeim HA. Acute efficacy of ECT in the treatment of major depression in the old old. Am J Psychiatry 1999; 156(12):1865–1870.

Thase ME, Frank E, Mallinger AG, Hamer T, Kupfer DJ. Treatment of imipramine-resistant recurrent depression, III: Efficacy of monoamine oxidase inhibitors. J Clin Psychiatry 1992; 53(1):5–11.

Trollor JN, Sachdev PS. Electroconvulsive treatment of neuroleptic malignant syndrome: a review and report of cases. Aust N Z J Psychiatry 1999; 33(5):650–659.

Weeks D, Freeman CP, Kendell RE. ECT: III: Enduring cognitive deficits? Br J Psychiatry 1980; 137:26–37.

Weintraub D, Lippmann SB. Electroconvulsive therapy in the acute poststroke period. J ECT 2000; 16(4):415–418.

Welch C. ECT in medically ill patients. In: CE Coffey, ed. The Clinical Science of Electroconvulsive Therapy. Washington DC: American Psychiatric Press, 1993, pp 167–182.

Welch C. Cardiovascular Effects of ECT. Convuls Ther 1989; 5(1):35–43.

Wengel SP, Burke WJ, Pfeiffer RF, Roccaforte WH, Paige SR. Maintenance electroconvulsive therapy for intractable Parkinson's disease. Am J Geriatr Psychiatry 1998; 6(3):263–269.

Wijkstra J, Nolen WA, Algra A, van Vliet IM, Kahn RS. Relapse prevention in major depressive disorder after successful ECT: a literature review and a naturalistic case series. Acta Psychiatr Scand 2000; 102(6):454–460.

Wingate BJ, Hansen-Flaschen J. Anxiety and depression in advanced lung disease. Clin Chest Med 1997; 18(3):495–505.

Zielinski RJ, Roose SP, Devanand DP, Woodring S, Sackeim HA. Cardiovascular complications of ECT in depressed patients with cardiac disease. Am J Psychiatry 1993; 150(6):904–909.

Zvara DA, Brooker RF, McCall WV, Foreman AS, Hewitt C, Murphy BA, Royster RL. The effect of esmolol on ST-segment depression and arrhythmias after electroconvulsive therapy. Convuls Ther 1997; 13(3):165–174.

12

Psychotherapy with Depressed Older Adults

Francesca Cannavo Antognini
McLean Hospital, Belmont, and Harvard Medical School, Boston, Massachusetts, U.S.A.

Back in the 1920s, Sigmund Freud made known his view of psychoanalysis with older adults (Freud, 1924, p. 258): "Near and above the fifties, the elasticity of the mental processes on which the treatment depends is as a rule lacking—old people are no longer educable, and on the other hand, the mass of material to be dealt with would prolong the duration of the treatment indefinitely."

This view still persists to some extent today, as one finds relatively few young practitioners—especially psychologists, who treat patients primarily through psychotherapy—specializing in geriatrics. However, the number is gradually increasing, perhaps in anticipation of the "graying boomers," as the oldest members of the largest generation in history now enter their mid-50s. Even beyond the issue of numbers and need, there are some other very important factors in considering the over-65 age group for psychotherapy. One is the nature of the challenges facing this group precisely by virtue of their age. Another is the efficacy of psychotherapy as an empirically validated treatment for depression at any age and for geriatric patients in particular.

OLDER ADULTHOOD AS A DEVELOPMENTAL STAGE

Erikson et al., (1986) and Muslin (1992), among others, have conceptualized older adulthood as a stage of life that carries with it the same complexity of developmental tasks presented by earlier life stages. Erikson, famous for his eight psychosocial stages of development (e.g., Erikson, 1982), in later years expanded on his treatment of old age as a time of conflict between integrity and despair (Erikson, et al., 1986). Erikson describes the older adult as challenged to integrate the strength and purpose necessary to maintain a sense of wholeness in the face of physical decline. Similarly, Muslin, in the theoretical framework of Kohut (1971), stresses the fragmentation of the self which threatens older adulthood. According to Muslin, older adults at risk of such fragmentation may be fixated on the younger self, unable to accept the transformations of self which come with age. As these individuals experience multiple age related failures and losses over time, such as role changes, loss of independence and occupational success, they experience aging as "truly tragic" (p. 34) and are at high risk for depression. The resulting fragmentation of self is accompanied by "disintegration anxiety," (p. 36) as psychological and physical drives, as well as body parts and organs, formerly integrated into a cohesive self, split off into a "free state" (p. 41) and become the object of obsessive focus. Offsetting or resolving these issues is a process involving considerable psychological resources, drawing in part on having successfully passed through previous developmental stages. The following is Muslin's conceptualization of a "crystallized" (as opposed to fragmented) elderly self (1992, p. 30):

> The elderly self is a self that has adapted, not adjusted, to its somatic limitations . . . [and] to the limitations imposed by the cultural institutions in the family, on the job, and in the reactions of the culture toward aging . . . unique values and unique ambitions that are particular to this specific group of aged persons who have passed through the described stages mark the person as a member of the elderly group in the culture to which he or she belongs . . . the badge signifying membership . . . is not age, but rather the fact that one has undergone the self transformations that mark one as elderly. . . .

Erikson et al., emphasizing the importance of wisdom, offer a slightly different focus (1986, p. 56):

> The elder is challenged to draw on a life cycle that is far more nearly completed than yet to be lived, to consolidate a sense of wisdom with which to live out the future, to place him- or herself in perspective among those generations now living, and to accept his or her place in an infinite historical progression . . . wisdom is detached concern with

> life itself in the face of death itself. It maintains and learns to convey the integrity of experience, in spite of the decline of bodily and mental functions. [Erikson et al., p. 37]

For Erikson, despair can "win out" in the older adult if wisdom is absent or not accessed.

Given the increased medicalization of conceptualizations of depression and its treatments, a question that naturally arises from these formulations is how the chances for successful long-term recovery from depression can be enhanced by psychosocial interventions, either as adjuncts or alternatives to psychopharmacological treatments, for what may be, at least in part, a psychologically determined illness.

THE EFFICACY OF PSYCHOTHERAPY IN THE TREATMENT OF GERIATRIC DEPRESSION

The efficacy of specific psychotherapeutic techniques in the treatment of depression for the adult population in general has been demonstrated repeatedly over the past 2½ decades. Some studies yield results demonstrating that cognitive behavior therapy is comparable to medication in alleviating depression (cited in McGinn, 2000). Others show that psychotherapy alone is as effective as psychotherapy plus medication in cases of mild depression, but that combined therapy is more effective for severe recurrent depression (Thase et al., 1997). Unfortunately there is a relative dearth of such studies for geriatric populations; the overwhelming percentage of studies of treatment for geriatric depression have focused primarily on medication (Gerson et al., 1999). However, those studies that have included psychotherapy as an independent variable—including cognitive behavior therapy, behavior therapy, psychodynamic therapy, interpersonal therapy, and problem-solving therapy—have yielded promising results. In a metanalysis of 17 published studies of the efficacy of various forms of psychotherapy with geriatric depressed patients in the absence of medication, Scogin and McElreath (1994) found an overall mean effect size of 0.78 for psychotherapy as compared to no treatment and to placebo control groups. Both individual and group therapy modalities were presented across the studies; treatment subjects showed significantly less posttreatment depression than those in control groups over all levels of depression severity (subclinical to major depressive disorder). In a subsequent meta-analysis of data published from 1974–1998 regarding treatment of patients over age 55 with depression, Gerson et al. (1999) stress the paucity of studies that include psychotherapy as a form of treatment. In those that did investigate the effectiveness of psychotherapy, behavior therapy, cognitive behavior therapy, and psychodynamic approaches were found to be significantly more effective than placebo; moreover, response rates to these nonpharmacological therapies did not differ significantly from those observed with antidepressants. The authors added, however, that direct comparison data were not sufficient to allow conclusive statements about comparative efficacy. In another study, three forms of psychotherapy alone (behavioral, cognitive, and brief psychodynamic) performed separately on three groups of geriatric patients with major depressive disorder had significant effects on subsequent maintenance of recovery (Thompson et al., 1987). A later study (Reynolds et al., 1999) on the effects of interpersonal psychotherapy and the antidepressant nortriptyline on recurrence rates in geriatric depressed patients over a 3-year period yielded the following recurrence rates across groups: 20% for patients treated with psychotherapy combined with medication, 43% for patients receiving medication only, 64% for psychotherapy-only patients, and 79% for the placebo group. These same authors conducted a study comparing responsiveness of "young old" patients (age 60–69) with middle-aged patients to the same forms of treatment (Reynolds et al., 1996). The results yielded no significant difference in responsiveness, although the younger patients recovered faster. In a related subsequent study, the results for patients above age 70 compared with those in their 60s were less promising, with "excellent" short-term response but significantly more long-term relapse in the older group (Reynolds, 1999). It is clear that there is a dearth of empirical data on psychosocial treatments with older depressed adults and a strong need for support of such research. The studies that have been done suggest that, at least in some cases, psychotherapy may be a viable alternative to medication for depressed older patients. However, as stated by one researcher of psychosocial treatments with depressed older adults, "these results notwithstanding, in clinical practice, combined treatment with both medication and psychotherapy is extremely common, and perhaps should be considered a standard of care" (Niederehe, 1996, p. 871). Clearly, an intervention cannot be justified based solely on its frequency of use. Interestingly, an expert panel of 50 geriatric psychiatrists recently endorsed psychotherapy as a first-line option in minor depressive disorder in older adults, and if the symptoms have persisted for 2–3 months, "their preferred strategy is to begin antidepressant medication in combination with psychotherapy, but they would also consider using medication or psychotherapy alone" (Alexopoulos et al., 2001, p. 27). For major depressive disorder in geriatric patients, these same experts recommend a combination of antidepressant medication and psychotherapy as the treatment of choice, with medication alone as another first-line strategy. The danger, however, is that given staff shortages and budget cuts, hospitals appear to be moving more and more in the direction of using pharmacotherapy alone and far less commonly adding adjunctive psychotherapy. This would be a lamentable trend, especially given the fact that the research does suggest that combined treatments are more effective. Indeed, as one major group of researchers states, "because few studies have compared psychosocial and pharmacologic therapies for geriatric depression, it seems premature to advocate one modality over another" (Scogin and McElreath, 1994, p. 73).

THE OLDER ADULT'S VIEW OF PSYCHOTHERAPY

In an illuminating article regarding the factors to consider in treating older adults, Knight (1999) stresses the importance of contextual and cohort based effects: "in many ways, working with someone from another cohort is like working with someone from another culture" (p. 930). Similarly, Zarit and Zarit (1998) stress the importance of generational differences: "The key to overcoming a client's current problems lies not within our generational framework, but in that of the client's" (p. 29). The people considered "old" today were born during the first 40 years of the twentieth century. Although this time span encompasses two generations, the entire cohort experienced catastrophic world events that affected virtually every household: the Great Depression and World War II. Whether as children or adults during one or both of these times of sociological and economic upheaval, these older adults as a group demonstrate a stoicism uncharacteristic of younger generations. Self-reliance was a most prized coping strategy during the Great Depression (Tice and Perkins, 1996), practiced by those who were young adults at the time and modeled for their children. Indeed, the tendency to minimize distress is so pronounced in this cohort that it is one factor which impedes the assessment of experienced pain in older patients; their stoicism in tending to underreport the intensity of pain makes pain management difficult (NARI, 1999). In response to asking older adults how they managed to get through "tough times" in their lives, one may hear: "we had no choice," "you did what you had to do," "that's just the way it was." There is marked de-emphasis on "feelings," perhaps precisely because to focus on emotion would have meant breaking through the adaptive denial that enabled them to "keep going" in their younger years during times of crisis. Generally, older adults seem to find it easier to express distress indirectly or somatically (Zarit and Zarit, 1998). When asked how they "feel," older adults tend to refer to physical rather than emotional states; in reporting depressive symptoms, older depressed adults more often express hypochondriacal concerns than do younger depressed adults (Brown et al., 1984).

While stoicism and discomfort with emotional expression may contribute to a hesitation to engage in psychotherapy, time may be an equally deterring factor for the aging adult. A reaction not unheard of from an older adult to a proposal of psychotherapy is: "I will be in my grave before it even starts to work." This is perhaps based on the outmoded view of psychotherapy as a process synonymous with psychoanalysis—years of involvement and "talk" with a very slow return (Mathiasen and Levert, 1997). A related assumption is that psychotherapy involves a major overhauling of the self, provoking a sense of hopelessness in the older adult: "I'm too old to change" (Thompson et al., 1992). A powerful factor in this cohort that further dampens enthusiasm for therapy is a stigmatizing view of mental illness. The older adults of today remember a time when "mental institutions" were filled with unmedicated patients, many of whom were likely suffering from manic or psychotic episodes and, in the absence of medication, had to be contained behind locked doors and barred windows (Gallagher-Thompson and Coon, 1996). Such memories may induce a feeling of shame and deter patients from even admitting that they are depressed. Thus, seeking psychotherapy may be viewed as part of a process along a continuum of "craziness." Indeed, many older adults seem to prefer the term *counseling*, with its implications of seeking advice in the form of "counsel," as one would from a lawyer.

While the barriers to the older adult's initiation of the therapeutic relationship appear daunting, these same factors may actually enhance the process once the older adult is engaged in psychotherapy. The focus away from feelings may motivate older adults more toward behavioral change, which flies in the face of the commonly held notion, especially among lay people, that psychotherapy is an indulgent process that only perpetuates self-preoccupation. While the physical limitations of older adults may necessitate frequent cancellations, older patients tend to be quite conscientious about responsible communication when such difficulties arise. Older adults tend to be compliant about the homework assigned in cognitive behavioral approaches, which, as noted earlier, are among the more effective forms of intervention. Additionally, the focus on family may actually serve to give family problems, when they arise, greater significance and therefore give patients more incentive to problem solve. Finally, the dictum of "keeping a stiff upper lip" may be motivating in that when stoicism fails, there is great pressure to do anything possible to restore even the pretense of effective coping, if only for the benefit of the outside world or family members.

Another factor that may serve to enhance the success of therapy with older adults is the wisdom of experience (Zarit and Zarit, 1998). Older adults, with the enormous fund of knowledge and insight that comes with longevity, may tend to be more realistic about the effort and work involved in change and not as quick to assume or expect a rapid "miracle cure," as do younger people. Moreover, paradoxically, the sobering realization of the finiteness of their existence gives older adults an ability to savor the "little things" in life, an appreciation that may generalize to an acceptance of the "microincrements" of improvement that tend to characterize progress in psychotherapy. This effect is enhanced by the fact that for this cohort and perhaps for older adults in general, patience and politeness are considered virtues. Indeed, it has been noted that the patience of the older adult in treatment may exceed that of the therapist (Finkel, 1991). While it might be argued that the latter two traits inhibit the patient's direct and candid interaction with the therapist (a valuable process for both therapist and patient), a nonconfrontational stance on the part of the patient may in the long run permit more objective processing of therapeutic input. Nuegaren and Schenider (1998) go so far as to say that as older adults become more inwardly focused, an observation originally made by Carl Jung (1939), they also become more reflective and philosophical, making them even more suitable for psychotherapy than are younger people.

AGE-RELATED FACTORS INHIBITING THERAPEUTIC PROGRESS

A number of additional factors to be considered in the therapy of older adults have to do less with beliefs and attitudes and more with the physical effects of aging. As noted earlier, the older adult tends to define feelings in somatic rather than emotional terms. While this is in part of a sociological and psychological phenomenon of this cohort, it also may derive from the fact that the somatic correlates of depression—gastrointestinal problems, insomnia fatigue, organically unexplained pain—may be more pronounced or exacerbated because of the physical effects of aging. Older adults tend much more than younger people to have coexisting mental and physical ailments (Sheikh, 1996). A significant period of therapeutic time with the older adult may be spent processing these physical complaints, at least in the early stages of therapy. Related to this, of course, are the physical and neurological concomitants of aging, which interfere on a purely logistical level. Hearing loss makes communication difficult at times (Thompson et al., in Myers, 1991). Short-term memory difficulties, whether simply age-related or secondary to depression or early dementia, may present problems with retention of information from one session to the next as well as tendencies on the part of the patient to repeat several times information previously communicated to the therapist. Prostatic hypertrophy in men or prolapsed bladder in women increases the urgency and frequency of bathroom visits, and aches and pains make sitting for prolonged periods uncomfortable. The degree to which these factors interfere with a patient's ability to sustain the therapeutic focus is, of course, in part dependent on personality factors and/or emotional state.

THE "GEROTHERAPIST" AND THE PATIENT: ENGAGING AND TREATING THE OLDER ADULT

Many older adults come to a psychotherapist at the behest of another—perhaps a primary care physician or a grown child. The first case contact may in fact be with a family member rather than the patient herself (Zarit and Zarit, 1996). The patient may arrive somewhat skeptical of the process, perhaps never having seen a therapist before or having had a history of negative experiences with the mental health system. The earlier-noted stigma of seeing a mental health professional may complicate matters further. There may be some anger at having been "coerced" into this visit, or at least some wariness or distrust of this professional, who may well be no older than the patient's children. And yet the politeness so characteristic of this cohort may inhibit expression of any of these feelings or reservations directly to the therapist, especially in the early stages of treatment. Mindful of the above, it is prudent for the therapist to assume that any or all factors may be at play, regardless of the patient's presentation. Furthermore, it is of paramount importance that the therapist be aware of his or her own attitudes and biases regarding aging. Newton and Jacobowitz (1999) point out that because so many older adults nowadays are segregated into senior centers, assisted living facilities, and nursing homes, less experienced geriatric therapists may have an impression of older adults based chiefly on relationships with parents and/or grandparents. Thus, beginning geriatric clinicians must educate themselves about various aspects of the aging process, distinguishing stereotype from fact. One strategy in remedying therapist ignorance about the phenomenological experience and behavioral manifestations of older adulthood is to grant the patient his or her expertise in issues of aging. Especially with respect to cohort issues, "the therapist must recognize the likelihood of his/her ignorance or misunderstanding, and must convey to the patient a sincere respect for assistance in remedying this ignorance" (Kivnik and Kafka, 1999; in Duffy, p. 114). Erikson et al. (1986) go so far as to assert that while the older patient is using therapy to rework and renew balances around a number of previously unresolved psychosocial stages, the lack of the therapist's own resolution of any of these psychosocial themes may undermine the success of the process.

Muslin (1992) outlines an approach to beginning therapy with the elderly client that, though formulated from a self-psychology model, can be adapted to any therapeutic approach. He recommends beginning with an "empathic diagnosis" to assess the patient's functioning in any areas of the self, from self-worth to self-values. Possible findings include a "mirror-hungry self," an "ideal-hungry self," or an "enfeebled or empty self" (p. 56). The development of the "self/self object bond" (p. 56) through the relationship with the therapist provides gradual restitution of the equilibrium of self. This requires constant attention on the part of the therapist to details of the interview as well as the creation of a safe haven for the patient to disclose his or her problems and to develop the necessary trust to incorporate the therapist's validation. To facilitate this, the therapist may bring in special objects of interest to the patient—such as books, magazines, and tapes—to further demonstrate the therapist's interest in the older adult as a unique individual. Kivnik and Kavka (1999) carry this one step further: "Elders often come for therapy because they are unable to secure the caring they feel they need from family sources. . . . the therapist must convey to the client a real sense of being cared about, and of having care to give, in return" (in Duffy, p. 122). Thus, older adults benefit not only from the caring of the therapist but also by reacquainting themselves with their own ability to care for another; through caring gestures toward the therapist, such as perhaps bringing gifts or educating the young therapist about historical events they have lived through. Brody (1999), expounding on Rollo May's existential approaches, offers the optimistic observation that "If the therapist accepts the existential view of humans as always in a state of 'becoming,' of being in a state of crisis without despairing, then a therapist can work with any cohort, including the elderly, in a participatory, helpful way" (p. 92).

THEORETICAL MODELS OF PSYCHOTHERAPY AND ADAPTATIONS FOR OLDER ADULTS

Various therapeutic approaches to treating depression have been developed. Four approaches have appeared in the literature most often in recent years: psychodynamic psychotherapy, cognitive behavioral therapy, and, more recently, interpersonal therapy and problem-solving therapy. The latter three are often termed *empirically validated treatments*, as they can be formalized and their effects quantified. While some studies indicate greater effectiveness of one of these approaches over another in the treatment of depression, cognitive behavioral therapy being perhaps the most often cited, other studies show relatively equal efficacy across all four approaches (see earlier cited studies). The few comparative studies done with older patients are consistent with these findings (e.g., Niederebe, 1996, Gallagher-Thompson et al., 1990). Of the four theoretical approaches, psychodynamic and cognitive behavioral therapy tend to be those forms of verbal intervention with which clinicians in today's mental health settings are most familiar and each is therefore treated in some detail in this chapter. The two other approaches—interpersonal therapy and problem-solving therapy—have appeared increasingly in the literature on older adults over the last 10 years.

Interpersonal therapy (IPT) was developed by Klerman and Weissman (1984) based on the interpersonal theories of Harry Stack Sullivan (1953). The premise is that disruption interpersonal relationships increases an individual's risk for depression. The theory argues further that major depressive disorder has damaging effects on the interpersonal relationships of the depressed person, which persist even into recovery. Development of interpersonal therapy for older adults is based on the finding that older patients with major depressive disorder who had a strained relationship with a spouse or adult child had poorer outcomes 1 year after leaving the hospital (Hinrichsen and Zweig, 1994). IPT addresses four possible interpersonal problem areas: grief (complicated bereavement), interpersonal disputes (conflict with significant other), role transition (significant changes in a life situation), and interpersonal deficits (lack of social skills). In the earlier noted series of studies of treatment efficacy with major depression in older adults, Reynolds et al. (1994, 1996, 1997, 1999) used interpersonal therapy as their psychosocial independent variable, with consistent success. This is an appealing form of treatment for older adults in that it is time-limited (16–20 sessions), focused on the present, and emphasizes action rather than exploration and insight (Markowitz et al., 1997).

Problem-solving therapy (PST) has a similar here-and-now focus. The premise is that depression results when deficits in problem solving lead to ineffective coping strategies in times of stress. Arean et al. (1993) outline an adaptation of problem-solving therapy for older adults that involves training in developing an appropriate orientation to coping with depression and its associated problems, labeling emotions as cues for problem identification, inhibiting automatic responses, better defining the nature of a problem, generating a range of alternative solutions, systematically evaluating the potential consequences of various solutions, and monitoring and evaluating the outcome after the chosen solution is implemented. These researchers compared the effects of problem-solving therapy and reminiscence therapy (RT) on major depressive disorder in geriatric patients. While both groups receiving therapy improved compared to a waiting list control group, PST was found to be significantly more effective than RT in relieving depressive symptoms.

Of all approaches studied, psychodynamic therapy is the oldest approach, having evolved from psychoanalysis. The theory behind this form of psychotherapy is that events which took place early in life have shaped one's current psychological state and should therefore be uncovered, explored, and worked through. Thus, relationships with parents become a focus of discussion, as well as the "transference"—i.e., the transferring of the patient's feelings about significant early relationships and objects into the therapeutic relationship and projecting them onto the therapist. "Insight" is achieved when the patient can meaningfully connect his or her current reactions with early experiences and resulting unconscious conflicts and in so doing come to realize that his or her current responses are outmoded. It is thought that at this point, change becomes possible. In the words of Leigh and Varghese (2001), "It has been argued that, as death draws closer, older individuals may become more reflective, more aware of life's vicissitudes, and have an increased need to get on with living. The process of psychodynamic psychotherapy involves helping the individual to understand and make sense of these vicissitudes, in order to get on with living" (p. 229). In contrast to Freud's earlier cited pessimism about the plasticity and responsiveness of older adults in psychotherapy, Myers (1991) argues that the defenses of the older individual are more malleable than the defenses of younger people. Indeed, when asked to recall their childhood years, many older adults will initially respond with: "Oh, that was a long time ago," but with some encouragement will go on to describe, in exquisite detail, recollections of their early years. The therapist takes care to emphasize the fact that therapy is not undertaken to assign blame to people in one's past but to understand the origins of one's feelings and behavior. It becomes important for the therapist to join the older adult in his or her schema of acceptance of parents and/or significant others and to avoid encouraging expressions of anger, especially early in the process, which could jeopardize the alliance with the patient. The older adult's successful engagement in the psychodynamic process can shed light on feelings and behaviors in current interpersonal relationships, such as those with grown children, which recapitulate old life themes. In the words of Nordus and Neilson (1999), who use an "integrative dynamic" model in short-term psychodynamic therapy with older adults, "In the client's attempt to satisfy need gratification or to establish and maintain satisfying relationships, he or she typically acts in ways that unintentionally elicit repetition of past traumatic experiences and disappointments" (p. 936). The following is a reconstruction of a psychodynamically oriented session with a 72-year-old widow, Mrs. R., admitted to the hospital with agitated depression and passive suicidal ideation a few months after bypass surgery:

Patient: I feel so anxious. I talk to my kids, they tell me to go walking every day for my heart, but I just don't feel like it.
Therapist: Do you connect your anxiety with these conversations?
Patient: Well, yes, sometimes. I feel guilty because I can't do it . . . they just don't understand . . . (tearfully) they're so good to me . . .
Therapist: It makes you sad when they reach out to you in this way.
Patient: They really care, but they have busy lives, and I don't want to burden them any more. They were there for me after the surgery . . . and now I'm depressed. No one else cares about me so much, and I'm always letting them down. How can I be so ungrateful?
Therapist: You say no one else cares so much. Have you always felt this way?
Patient: Well, at least since my husband died. He did everything for me, but I was his whole life. And he was mine, of course. The kids shouldn't have to worry about me (tearful). I'm becoming such a burden that they may just wind up burning out on me.
Therapist: It seems like it's hard for you to feel OK about being cared for when you can't give anything in return. But wasn't there a time when you were there for your children?
Patient: That was different. I was their mother; it was my job. I gave them a lot, and now I can't give them anything (tearful).
Therapist: You worked very hard as a parent.
Patient: I was determined to give them everything I missed out on.
Therapist: Such as?
Patient: Well, I don't know . . . (pause) . . . my mother got so depressed

after my father left her. They had no medicine for it back then. She would be in bed for days. I did all I could to help her, but I was so young. When my brothers went off to war it was just me and her. I couldn't do much.

Therapist: How did her depression affect her caretaking of you?

Patient: I don't know . . . she did the best she could. I tried to stay out of her way. It was hard sometimes. But she was always building me up, telling me how good I was and how I'd make a great wife and mother someday.

Therapist: How about when you just behaved like a child? Or when you needed support yourself?

Patient: I don't remember . . . it was a little lonely . . . I don't remember misbehaving. . . . Actually it would have been unthinkable (laugh).

Therapist: How so?

Patient: I'm not sure, really . . . she might have given up on me . . . well, thought less of me, I don't know.

Therapist: So it was hard to feel that you could just be a kid and have your mother feel as good about you as she did when you were helpful and did what you were told.

Patient: Yes, but if she weren't depressed . . . if my father had stayed . . . everything would have been different. She loved me in her own way.

Therapist: Yes, that's probably true. But I wonder if your experience of your mother's depression is having some impact on your feelings about your own depression.

Patient: What do you mean?

Therapist: Well, I have two thoughts. One is that you may fear that your depression is causing the same pain for your children that your mother's depression caused for you. And secondly, you may be afraid that if you don't do what you're told by your children, they will give up on you, just as you feared your mother would, if you disobeyed or misbehaved.

Patient: I don't know. . . . I think I'm different from my mother. I've tried to be there for them always, even when I was depressed before. My mother couldn't help herself. I guess . . . well, maybe I'm being a little hard on myself. Is that what you're thinking?

Cognitive behavior therapy (CBT) is a form of treatment based on the premise, formulated by Aaron Beck (1979), that negative feelings such as depression and anxiety derive from maladaptive thought patterns. A triggering event produces a reaction in the form of a "dysfunctional automatic thought," which in turn generates a feeling. Habitual negative thoughts can result in chronic depression and/or anxiety. According to Beck, depression develops in the context of an individual's "cognitive triad" of negative beliefs ("schemata") about self, environment, and future. CBT, through mood monitoring (recording of dysfunctional thoughts and resultant feelings) and exploration of more adaptive cognitions, has been widely employed in ameliorating anxiety and depression. In the behavioral component of CBT, a variety of techniques—including assertiveness, social skills training, and behavioral scheduling—are used to modify dysfunctional behaviors that may result from maladaptive thoughts. In the first study to demonstrate the efficacy of a psychosocial treatment over medication in the treatment of depression, Rush et al. (1979) found CBT to be more effective than tricyclic antidepressants in patients suffering from clinical depression. The Rush study later came under criticism for methodological flaws; however, other studies have continued to demonstrated that CBT holds up well when compared to psychopharmacological interventions (McGinn, 2000). A number of studies have demonstrated the effectiveness of CBT, using a few modifications with older adults (e.g., Scogin et al., 1994; Teri et al., in Dick-Siskin, 2002). The treatment can be performed individually or in groups. Dick-Siskin (2002) recommends that before beginning CBT, the geriatric patient should be evaluated on a measure of gross cognitive functioning, such as the Folstein Mini-Mental State exam (Folstein, 1975), to provide a baseline with which to compare suspected changes in cognitive function as well as a guide regarding the volume of material that can be covered in one CBT session and the feasible complexity of homework assignments. She goes on to recommend the use of large-type handouts, audiotaping of sessions for older adults with mild cognitive impairment or anxiety, and providing frequent breaks in the session to summarize the material. Therapists administering CBT to geriatric patients should also be sensitive to the feelings of infantilization (at times so poignant but unexpressed in older adults) that might be engendered by the assignment of homework, as in the case of the occasional patient who will comment, "It feels like I'm back in third grade." However, we find that older adults take well to cognitive behavioral therapy, given its focus on the present, its educational component, and its time-limited, goal-oriented approach. The following session is a hypothetical reformulation of the session presented in the previous section as it would proceed from a cognitive behavioral approach:

> *Patient*: I don't know—I feel so anxious. I talk to my kids on the phone, they tell me to do all these healthy things—go walking for my heart, every day, clean the house, stay on a diet—but I just don't feel like doing it all.
>
> *Therapist*: What do you think to yourself after those conversations?
>
> *Patient*: I think that I don't want to do it all, I can't, but they won't be happy if I don't.

Therapist: And if they're not happy?
Patient: Well . . . they might get fed up with me. They might just say, "she's hopeless" and give up on me.
Therapist: So, if you don't follow a suggestion they make, they will just give up on you. Do you detect some catastrophic thinking there?
Patient: I guess so. But they keep making these suggestions—they love me, how can I let them down? They have their own busy lives. I'm such a burden.
Therapist: So the fact that you don't follow their suggestions makes you a burden.
Patient: Well, I tell them I'm going to do what they say—I promise to, and then they call to check and I haven't done it. So they keep worrying, but soon enough they're going to get tired of worrying.
Therapist: If you know you are going to have difficulty doing all those things, what makes you promise to do them? Do you have a specific thought that makes you promise, rather than just saying you don't think you can?
Patient: They might get angry. Or they might think I don't respect their opinion. "You don't bite the hand that feeds," my mother always said.
Therapist: So they might get angry. What would that mean for you?
Patient: Oh, God, it would be awful to have my children angry at me. I can't imagine what it would be like.
Therapist: Well, how do they react when you tell them you haven't done what they wanted?
Patient: I don't know . . . they get impatient, they sigh, they sound exasperated with me.
Therapist: It doesn't sound like they actually get angry, though. Or fed up, as you fear. They do keep calling.
Patient: Yeah, I guess. But I try to avoid their calls when I haven't done the things they want me to do. And then I feel more guilty.
Therapist: I wonder if you would feel less like avoiding them if you told them that you weren't yet ready to do all the things they suggest.
Patient: I can't seem to get myself to be, well, assertive. I just agree, and then hide.
Therapist: When your children call and suggest you do something, you have, up to now, been thinking to yourself that you can't disagree, because they might get angry and give up on you. But what's the evidence for that?
Patient: None, I guess. It hasn't happened yet. But I'm afraid it will.
Therapist: Let's assume the worst, that they do get angry. What would happen then?

Patient: Well they might not want to see me and then I would really be alone.

Therapist: Do you think that you would be alone for a long time?

Patient: Well, they might get fed up with me—I don't know. You know, my mother was depressed too, and she always expected a lot of me. And now it's my kids. I guess I'm getting kind of fed up too.

Therapist: So I wonder if you think to yourself: "this sounds like my mother, telling me to do something I don't want to do. If I say no, I'll be letting them down, just like I let her down."

Patient: Yeah, something like that, I guess.

Therapist: Can you think of a more adaptive thought? Something more related to the here and now, which would help you ask them not to expect you to do something you're not quite ready to do, and to tell them that that you will get to it in your own time?

Patient: Gee, that sounds great, when you say it. But I don't know if I can. I don't know what to think to help myself. That old fear keeps popping up.

Therapist: You remember that we have often talked about how depression involves a feeling of helplessness, and how assertiveness helps with that feeling.

Patient: Yes.

Therapist: So, it might help your depression to be assertive in this situation as well.

Patient: Yes, but if they get angry it will depress me more.

Therapist: Earlier, you said the worst thing about your children getting angry would be they might not want to see you.

Patient: Yes.

Therapist: And then?

Patient: Well . . . I'll feel lonely.

Therapist: How often do you see your children?

Patient: Well, maybe once every two weeks or so.

Therapist: And how do you make out when they're not visiting?

Patient: Oh, of course I'm okay. I have friends in the building, we play bingo and bridge. There's always something to do. Although lately I don't feel like it so much.

Therapist: Do you think your children would never want to see you again if you asserted yourself?

Patient: (chuckling) I guess that's kind of silly. No, I imagine they'd get over it eventually.

Therapist: So what can you say to yourself to help yourself be assertive when they tell you what to do?

Patient: Well . . . first, I guess, I could tell myself that its important to be assertive so I can feel less depressed. And then, that they probably won't really be all that angry, but if they are, I'll survive—I guess (laugh). And maybe I won't have to avoid their phone calls and feel so guilty if I don't do the stuff they want me to do. How's that, Doctor? Actually, it doesn't seem so bad; I think I could do it.

TOWARD AN INTEGRATIVE APPROACH

It is not uncommon for therapists who have been trained in a specific approach to use that approach almost exclusively, sometimes with good outcome, but at other times with the unfortunate result that the patient has been forced into a "therapeutic" Procrustean bed. Clearly, the theory must be adapted to fit the patient, rather than the other way around. With older patients in particular, flexibility is a major factor in therapeutic success. Some older patients loathe dwelling on the past for any length of time and may resist a solidly psychodynamic approach. Others object to the "intellectual" nature of cognitive behavior therapy, especially when the treatment is presented in formulaic fashion, as is the case when less experienced therapists employ the many treatment manuals that are now on the market. In the author's clinical experience with this population, an approach that considers both the events of the past and the beliefs and assumptions of the present, moving flexibly back and forth between the two as needed, is quite effective. I call this approach *gerodynamic psychotherapy*. "Looking back" with the patient to identify and consider the impact of certain early experiences on his or her current belief system and then working in the here-and-now from a CBT framework toward modifying "outmoded" or "obsolete" maladaptive cognitions and behaviors provides a solid foundation for change. As noted earlier, it should be stressed to the patient that in looking back and identifying contributing factors, the purpose is to explain, not to blame. Returning to the case of Mrs. R., above, a gerodynamic approach would involve a more deliberate integration of the material in the psychodynamic session and the CBT session, elucidating for the patient how her childhood experiences with a depressed mother contributed to her current maladaptive assumptions about her own children, generating a spiral of self-defeating behaviors. It should be noted that while the "looking back" component of gerodynamic psychotherapy is formulated psychodynamically, the "here-and-now" work need not be restricted to CBT but might also include approaches from other theoretical models, such as IPT and PST. What makes the integrated approach especially relevant to older adults is that it can be used flexibly, with as little or as much stress on the past as the patient can tolerate and with a less concentrated, slower pace in the CBT phase that replaces the intense, task-oriented focus one might attempt with younger adults with a more gradual, "microincremental" approach tailored to the patient's capabilities. (An extensive treatment of gerodynamic psychotherapy is in progress for future publication by the author.)

OTHER TREATMENT MODALITIES

Group Therapy

Why would group therapy be considered a useful approach with older adults, many of whom prefer a context of individual attention? Group therapy has many benefits and, given its greater cost-efficiency in this era of managed care, is increasingly becoming the most common form of psychotherapy on inpatient units with patients of all ages. It is also a less costly form of outpatient therapy, which is of benefit to those older adults with modest incomes. Group therapy has in fact been shown to be an effective form of treatment for depression in older adults (e.g., Thompson et al., 1983; Steuer et al., 1984; Beutler et al., 1987; Lewisohn et al., 1992). Contraindications to group interventions with older people include severe hearing loss, evidence of personality disorder, and a prior history of poor response to group treatment (Zarit and Zarit, 1998). For most older adults, however, group therapy has a variety of advantages over individual therapy. Moberg and Lazarus (1990) expound on these benefits—namely, the opportunity for personal feedback, given the tendency of older adults to emphasize faults and minimize strengths; the importance of "resocialization" and "remotivation" to combat loneliness and facilitate relationships; the enhancement of self-esteem through realization that the problems of aging are not unique to oneself; and the emotional catharsis involved in allowing isolated older adults to express feelings of self-pity, guilt, and failure (p. 404). Moberg and Lazarus cite the opportunity to express and share existential concerns—including anxiety about death and the wish to find meaning in life—as being of particular value. Citing an unpublished work by Davis and Williams, Moberg and Lazarus comment on the benefits of inpatient group treatment for depressed older adults: "Universality and instillation of hope are particularly curative factors in inpatient settings, where patients often feel isolated and hopeless in the midst of severe mental illnesses" (p. 404). Once the initial resistance has passed, older patients in group therapy often bond quite intensely with each other. This is facilitated by group therapy's focus on concerns that are unique to older adults: physical decline, losses, and changing family relationships. The group becomes a haven for commiserating about these inevitable changes, and this process becomes invaluable in reducing feelings of isolation and uniqueness. Especially in outpatient groups, patients share ideas and resources with each other on how to cope with the various challenges of aging.

One may speculate that the characteristics of the current cohort of older adults described earlier, namely their hesitancy to reveal personal problems and their view of mental illness as a stigma, might diminish their receptiveness to group therapy, especially in the early stages of the process. However, these very characteristics may make group therapy especially important for older adults, as the group shares and demystifies problems that may seem unique and shameful, thus mitigating the stigma associated with depression. In the author's treatment settings, for example, where patients are transitioned through progressively less restrictive levels of care, those who have been hospitalized become well acquainted and eventually quite comfortable with the process of group therapy, so that they experience their involvement in outpatient groups as a natural transition from more intensive treatment. For newcomers to the process, group therapy may be a more appealing alternative to the stigma older adults associate with seeing a psychiatrist. In our experience, the older adult, perhaps as a form of rationalization, often views group therapy more as an educational experience, referring to the group as a "class." Other cohort characteristics, such as politeness, may result in fewer challenges for the geriatric group therapist. Older adults in groups tend to be more supportive then confrontational. Myers (1991) cites studies showing that older adults are more tolerant of silence and of "monopolists," holding onto the belief that they each get a turn if they wait. Competitive issues are not as common as they are in younger groups and, if present, are less likely to be expressed. In our experience, one benefit of this tendency toward greater tolerance and patience among older adults is a reduced need for the therapist to attend to group process issues, permitting a more direct focus on substantive clinical and life problems. This may seem a departure from traditional views about what the focus of group therapy should be (i.e., analysis of group dynamics as a microcosm of social interaction). However, the fact that group therapy is no longer offered primarily as an adjunct to individual therapy to assist a patient in resolving social issues, but is, for economic reasons, becoming the primary if not the only available form of psychotherapy in many treatment settings demands some rethinking of group focus and goals, especially with older adults. This trend also has some impact on the structure of group therapy itself. Given that group psychotherapy may be the only mode of treatment aside from pharmacological intervention, the primary goal remains relief of depression for each group member. "Contact work" (Yost et al., 1986)—i.e., serial focus on each individual within the context of the group—often becomes an integral part of the treatment, while the other group members are invited to offer their own relevant experience and feedback to the patient who is "on." In supportive group therapy, the contact work may take the form of speaking about a particular problem or "challenge" that presented itself in a patient's life since the last session and/or reporting on progress toward a goal. Ideally, all the members will receive a turn, although in the case of large groups this requires some skill on the part of the therapist to direct and limit the sharing. The following is an example of contact work in a partial hospitalization therapy group with Mrs. D., a depressed, somatic patient who developed severe but medically unexplained foot pain after her daughter began working full time and became less available:

Mrs. D.: I can't function. I'm nobody now. It's no use; I can't do anything.
Patient 1: You got here today!
Mrs. D.: You didn't know me before. Coming here is nothing; I come by cab. It's a far cry from what I used to do. I can't walk on these feet. And I can't find the right shoes anywhere. I don't know how many pairs I've had to return. They feel all right in the store, but then when I get home and wear them awhile they're just not right. . . . Janice has been taking me to shoe stores on her lunch hour on Thursdays, a half hour here, an hour there when she has the time. I know when I find the right shoes I'll be able to get around better and not rely on her so much. Now I have to rely on my neighbor to take me with her to the supermarket. Janice helps with the shoes because it's a medical issue. She has no time for food shopping any more on Saturdays, what with the job and the kids.
Patient 2: Reminds me of my daughter. They're so busy, carting the kids here and there.
Therapist: The pain in your feet must be very distressing. You have to deal with two things at once, the pain itself and the fact that you can't get around on your own any more.
Mrs. D.: I feel like my life is over. I can't get around, Janice has no time, what's there left?
Therapist: Back before all this pain started, and before your daughter was working, what was it like?
Mrs. D.: Well . . . I felt well. Janice and I would go to Star Market on Saturday morning, then on the way back we would pick up sandwiches at this deli nearby and after she helped me put the food away we would sit in the kitchen and eat together . . . they made the best pastrami sandwiches outside New York . . . all together we had just an hour or two to talk. But she's very busy now. She has a very responsible job. My daughter's very talented. My son-in-law does more around the house now, which is good for Janice. He even answers the phone now . . . it used to be her. The kids are teenagers, and they're helping too.
Patient 3: You know we did so much for our kids, but now that we're old . . .
Mrs. D.: Sorry, I don't see it that way. We did what we had to do. They don't owe us anything.

Patient 2: Well, but don't you feel like, well, she should have time for you? You are her mother.
Mrs. D.: Well . . . the kids need her more. Although I guess I need her just a little bit now . . . you know, for the shoes.
Therapist: We all need our loved ones. You must miss those Saturdays with her.
Mrs. D.: Oh, for sure. I don't know what to do with myself. Going with my neighbor is all right, but she's not interested in lunch. Anyway, she's Chinese and she probably doesn't like pastrami (laughter). But I'm having more trouble going with her now that my feet are really bad.
Patient 1: Does your daughter know how much you miss that Saturday time?
Mrs. D.: She must know. But she can't do anything about it.
Patient 1: Have you told her?
Mrs. D.: What's there to tell? She works now and can't be bothered. And I can't bother her with my troubles.
Patient 2: I don't mean this badly, but aren't you already bothering her about your shoes?
Mrs. D.: Well that's something I really need. I don't need to be more of a burden by telling her how much I miss her.
Therapist: You feel it would burden her to know how much you valued your time with her. Does anyone else have any thoughts about that?
Patient 4: My daughter tells me it drives her crazy when I don't tell her how I feel. She tells me I hold grudges. I don't but she says I'm not direct enough.
Patient 3: They're too busy with the kids to be bothered. I don't want to be a bother, and I'm sure (Mrs. D.) feels that way too.
Patient 1: Why is it so easy for us to ask them to do things for us, but when it comes to telling them we just want to see them more, or maybe that we're just lonely, we can't?
Mrs. D.: Well in my case, the shoes are very important because without them I won't be able to walk anywhere. I have to ask her to help me find the right ones. They used to have these Space Shoes. Janice and I can't find them anywhere.
Therapist: So let's look at all this for a minute. A number of you seem to agree with the idea that it is easier to ask for help with practical things than to let your children know that you are lonely, or that you wish you could see them more. I wonder if that makes it easier to feel the physical needs more than the emotional.
Mrs. D.: So you're saying my feet don't really hurt?
Therapist: Not at all. Your pain is very real. But I think it's a lot easier

to allow yourself physical than emotional feelings. As Mrs. A (Patient 1) said, its easier to let your children know about the physical needs than the emotional needs.

Mrs. D.: Well I should be stronger. I shouldn't need my daughter so much.

Therapist: Reactions from the group?

Patient 1: I feel that way too sometimes. But I don't think my daughter feels that way. She actually sounds more sympathetic when I tell her how lonely I am. She has very little time, like your daughter, but she softens a little when she hears me say that. I can hear it in her voice and just that helps, even if she can't see me much. Don't you think so?

Mrs. D.: I don't know. I've never really told her. She's really very good about the shoes. But if she really wanted to be there for me on Saturday I guess she could still make the time.

Therapist: So maybe you're a little miffed with her too?

Patient 2: I would be. She dropped you like a hot potato. That's what we get for all the time we put in when they need us. My kids are scattered around the country, they never even call. You're lucky—at least she takes you shoe shopping (laughter).

Therapist: Listening to all the feedback you've gotten, Mrs. D., what do you think?

Mrs. D.: I guess I could tell her. Maybe if she just sees me for lunch on Saturday. . . . maybe not every Saturday, even just once a month, for the pastrami sandwich!

Patients: Forget the food shopping! (laughter)

Group therapy may be performed from a particular theoretical framework. CBT in group format is increasingly becoming a popular treatment with older adults on inpatient units, as it is considered an effective form of short-term intervention (see the discussion of CBT above). In group CBT, a "lecturette" on a particular topic may precede serial contact work (Yost et al., 1986). The topic is usually a theme universal to older depressed patients: coping with transitions, loss, aging, family issues, etc.—all discussed from a cognitive behavioral approach focusing on the modification of maladaptive cognitions that can produce change in these areas (see earlier section on individual CBT). Homework is often assigned to help a patient track and modify dysfunctional thoughts ("mood monitoring") between sessions. During contact work, the individual focus is often made relevant to the topic; patients may be asked to share completed homework or share their thoughts and experiences regarding the topic at hand.

Reminiscence therapy (RT) is a form of group therapy undertaken almost exclusively with older adults. This form of therapy, also called *life-review therapy*, has been shown to be moderately effective for late-life depression (Molinari, 1999). Based on the idea that looking over one's life can result in an enhanced sense of identity and accomplishment, patients are asked to recall and share meaningful events in their lives. A structured modification of life-review therapy for use with depressed older adult inpatients and for older adults with mild cognitive impairment, which the author has developed and called *retrospective focus therapy* (RFT), involves having patients recall and share challenging events in their lives that they dealt with successfully and then helping them to identify the personal qualities in their "character" that helped them to cope at the time. This is designed to bring depressed patients in touch with their strengths, which become the object of focus as enduring personality traits that persist despite depressive episodes, raising hope, decreasing "learned helplessness" (Seligman, 1975), and enhancing self-esteem and a sense of identity—particularly important for the patient in cognitive decline. In more long-term groups, this may be facilitated by having patients construct a "time/lifeline" that can be referred back to at each session to facilitate recall of additional events. For more detailed consideration of specific theoretical models of group therapy with older adults, including cognitive behavioral and psychodynamic group work, the reader is referred to a number of informative articles (see the references at the end of this chapter).

Couples Therapy with Depressed Older Adults

Couples therapy, a rewarding and productive modality of treatment for older adults, has received little attention in the literature. The issue of couples therapy for depressed older adults is more fully addressed in chapters on caregiver burden and case management in this volume; is it therefore treated here in limited scope. While one may not often encounter older adults seeking marital therapy as self-referred outpatients, it is not uncommon for the need for couples therapy to emerge as a result of the treatment of one member of the couple, either in an inpatient or partial hospitalization program. The recommendation may be made for a variety of reasons: perhaps the patient's spouse is having difficulty managing stress as a consequence of the patient's depression, perhaps the well spouse is having difficulty understanding the nature of the illness and is withdrawing from or criticizing the patient, or perhaps the patient has something to address in the relationship that is contributing to his or her distress. This section focuses on the long-married or cohabitating couple in which one member has become depressed. The older couple seeking therapy in such cases is dealing with change, perhaps of crisis proportions, that derives from the illness of one of the partners. Expectations must change, including perhaps the long-awaited enjoyment of the retirement years, as the depressed spouse's illness "may impose a lifestyle that is increasingly restricted to the home and limited to the activities of self and domestic maintenance" (Gilleard, 1996, p. 567). Historically successful patterns of functioning between the members of the couple may be breaking down or no longer working. Furthermore, the illness may be accentuating longstanding difficulties that have, over the years, been dealt with in a dysfunctional but lasting equilibrium, now destabilized by the imbalance of the illness of one spouse. For example, one may observe a "historic lack of reciprocity in sharing tasks, absence of any shared outlook on the nature of marital life, and a chronic inability or unwillingness of one or both to understand the perspective of the other" (Gilleard, 1996).

It is most useful, initially, to involve the older couple in an assessment of their strengths, their perceptions, and their handling of the current problem as well the resources that they have available (family, friends, other treaters or caretakers). The evaluative phase can also be therapeutic, as the assessment of the relationship's assets will include emphasis on the longevity of the relationship as a sign of success and strength. Therapy ideally begins with acknowledgment and reinforcement of this fact. A relationship of 50 years is a demonstration of long-term equilibrium, regardless of how dysfunctional that equilibrium may appear to the outside observer or even to the partners themselves! In the context of this focus, the couple's successful coping mechanisms are identified and explored. Since the couple is seeking help, it is appropriate to point out that some sort of breakdown has occurred but to attribute it to the situational change rather than to the personal failure of either or both members. This can also serve to move the couple away from blame and unite them around a problem they are attempting to deal with together, albeit with difficulty. The therapist should then proceed to work on the problem at hand and avoid wandering into other territory, despite the temptation to change certain patterns, especially if they are longstanding. As Rosowsky (1999) points out in her informative essay on couple therapy with older adults, the old adage "If it ain't broke, don't fix it" is a good general rule in treating elderly couples; in doing otherwise the therapist risks losing the alliance and ultimately, the couple. The same author introduces a useful metaphor: "boat and baggage," referring "to the vessel the couple are in, together, negotiating the uncharted waters of old age. The baggage refers to their old resentments and hurts, which they can choose to unload to lighten their load and enhance the safety and comfort of their passage" (p. 264).

As a final word, it is important to note that depression may be accompanied by a reduction or impairment in a couple's sexual relationship and that this may become a factor motivating the couple to pursue therapy. Such couples may be referred by a primary care physician; however, the sexual dysfunction, although deeply troubling to both individuals, may be difficult for them to discuss openly. This becomes relevant especially for patients on certain antidepressant medications, which may affect sexual desire and functioning. Although a discussion of this important form of couples therapy with older adults is beyond the scope of this chapter, the reader is referred to a sensitive and informative work by Helen Singer Kaplan (1991), the renowned expert in sex therapy with older adults, who underscores the need for attention to this often neglected dimension of the older couple's relationship:

> Though it is widely believed that sex no longer matters as an individual gets older, the opposite is often true. Sex may become more important in a person's life with the passage of time because sexuality is among the last of the pleasure-giving biological processes to deteriorate. It is a potentially enduring source of emotional well-being at a time when more and more losses must be accepted and fewer and fewer gratifications remain available. [Myers, p. 37]

Family Therapy

As with couples therapy, family interventions are treated more extensively elsewhere in this volume; however, a discussion of psychotherapy would not be complete without some mention of this important modality, especially with the older adult. The literature on the structure and efficacy of family therapy with older adults is scanty. Family work with a depressed older adult as the identified patient can take the form of either didactic, psychoeducational interventions or the more traditional family therapy approaches that view the family as a system containing both the problem and the resources for its solution (Gilleard, 1996). Common presenting themes in family treatment with depressed older adults include marital difficulties (see preceding section); caregiver burden; major transitions and losses, such as a move to an assisted-living facility or the death of a spouse; and/or intergenerational issues, most commonly relationships with grown children. Family therapy is rarely sought directly by the depressed older adult but is most often initiated by a grown child, spouse, individual therapist, or other involved treater. In an informative essay on family therapy with the older adult, Qualls (1999) identifies the last stage of the family cycle as the time, following the "launching" of grown children, when adults recognize the growing dependence of their own parents. She goes on to point out that grown children are often in denial about the degree of decline in an elderly parent because to recognize it would mean facing changes in their own roles and acknowledging their own mortality as they move closer to becoming the "omega generation" (Hagestaad, 1998)—i.e., the next generation of the family in line to die. Qualls proposes several foci of family intervention with the older adult, including labeling and educating, that facilitate the identification of problems and revision of expectations. Thrust into "filial maturity" by the parent's decline, a grown child may be forced to "take the reins" in a role reversal, which may involve an adjustment to the fact that the ill parent is no longer in an advising, supportive, or caretaking role. Clearly, relinquishing the parental role may be at least as hard for the depressed older adult as its effects are for the grown child, especially considering the Depression-era cohort's view of self-reliance as a prized virtue (see earlier section). In our experience, it is helpful for members of both generations to share their discomfort with and distress over such role reversals in a safe therapeutic context, as this provides a common ground on which to base mutual coping strategies and ongoing communication.

Gilleard (1996) stresses the importance of family assessment, which also serves as an intervention. Citing the work of Neidhart and Allen (1992), he identifies four stages of family evaluation: [1] identification of past history and future possibilities, using a life-events calendar to identify emergence of the problem in the context of the family's own life cycle to pinpoint key transitions within the family history and acknowledge the family's hopes and fears for the future; [2] identification of family structure and boundaries through the use of a genogram; [3] identification of communication patterns through clinical first-hand observation of the family; and [4] discovery of the "hidden dynamics" that are creating, maintaining, or intensifying the family's problems. Regarding the process of family therapy itself with the older adult, Benbow (1993) distinguishes between direct and indirect therapeutic techniques with families where the older adult is the identified patient. Indirect techniques include circular questioning, positive reframing, restraining change, and paradox, while direct techniques include genogram interpretation, communication work, advice giving, and recommendations. Pointing out that the noted "indirect techniques" are the essence of family therapy as opposed to "family work," Gilleard (1996) asserts that "there is a need for greater research to demonstrate the benefits of systemic approaches (with older adults) over and above those associated with informing and advising the family" (p. 572).

SPECIAL APPLICATIONS

The Depressed Older Man in Psychotherapy

It is widely acknowledged that depression affects greater numbers of women than men, in a ratio of roughly 2 to 1. On geriatric inpatient units, females tend to predominate, and therefore much of the experience gained by clinicians doing therapy with geriatric patients has been with women. However, older men have a greater percentage of suicides than any other group (Pollack, 1999); therefore, from a preventive point of view, this high-risk group deserves special attention. Pollack, writing from a psychoanalytic framework, traces the roots of depression in men to the abandonment by the nurturing mother necessitated by the healthy resolution of the Oedipus conflict: "Unearthed from beneath layers of repression and anger, a deep sadness often comes forward, a delayed mourning for a tragic loss. This premature push for separation in boys is not a healthy form of self-differentiation but rather a traumatic disruption of their early holding environment" (p. 208). In contrast, the female's resolution of her early attachment to her father necessitates a continuing, socially acceptable bond with the nurturing mother, so there is no such disruption. One wonders about the possible connection between the early "abandonment depression" in males and the fact that the death of a spouse has been associated with increased mortality for the older male (Jacobs and Ostfeld, 1977). Further complicating the situation for males, Pollack adds, is the fact that boys are shamed into the suppression of all vulnerable emotions. In treating depression in older men, Pollack asserts, special attention must be given to symbolically recreating the holding environment originally provided by the lost mother, as well as being sensitive to the shame harbored by the male for both his unresolved dependency and his resultant depression. The latter may well be exacerbated for today's older male, as the current cohort of elders tend to feel that suffering from depression, as well as direct expression of emotion, stems from weakness. The majority of these men were the family breadwinners and, as noted earlier, stoicism was a favored response to distressing circumstances. To be incapacitated by what they regarded as an emotional disturbance meant to fail rather than to fall ill. And to visit a therapist was an admission of that failure. In defense against these feelings of shame and failure, depressed men may experience and express their distress somatically to justify obtaining the support they need (Huyck and Guttman, 1999). And for older depressed men with legitimate pre-existing somatic concerns, this may be an easy albeit maladaptive form of avoidance. Huyck et al. stress that it is important for the therapist to be aware of this defensive maneuvering and "to suggest, by an accepting, concerned manner, that the patient will not be shamed or rebuffed if he dispenses with the somatic defense and brings his depressed, hungry feelings into the treatment" (p. 89). Sprenkel (1999), in a discussion of group therapy with older men, recommends reframing the goal of therapy as "doing better" rather than "feeling better." Engaging the older male patients in active problem solving can move the overt agenda away from emotion while empowering the man to take charge of his own situation and, in the context of group therapy, help others to do so as well.

In the treatment of older men, seemingly superficial topics can catalyze discussion of more emotionally laden issues. For example, many older men are eager and willing to talk about their working years. This not only enhances self-esteem in a depressed older man but can serve as a jumping-off point for discussions about the experience of retirement, which is not uncommonly a trigger for a depressive episode, and feelings about providing for family, which many older men continue to strive to do through helping their grown children with the purchase of homes and the education of grandchildren. While addressing work issues, the therapist can reinforce the patient's sense of competence by reminding him of his accomplishments in the past, which still count, and the impact that the sharing of his wisdom and experience can have on his children and grandchildren. In individual and/or group therapy, this can often be accomplished by asking older men to recall a time in their lives when they faced a very difficult challenge and how they coped with or resolved the situation. In response to this, men will often share their experiences during World War II or the Korean War or even memories of working as adolescents to help their families during the Depression years.

The Suicidal Older Patient

The older patient with suicidal ideation is often seen on an emergency basis and perhaps ultimately admitted to an inpatient unit as the result of overtly expressed suicidal intent or an actual suicidal gesture or attempt. Of course, he or she may also initially present in an outpatient setting. Clinicians working with older adults may notice that the experience of a depressive episode can in itself induce a "metadepression," resulting in suicidal ideation as the older person feels that this is the "end of the road" and his or her loss of functioning is permanent.

The patient with suicidal ideation presents a crisis of sorts for the evaluating clinician, particularly for the less experienced therapist. Feeling a tremendous responsibility bordering on panic, the therapist may rush to "contract for safety" with the suicidal patient. While this is an important move and its outcome may determine whether the patient is hospitalized, its timing is equally important. (The assessment of suicidality is treated elsewhere in this book.) Asking a patient immediately to verbalize assurance that he or she will not commit suicide in the next 24 hours may serve more to relieve the therapist's anxiety than to guarantee the patient's safety. Attention has been given recently in the literature to the importance of giving the patient the time and encouragement to share fully with the therapist his or her intense emotional pain or "psychache" (Schneidman, 1996) and for the therapist to attempt to "empathize with the patient's pain experience to such a point that he/she can 'see' why suicide is the only alternative" (Orbach, 2001, p. 173). Indeed, it has been shown that the factor that correlates most strongly with suicide potential is an extreme sense of hopelessness (Beck et al., 1974, 1990, 1993). Older people, facing the numerous forms of irreversible decline and loss as they age, are particularly prone to feelings of hopeless and helpless (McIntosh et al., 1994). Sharing these feelings with a therapist is a form of reaching out, however feeble, indicating some degree of hope that help may be offered. The patient must be assured both that the therapist understands and appreciates his or her despair and, at the same time, that there is some reason to go on living. The following is an excerpt from a session with a 68-year-old widow hospitalized after overdosing on lorazepam on the 2-year anniversary of her husband's death:

> *Patient*: I was fine for awhile. Everyone stepped in—the kids, Sam's family . . . they were all there. I didn't have to lift finger for the funeral.

For awhile, they all called. I got invited by our friends. You know, most of them are still around. Sam died young. Too young. We could have had another 20 years together. Anyway, they were always calling. Then there was the financial stuff to deal with. Unfortunately, our finances were a mess. Sam loved good times, and he was so much fun to be around . . . everyone loved him, but he wasn't much of a planner. So I spent time talking to lawyers, accountants . . . there was so much to do.

Therapist: So you're saying that in the first few months after his death, you had a lot of support from family, and friends called for awhile after that. And settling the finances kept you busy for quite some time also.

Patient: Yes, but that's all over now. Its all settled. My children are busy with their own lives now. Sam's family I don't hear from much any more. And the friends . . . it feels like they've forgotten about me. You know, I'm just a fifth wheel now, the odd person out with no husband. So whom do I have? Nobody. Nobody called on Sunday, his anniversary. That was the last straw. Nobody remembered. Nobody cared if I was dead or alive.

Therapist: You must have felt very alone. Did you think of calling someone yourself?

Patient: I shouldn't have to. They know I'm there. They know I've had anxiety and depression. They just don't care. Now that I'm in the hospital they're all concerned and calling. But its too late. No matter what they do, I don't want to go on.

Therapist: I imagine that you must on some level feel pretty angry at your family.

Patient: Angry? Well, upset, I suppose. Wouldn't you be? But then again, they have their own lives. Their kids are more important than an old lady like me (crying). How can you or anyone possibly understand? Its no use.

Therapist: You feel you don't matter any more, your life doesn't matter any more.

Patient: (relieved) That's exactly how I feel.

Therapist: I don't know what your pain feels like, because I'm not you, but I'd like to try to understand, so that we can work together to help you feel better. You have taken a good first step in sharing your thoughts and feelings so honestly today. Together, you and I and the rest of your team will work toward a solution that you will come to see as preferable to ending your life. We don't know what that is yet, but it will become clearer as we work together.

Notice that the therapist encourages some expression of anger—which is not infrequently a covert component of suicide. The therapist also reduces the patient's profound sense of aloneness through a number of "we" statements and attempts to empower the patient through reinforcement of her ability to express her feelings. Finally, the promise of a better "solution" gives the patient a sense of hope. In subsequent sessions, patients may be asked to make lists of things they have to live for. The therapist can and should assume a very proactive stance in this, as the patient herself may be at a loss. As a final word, it is often useful to educate the patient about the impact of a successful suicide on other family members, in particular the increased likelihood that close relatives may see suicide as a solution. While some may object that this may engender guilt feelings in an already depressed patient, it should be remembered that, since the suicidal act was not successful, any guilt is usually temporary and may be replaced by motivation to avoid a repetition of the behavior.

Clearly, family involvement is an important component of treating suicidality in the elderly, both for the benefit of the family in dealing with the depressed member and to mobilize the patient's support network and facilitate the patient's direct communication of his or her needs and feelings with loved ones. Bringing in family members also permits a thorough assessment of the family's functioning, which is also helpful in understanding the precipitants and outcome of a suicidal act. Richman (1996), in a discussion of family therapy with suicidal elderly, states: "To understand suicide we must explore at least three generations, especially how the family deals with loss and bereavement . . . suicidal events may be inseparable from the relationships between the generations . . . unresolved mourning can usually be traced back to at least three generations in depression and suicide-prone families" (p. 655). Underscoring the importance of the family's response to a suicidal gesture, he cites the work of Stengel (1964), who argued that the outcome of a suicidal act depends upon its consequences: "if it brings people closer, no further suicidal or other self destructive behavior will take place. If nothing changes, or if the situation becomes worse, the result is further suicidal behavior and completed suicides" (Duffy, p. 653). Finally, treatment of the family becomes important when one remembers that family members of a patient who has completed suicide are at risk for suicide themselves (McIntosh, 1994).

A variety of theoretical approaches have been employed to treat the suicidal adult. Studies suggest that psychosocial treatments such as CBT and interpersonal therapy are effective in reducing feelings of hopelessness in suicidal adults (Szanto et al., 1998). Aaron Beck, who, with his colleagues, developed the Beck Hopelessness Scale to assess suicide potential in adults (Beck et al., 1974), is a strong proponent of CBT in the treatment of suicidal ideation. In this schema, feelings of hopelessness derive from negative thoughts, such as

"It's all over for me," "I will always feel this lonely," "no one cares about me," etc. According to Beck (1974) the patient may, for example, engage in catastrophic thinking and overgeneralization in coming to maladaptive and inaccurate conclusions about his or her situation. This can occur at any age, but older adults, with their vulnerability to a variety of losses, are particularly at risk. Through examining the evidence for their conclusions, patients can begin to question their negative thinking, generate more realistic thoughts, and reduce their feelings of hopelessness.

The Depressed Older Adult with Personality Disorder

Patients with personality disorders present significant challenges in the therapeutic process. There are many types of personality disorders, and a discussion of psychotherapy with these patients could fill an entire volume. Here, some connections between personality disorder and depression in older adults are addressed in order to discuss their implications for psychotherapy.

Researchers have observed that there is a significantly greater proportion of personality disorders among older adults with a history of depression (Abrams et al., 1987). Sadavoy (1999) identifies the "immature" personality disorders involving impulsive behaviors—antisocial, borderline, and histrionic—as those that tend to diminish behaviorally by middle age, although the underlying psychodynamics may remain the same. Thompson et al. (1988) found that two-thirds of their sample of depressed patients met criteria for personality disorders during the depressive episode, but only one-third did so after remission. They argue for caution in the diagnosis of a personality disorder during an acute depressive episode. Other theorists emphasize the importance of determining the presence of a personality disorder in the depressed older adult, as such disorders are frequently associated with prolonged treatment or treatment failure and relationship complications (Sadavoy, 1999). Thompson et al. (1988) found that elderly patients with personality disorders benefit less from short-term therapy than patients with no clear personality disorder. Following short-term treatment with CBT, behavior therapy, or brief psychodynamic therapy, depressed patients without a diagnosed personality disorder had a tenfold rate of success compared to those with personality disorder. Noting that there are no published outcome data on the psychotherapeutic treatment of personality disorders in older adults, Lynch (2002) has proposed an adaptation of dialectical behavior therapy (DBT)—a form of CBT developed for patients with borderline personality disorder (Linehan, 1993)—for older adults with personality disorder. He has already used a variant of DBT to treat depressive illness in older adults, with some success.

Zarit and Zarit (1998), in discussing the difficulties of the depressed personality-disordered patient, point out that older adults with personality disorders are more isolated, partly because of poor social skills and partly because of burnout in their social networks. Estrangement from grown children is not uncommon among these patients, and their risk for suicide is high. These authors assert that such patients require longer-term psychotherapy, and treatment is often a "balancing act" between preventing crises and building more adaptive behaviors. However, while personality-disordered patients may initially be mistrustful of and even hostile toward the therapist, they may eventually benefit from treatment if good rapport is established. Termination with the depressed personality-disordered patient may be problematic, however, because it may mean severing the only meaningful relationship the patient has. The authors therefore recommend that the therapist, rather than terminating completely, maintain regular albeit infrequent follow-up contact with the patient.

It is important to emphasize that in treating the personality-disordered older adult with depression, the goal is not to "cure" the personality disorder but to treat the depression. By adhering to such an expectation, the clinician may avoid the burnout that is not uncommon among the treaters and caretakers of these patients. In attempting to engage the personality-disordered patient, the therapist should be mindful of two dangers: the possibility of getting so pulled into the vortex of the patient's distress that he or she unwittingly becomes a collaborator in perpetuating the problem, and the risk of negative countertransference. Thus, the therapist must achieve a balance between providing genuine empathy, maintaining neutrality and firm boundaries, and carefully structuring the therapy around clear, concrete goals. In our experience, many patients with personality disorders are ultimately able to develop a strong, healthy therapeutic alliance when they discover that the therapist has the strength to remain neutral and objective.

Psychotherapy of the Depressed Older Adult with Cognitive Impairment

The patient newly diagnosed with Alzheimer's disease or the patient in the early stages of vascular dementia is acutely aware of the decline in his or her cognitive functions, especially memory. In these cases, depression may be a concurrent, seemingly independent disorder, or it may be reactive to the patient's self-perceived diminishing capacity. Nonetheless, while the literature is replete with behavioral and therapeutic approaches for the patient with advanced dementia, it is relatively deficient in studies of psychotherapy with depressed patients who are in the early stages of dementing diseases. Clearly, such patients need support not only in dealing with the sense of loss in receiving a devastating diagnosis but also with the progressive practical consequences of loss of function. For similar reasons, the family and other caregivers clearly need support and possibly treatment as well. Treatment of caregiver burden is discussed in another chapter in this volume.

Teri and Thompson (1991) have developed a program of cognitive behavioral interventions for the treatment of depression in early Alzheimer's patients. They outline a set of guidelines for cognitive therapy for patients with mild impairment and behavioral interventions for patients with moderate to severe impairment. In the first group, patients are helped to identify maladaptive cognitions that increase their sense of hopelessness and helplessness. A modified dysfunctional thought record is used by the patient to record cognitions resulting in negative feelings, such as ruminations about the future or magnification of current deficits. The therapist then helps the patient challenge these thoughts and explore more adaptive alternatives, such as focusing on what the patient is able to do rather than what he or she cannot do and staying grounded in the present. Patients are also asked to rate their feelings before and after generating adaptive thoughts, which gives them a sense of control and accomplishment. Although older adults with early dementia need considerable practice to develop these skills, they find the interventions of a patient therapist quite beneficial. For more severe levels of impairment, these authors use a modification of behavior therapy based on the theory that depression is in part maintained by a lack of pleasant experiences in the patient's life. Thus, the treatment involves increasing the number of pleasant events and interactions in the older adult's life and decreasing the negative ones. As the patient declines further, caregivers are increasingly involved in the therapeutic process to facilitate implementation of the plan. While this approach may seem simplistic, it actually involves a thorough analysis of behaviors and situations that are maintaining the patient's depression.

Yale (1991) uses here-and-now experiences in group therapy to build coping strategies in patients with mild to moderate cognitive impairment. For example, if one patient in the group loses the thread of a problem being discussed, Yale asks other group members to report similar difficulties. He also stresses the adaptiveness of denial in patients with progressive dementia and recommends that the therapist be cautious and hesitant about breaking through their denial.

Other approaches have been developed for the treatment of depression in patients with dementia. Validation therapy (Feil, 1989) employs a variety of nonverbal techniques to help the patient with severe cognitive impairment to express and process feelings and needs triggered by their still intact remote memory. In resolution therapy (Stokes and Goudie, 1990), the therapist, through empathic listening, helps the patient to identify feelings in the here and now while modifying the environment, if possible, to meet the patient's needs.

Clearly, more work is needed in the psychosocial treatment of patients with early-stage dementia, especially in view of the finding that depression adds a layer of impairment, termed *excess disability*, to the functioning of patients with Alzheimer's disease (Reifer and Larson, 1989), 30% of whom meet criteria for major depressive disorder.

CROSS-CULTURAL CONSIDERATIONS IN PSYCHOTHERAPY WITH OLDER ADULTS

In a study of factors motivating caregiving behavior among Korean Americans and Caucasian Americans, obligation, affection, and reciprocity were the three motivational responses offered most frequently by both groups. However, respect for parents, family harmony, and filial sacrifice were important motivational responses only for the Korean American caregivers (Sung, 1994; Wong and Ujimoto, 1994). This finding clearly highlights differing cultural values that may translate into significant cultural differences in intergenerational expectations. Holzberg (1982) stressed the importance of considering "how these expectations and structural pressures actually mold the way in which a person perceives, defines, and seeks solutions to problems associated with aging" (Wong, p. 169).

The purpose of this section is not to acquaint the reader with specific cultural characteristics and differences but to underscore the importance of being aware of them in treatment planning and goal setting with culturally diverse older adults. Culture has been defined as "the totality of learned, socially transmitted behavior of a group that emerges from its members' interpersonal interactions" (Morales, 1999). Thus the earlier noted cohort differences between today's older adults and succeeding generations may be considered an example of cultural variation. And just as cohort differences have an impact on an individual's receptivity to psychotherapy and his or her behavior in a therapeutic context, so can ethnic differences, especially among newly arrived and first-generation Americans. In an extensive treatment of the topic, Morales (1999) discusses characteristics common to a number of ethnic groups that may impact on the older adult's engagement in the therapeutic process. She expounds on the following tendencies and patterns of older adults from four cultural groups (Asian American, Native American, Hispanic American, and African American) that cut across ethnic lines: mistrust and suspicion of the dominant culture, greater entrenchment in religious institutions, greater respect and reverence of parents and grandparents as teachers of culture and oral history, and strong family bonds, resulting in attempts to solve problems within the family. What derives from these differences is some speculation about how older adult members of these cultural groups might respond to sharing their personal problems with a therapist, how they might view their relationships with their grown children, and how they might feel about involvement in a senior center, placement in a nursing home, or admission to a psychiatric hospital. At the same time, the clinician must take care to avoid overarching assumptions about a large ethnic group. Wong and Ujimoto (1994), for example, discuss the concept of "filial piety" in the Asian culture—i.e., the expectation that grown children will honor and respect their parents. However, they emphasize the fact that this phenomenon is expressed differentially in Japan, China, and Korea. Morales (1999) similarly stresses the importance of acknowledging differences between various tribes of Native Americans. Thus the clinician must walk a fine line between factoring in cultural differences and avoiding blanket generalizations about ethnic groups, which might compromise not only the patient's ethnic uniqueness but his or her individuality. With a view toward maintaining a balanced, informed approach, it behooves the clinician working with a "culturally different" older adult to become familiar with some of the beliefs and traditions of the particular ethnic group through reading or, perhaps even better, by seeking education directly from the patient or family. The following case example underscores the importance of this:

> Ms. P., an Asian-American older adult, was attending a partial hospitalization program for treatment of depression. Upon further assessment, it was discovered that after moving from another state to live with her grown daughter in her rural home, Ms. P. had become increasingly lonely and overworked, as she spent her days in the house cleaning and cooking while the daughter was at work. The therapist attempted to work with Ms. P. on asserting herself with her daughter about her need for transportation and her desire to cut back a bit on the household chores. Despite the employment of various assertiveness training techniques, Ms. P. could not bring herself to have the recommended "talk" with her daughter and furthermore could not explain why. During the treatment of the patient, the therapist happened to attend a lecture on cross-cultural issues with patients. Suspecting that cultural factors might be at play, the therapist in the next session gently explored the reasons for the patient's reluctance to talk with her daughter, offering some speculations from what she had learned. Encouraged by the therapist's genuine interest, the patient informed the therapist that in her particular culture, the grown child assuming the caretaking role became the authority; it was therefore inappropriate for Ms. P. to "challenge" her daughter. Moreover, the patient admitted that she had not wanted to share this information with the therapist because it would also be inappropriate to challenge another caretaker, the doctor; to do so would undermine the therapist's authority. Thus, the patient had felt stymied, both with her daughter and with her therapist. As a result of this discussion, the therapist arranged a family meeting with mother and daughter in which communication was gently and sensitively facilitated between parent and grown child, with productive results.

CONCLUDING REMARKS

The purpose of this chapter has not been to train the reader in psychotherapeutic techniques with older adults but rather to emphasize the responsiveness of older adults to psychotherapy and to help familiarize the clinician with the special issues of aging that affect therapeutic process and outcome. This knowledge will become more important in the next decade, as the population begins to swell with older adults as the oldest of the post–World War II baby-boom generation reach retirement age. It is lamentable that the literature on psychotherapeutic techniques with older adults lags seriously behind psychopharmacological treatment studies, since "boomers," tending to be more comfortable with direct expression of emotion, may well be greater consumers of psychotherapy and perhaps not as quick as their parents to comply with pharmacological interventions. At the same time, it is hoped that the reader will come away with the realization that there are more similarities than differences in therapeutic technique and efficacy across adult age groups, reflecting the fact that older people are, first and foremost, adults in every sense of the word.

REFERENCES

Abrams RC, Alexopoulos GS, Young R (1987). Geriatric depression and DSM-III-R personality disorder criteria. J Am Geriatr Soc 35:383–386.

Alexopoulos GS, Katz IR, Reynolds CF III, Carpenter D, Docherty JP (2001). Pharmacotherapy of depressive disorders in older patients. Postgrad Med Spec Rep October, pp. 24, 27.

Arean PA, Perri MG, Nezu AM, Schein RL, Christopher F, Joseph TX (1993). Comparative effectiveness of social problem-solving therapy and reminiscence therapy as treatments for depression in older adults. J Consult Clin Psychol 6(6):1003–1010.

Beck AT, Weissman A, Lester D, Trexler L (1974). The measurement of pessimism: The Hopelessness Scale. J Consult Clin Psychol 42:861–865.

Beck AT, Rush J, Shaw B, Emery G (1974). Cognitive Therapy of Depression. New York: Guilford Press.

Beck AT, Weishaar ME (1990). Suicide risk assessment and prediction. Crisis 11:22–30.

Beck AT, Steer RA, Beck JS, Newman CF (1993). Hopelessness, depression, suicidal ideation, and clinical diagnosis of depression. Suicide Life Threat Behav 23:139–145.

Benbow SM, Marriott A, Morley M, Walsh S (1993). Family therapy and dementia: review and clinical experience. Int J Geriatr Psychiatry 8:717–725.

Beutler LE, Scogin F, Kirkish P, Schretlen D, Corbishley A, Hamblin D, Meredith K, Potter R, Bamford DR, Levenson AI (1987). Group cognitive therapy and alprazolam in the treatment of depression in older adults. J Consult Clin Psychol 55(4): 550–556.

Blazer D (1994). Intervention Strategies for Emotional Problems in Later Life. Northvale, NJ: Jason Aronson.

Brody CM (1999). Existential issues of hope and meaning in late life therapy. In: Duffy M, ed. Handbook of Counseling and Psychotherapy with Older Adults. New York: Wiley, pp 91–106.

Brown R, Sweeney J, Loutsch E, Kocsis J, Frances A (1984). Involutional melancholia revisited. Am J Psychiatry 141:24–28.

Dick-Sisken L (2002). Cognitive behavioral therapy with older adults. The Behavior Therapist, 25(1):3–6.

Duffy, M, ed (1999). Handbook of Counseling and Psychotherapy with Older Adults. New York: Wiley.

Erikson EH, Erikson JM, Kivnick HQ (1986). Vital Involvement in Old Age. New York: Norton.

Erikson E (1982). The Life Cycle Completed. New York: Norton.

Feil N (1989). Validation: an empirical approach to the care of dementia. Clin Gerontol 8:89–94.

Finkel SI (1991). Group psychotherapy in later life. In: Myers WA ed. New Techniques in the Psychotherapy of Older Patients. Washington, DC: American Psychiatric Press, pp 223–224.

Folstein M, Folstein S, McHugh P (1975). "Mini-Mental State"—A practical method for grading the cognitive state of patients for the clinician. J Psychiatr Res 12: 189–198.

Gallagher-Thompson D, Coon DW (1996). Depression. In: Sheikh JI, ed. Treating the Elderly. San Francisco: Jossey-Bass, pp 1–44.

Gerson S, Belin TR, Kaufman A, Mintz J, Jarwik L (1999). Pharmacological and psychological treatments for depressed older patients: a meta-analysis and overview of recent findings. Harvard Rev Psychiatry, 7(1):1–28.

Gilleard C (1996). Family therapy with older clients. In: Woods RT, ed. Handbook of the Clinical Psychology of Ageing. Chichester, UK: Wiley, pp 561–574.

Hegestad GO (1988). Demographic change and the life course: some emerging trends in the family realm. Fam Rel 37:405–410.

Hinrichsen GA (1999). Treating older adults with interpersonal psychotherapy for depression. JCLP/In Session: Psychother Pract 55(8):949–960.

Holzberg CS (1982). Ethnicity and aging: anthropological perspectives on more than just the minority elderly. Gerontologist 22:249–257.

Huyck MH, Gutmann DL (1999). Developmental issues in psychotherapy with older men. In: Duffy M, ed. Handbook of Counseling and Psychotherapy with Older Adults. New York: Wiley, pp 77–90.

Jacobs S, Ostfield A (1977). An epidemiological review of the mortality of bereavement. Psychosom Med 39:344–357.

Kaplan HS (1992). Sex therapy with older patients. In: Myers WA, ed. New Techniques in the Psychotherapy of Older Patients. Washington, DC: American Psychiatric Press.

Kivnik HQ, Kafka A (1999). It takes two: therapeutic alliance with older adults. In: Duffy M, ed. Handbook of Counseling and Psychotherapy with Older Adults. New York: Wiley, 107–132.

Klerman GL, Wiseman MM (1993). New Applications of Interpersonal Psychotherapy. Washington DC: American Psychiatric Press.

Knight BG (1999). The scientific basis for psychotherapeutic interventions with older adults: an overview. JCLP/In Session: Psychother Pract 55(8):927–934.
Kohut H (1971). Analysis of the Self. New York: International Universities Press.
Leigh R, Varghese F (2001). Psychodynamic psychotherapy with the elderly. J Psychiatr Pract 7(4):229–237.
Lewisohn PM, Munoz RF, Youngren MA, Zeiss AM (1992). Control Your Depression, rev ed. New York: Simon & Schuster.
Linehan MM (1993). Cognitive-Behavioral Treatment of Borderline Personality Disorder. New York: Guilford Press.
Lynch TR, Morse JQ, Vitt CM (2002). Dialectical behavior therapy for depressed older adults. The Behavior Therapist, 25(1):7–8.
Markowitz JC (1998). Is IPT time-limited psychodynamic psychotherapy? J Psychother Pract Res 7(3):185–195.
Mathiasen P, Suzanne L (1997). Late Life Depression. New York: Bantam Doubleday.
McGinn LK (2000). Cognitive behavioral therapy of depression: theory treatment and empirical status. Am J Psychother 54(2):257–261.
McIntosh L, Santos JE, Hubbard RW, Overholser JC (1994). Elder Suicide: Research, Theory and Techniques. Washington, DC: American Psychology Association.
Moberg P, Lazarus L (1990). Psychotherapy of depression in the elderly. Psychiatr Ann 20(2):92–96.
Molinari V (1999). Using reminiscence and life review as natural therapeutic strategies in group therapy. In: Duffy M, ed. Handbook of Counseling and Psychotherapy with Older Adults. New York: Viking, pp 154–165.
Morales P (1999). The impact of cultural differences in psychotherapy with older clients: sensitive issues and strategies. In: Duffy M, ed. Handbook of Counseling and Psychotherapy with Older Adults. New York: Wiley, pp 132–153.
Muslin HL (1992). The Psychotherapy of the Elderly Self. New York: Brunner/Maezel.
Myers WA, ed (1991). New Techniques in the Psychotherapy of Older Patients. Washington, DC: American Psychiatric Press.
Myers WA (1991). Psychoanalytic psychotherapy and psychoanalysis with older patients. In: Myers WA, ed. New Techniques in the Psychotherapy of Older Patients. Washington, DC: American Psychiatric Press.
National Ageing Research Institute (NARI). (1999). Older people to benefit from diagnosis and treatment. Ageing Well March 18, 1999.
Neidhardt ER, Allen JA (1992). Family therapy with the Elderly. London: Sage.
Newton NA, Jacobowitz J (1999). Transferential and countertransferential processes in therapy with older adults. In: Duffy M, ed. Handbook of Counseling and Psychotherapy with Older Adults. New York: Wiley, pp 21–40.
Niederehe G (1996). Psychosocial treatments with depressed older adults. Am J Geriatr Psychiatry 4(suppl 1):866–878.
Nordhus IH, Nielsen GH (1999). Brief dynamic psychotherapy with older adults. JCLP/in Session: Psychother Pract 55(8):935–947.
Orbach R (2001). Therapeutic empathy with the suicidal wish: principles of therapy with suicidal individuals. Am J Psychother 55(2):166–184.
Qualls SH (1999). Realizing power in intergenerational family hierarchies: family reor-

ganization when older adults decline. In: Duffy M, ed. Handbook of Counseling and Psychotherapy with Older Adults. New York: Wiley, 228–241.
Pollack WS (1999). The tortures of Job: diagnosing and treating hidden depression in older men. J Geriatr Psychiatry 32(2):195–222.
Reifler BV, Larson E (1989). Excess disability in dementia of the Alzheimer's type. In: Light E, Lebowitz BD, eds. Alzheimer's Disease Treatment and Family Stress: Directions for Research. Rockville, MD: National Institute of Mental Health, pp 363–397.
Reynolds CF III, Frank E, Dew MA, Houck PR, Miller M, Mazumdar S, Perel JM, Kupfer DF (1999). Treatment of 70+ year olds with recurrent major depression. Am Geriatr Psychiatry 7(1):64–66.
Reynolds CF III, Frank E, Houck PR, Mazumdar S, Dew MA, Cornes C, Buysee DJ, Begley A, Kupfer DJ (1997). Which elderly patients with remitted depression remain well with continued interpersonal psychotherapy after discontinuation of antidepressant mediation? Am J Psychiatry 154(7):958–962.
Reynolds CF III, Frank E, Kupler DJ, Thase ME, Perel JM, Mazumdar S, Houck PR (1996). Treatment outcome in recurrent major depression: a post hoc comparison of elderly ("young old") and midlife patients. Am J Psychiatry 153(10):1288–1292.
Reynolds CF III, Frank E, Perel JM, Miller MD, Cornes C, Rifai AH, Pollock BG, Mazumdar S, George CJ, Houck PR, Kupfer DJ (1994). Treatment of consecutive episodes of major depression in the elderly. Am J Psychiatry 151(12):1704–1743.
Reynolds CF III, Frank E, Perel JM, Imber SD, Cornes C, Miller M, Mazumdar S, Houck PR, Dew MA, Stack JA, Pollock BG, Kupfer DJ (1999). Nortriptyline and interpersonal psychotherapy as maintenance therapies for recurrent major depression. JAMA 281(1):39–45.
Richman J (1999). Psychotherapy with the suicidal elderly: a family oriented approach. In: Duffy M, ed. Handbook of Counseling and Psychotherapy with Older Adults. New York: Wiley, pp 650–661.
Rosovsky E (1999). Couple therapy with long-married older adults. In: Duffy M, ed. Handbook of Counseling and Psychotherapy with Older Adults. New York: Wiley, pp 242–266.
Rush A, Beck AT, Kovacs M, et al (1979). Comparative efficacy of cognitive therapy and imipramine in the treatment of depressed patients. Cogn Ther Res 1:17–37.
Sadovoy J (1999). The effect of personality disorder on Axis I disorders in the elderly. In: Duffy M, ed. Handbook of Counseling and Psychotherapy with Older Adults. New York: Wiley, pp 397–413.
Schneidman E (1996). The Suicidal Mind. New York: Oxford University Press.
Scogin F, McElreath L (1994). Efficacy of psychosocial treatments for geriatric depression: a quantitative review. J Counsel Clin Psychol 62:69–74.
Seligman MEP (1975). Helplessness: On Depression, Development, and Death. San Francisco: Freeman.
Sheike JI, ed (1996). Treating the Elderly. San Francisco: Jossey-Bass.
Sprenkel DG (1999). Therapeutic Issues and Strategies in Group Therapy with Older Men. In: Duffy M, ed. Handbook of Counseling and Psychotherapy with Older Adults. New York: Wiley.

Stengel E (1964). Suicide and Attempted Suicide. Baltimore: Penguin.
Steuer JL, Mintz J, Hammen CL, Hill MA, Jarvik LS, McCarley T, Motoike P, Rosen R (1984). Cognitive-behavioral and psychodynamic group psychotherapy in treatment of geriatric depression. J Consult Clin Psychol 51:180–189.
Stokes G, Goudie F, eds (1990). Working with Dementia. Bichester, UK: Winslow Press.
Sullivan HS (1953). The Interpersonal Theory of Psychiatry. New York: Norton.
Sung TK (1994). Cross-cultural comparison of motivations for parent care: the case of Americas and Koreans. J Aging Studies 8:195–209.
Szantos K, Reynolds CF, Conwell Y, Begley AE, Houck P (1998). High levels of hopelessness persist in geriatric patients with remitted depression and a history of attempted suicide. J Am Geriatr Soc 46:1401–1406.
Teri L, Gallagher-Thompson D (1991). Cognitive-behavioral interventions for treatment of depression in Alzheimer's patients. Gerontologist 31(3):413–416.
Teri L, Lewinsohn P (1982). Modifications of the pleasant and unpleasant events schedules for use with the elderly. J Consult Clin Psychol 55:444–445.
Thase ME, Greenhouse JB, Frank E, Reynolds CF III, Pilkonis PA, Hurley K, Grochocinski V, Kupfer DJ (1997). Treatment of major depression with psychotherapy or psychotherapy—pharmacotherapy combinations. Arch Gen Psychiatry 54: 1009–1015.
Thompson LW, Gantz F, Florshein M, Del Maestro S, Rodman J, Gallagher-Thompson D, Bryan H (1991). Cognitive behavior therapy for effective disorders in the elderly. In: Myers WA, ed. New Techniques in the Psychotherapy of Older Patients. Washington DC: American Psychiatric Press.
Thompson LW, Gallagher D, Breckenridge JS (1987). Comparative effectiveness of psychotherapies for depressed elders. J Consult Clin Psychol 55(3):385–390.
Thompson LW, Gallagher D, Czirr R (1988). Personality disorders and outcome in the treatment of late-life depression. J Geriatr Psychiatry 21:133–146.
Tice CI, Perkins K (1996). Mental Health Issues and Ageing. Pacific Grove, CA: Brooks/Cole.
Wong PT, Ujimoto KV. The elderly: their stress, coping, and mental health. In: Lee LC, Zane NWS, eds. Handbook of Asian-American Psychology.
Woods RT, ed (1996). Handbook of the Clinical Psychology of Ageing. New York: Wiley.
Yale R (1991). A Guide to Facilitating Support Groups for Newly Diagnosed Alzheimer's Patients. San Francisco: Alzheimer's Association, Greater San Francisco Chapter.
Yost EB, Bentler LE, Corbishley MA, Allender JR (1986). Group Cognitive Therapy: A Treatment Approach for Depressed Older Adults. New York: Pergamon Press.
Zarit SH, Zarit JM (1998). Mental Disorders in Older Adults. New York: Guilford Press.

13

Late-Life Suicide

Ashok J. Bharucha
University of Pittsburgh School of Medicine, Pittsburgh, Pennsylvania, U.S.A.

INTRODUCTION

Suicide remains an all too common solution to intolerable psychological and physical suffering in the elderly. It can best be described as a multidetermined process, articulated by Havens as "the final common pathway of diverse circumstances, of an interdependent network rather than an isolated cause, a knot of circumstances tightening around a single time and place" (1). No other segment of the population epitomizes this description more clearly than the elderly. It is the objective of this chapter to highlight the high rates of suicide; the interdependent network of physical, psychiatric, and personality dimensions that contribute to late-life suicide; and potential intervention strategies, particularly in primary care practices.

EPIDEMIOLOGY

According to the latest report of the National Center for Health Statistics (2000), the 1998 suicide rate for the general population was 11.3 per 100,000 (2). More specifically, the rate peaked in the bracket of 80–84 year olds at 22.9 per 100,000. Put another way, the elderly accounted for 19.0% of the suicides while constituting only 12.7% of the population (3). Of the demographic factors, disparity along gender lines is the most striking, with males being at consistently higher risk of completing suicide than females. Historically, suicide risk is incremental with advancing age in white males; consistent with this trend, white males aged 85 and older completed suicide six times more frequently than the age-adjusted national rate in 1998, making them the highest-risk group. In contrast, suicide rates for nonwhite males (Hispanics, African Americans, and Native Americans) tend to peak in early adulthood and to decline thereafter (4). With the exception of young widowers, suicide rates in each marital category tend to be higher for the elderly as well (4).

The most common method of suicide in the elderly involves the use of a firearm. In 1992, a total of 68.7% of elderly suicides were completed with firearms, compared with 60% of all U.S. suicides (5). Males used firearms seven times more frequently than females. The more violent and definitive nature of late-life suicide explains in part the finding that the ratio of attempted to completed suicide drops precipitously from 200:1 in the young to 4:1 in the elderly (6). The first suicide attempt among elderly patients may well be the last, given their compromised physical functioning, social isolation, and lack of communication of suicidal intent (4). Indirect self-destructive behaviors such as refusal of medication and food may also be suicidal in nature; however, such factors are infrequently taken into account in the medical examiners' determination of cause of death, thus substantially underestimating the actual number of late-life suicide deaths (7). The urgent need for the development and implementation of effective interventions is evident in the fact that demographers expect the elderly to account for one-third of all suicides in the United States by the year 2030 if current trends continue (4).

PHYSICAL ILLNESS

Age-related variations in recent life events preceding suicide suggest family, occupational, and financial problems to be most salient in the younger age groups, while physical illness has been noted to be a more common and critical element among both late-life suicide completers as well as attempters (8–11). The evidence pointing to an association between physical illness and suicide, however, comes largely from studies that lack age- and sex-specific control groups, that do not use standardized measures of physical illness burden, and that do not assess functional impairment. The increased morbidity and mortality due to the impact of psychiatric illness on some of the most common chronic medical conditions such as coronary artery disease also confounds this association (12). Also of note, alcoholism is overrepresented in the older studies attempting to establish an association between physical illness and suicide (13). Conwell et al. recently reported their findings from a case-control study in which psychological autopsy data on those primary care patients who had completed suicide within a month of visiting their primary physician ($N = 42$) were compared with prospective data on a representative control sample of older patients in primary care from that region ($N = 196$) (14). The authors noted significantly higher rates of physical and functional deficits and disability in individuals completing suicide, a point of great relevance both in terms of improving the quality of life of older patients and curbing late-life suicide rates. Since a vast majority (> 70%) of elderly who complete suicide visit their primary care physician within the last month of their life, primary care practices appear to be a natural site for collaborative preventative strategies targeting both physical and mental health (15).

PSYCHOPATHOLOGY

The ubiquitous presence of psychiatric illness (> 90% of cases) in those who complete suicide is well documented, with the nature of the psychopathology varying with age (16–18). Older persons who commit suicide are most often in the middle of their first lifetime episode of nonpsychotic major depression, with a smaller minority also abusing alcohol (19,20). In contrast to the younger age groups, primary psychotic illnesses, substance abuse (other than alcohol), and personality disorders are infrequent in late-life suicide (19). Conwell et al.'s controlled study of completed suicide among older primary care patients sheds more light on the salient issues at hand (14). Consistent with prior reports, major depression was not only significantly more common in suicide completers but was also more severe according to the Hamilton Depression Rating Scale (17,19). When only the depressed subgroup of suicide completers and the prospective control subjects were examined, physical health measures failed to distinguish the groups. Ironically, in spite of the fact that antidepressants were prescribed at significantly greater rates to the suicide completers than to the prospective cohort, only 14.6% were in mental health treatment at the time of death. The depressed subgroups of subjects in both cohorts were prescribed antidepressants with equal frequency despite the greater severity of mental illness in the suicide completers. The minority of patients from both groups who were in psychiatric treatment at the time of death were clinically indistinguishable.

Axis I psychopathology in late-life suicide has been described with considerable consistency in the literature (17,19). In contrast, there is a dearth of controlled studies using standardized personality inventories to determine personality traits that may confer vulnerability to late-life suicide. While categorical personality disorders are thought to be rare, certain traits may be instrumental in the biopsychosocial pathway leading to suicide. Duberstein and colleagues have conducted the only controlled study using the NEO Personality Inventory addressing subjects over the age of 50 years (21). They report greater levels of neuroticism (N) and lower "openness to experience" (OTE) in suicide completers compared to age-matched controls. Low OTE may indicate diminished adaptive capacity in a season of losses coupled with potential lack of communication of internal affective and cognitive states. It is well known that the elderly rarely communicate suicidal intent (22).

One cognitive stance that is thought to be predictive of suicidal ideation and eventual suicide is hopelessness, defined by Beck as a state of negativism and pessimism unrelated to medical or psychiatric prognosis per se (23–25). Although Beck's sample consisted largely of younger individuals, similar impact of hopelessness on suicidal ideation and completed suicide has been reported in the elderly as well (26,27). Even after resolution of depressive symptoms, high levels of hopelessness may persist in depressed elderly who have already attempted suicide and may contribute to treatment noncompliance and eventual suicide (28). Independent of depression, hopelessness has been found to be a significant predictor of desire for physician-assisted suicide in a sample of terminally ill cancer patients treated in an academic facility specializing in the management of cancer patients (29).

Identification of individual factors that confer vulnerability to late-life suicide is an important starting point. However, the ultimate goal must be to elucidate the mechanisms by which the complex interplay of these biopsychosocial factors results in this tragic outcome.

PREVENTION

Primary Care Practice

The scenario of late-life suicide most often involves an elderly white, widowed male in the middle of his first episode of nonpsychotic major depression who has access to firearms. Of the modifiable risk factors, early and accurate diagnosis and treatment of major depression in the primary care setting appears to be critical. The fact that a vast majority of older suicide victims have visited their primary care physician within a month of their death highlights the importance of this treatment setting in averting late-life suicide (15). Furthermore, most older adults do not seek treatment from mental health professionals or utilize general suicide hotlines (30,31). The underdiagnosis and subtherapeutic treatment of depression by primary care physicians is, however, well recognized (32,33). The scope of the problem may be vastly underestimated considering the functional impairments and morbidity associated with even subthreshold depression, which is likely to elude the primary care physician (34). Providing primary care physicians with the knowledge and skills to effectively diagnose and manage depression and recognize agist biases and negative countertransference must become a high priority. In addition, implementation of depression practice guidelines and the routine use of short depression screening instruments such as the Geriatric Depression Scale and the Center for Epidemiologic Studies Depression Scale, which have been validated in the primary care setting, appears prudent (35–37). The primary care physician, of course, is also in an opportune position to minimize the functional impairments, dependence, and demoralization associated with chronic medical conditions. Collaborative care models in which mental health professionals provide on-site or telephone consultation show promise in optimizing management of depression in primary care practices; however, no study of such a model has addressed the elderly specifically (38). Referral to a psychiatrist should be strongly considered under the following conditions: atypical presentation, vague symptoms or multiple somatic complaints not well accounted for by a comprehensive medical workup, comorbid psychiatric conditions, polypharmacy, and active substance abuse.

Community Interventions

Several innovative community outreach programs have been developed to address the fact that older adults rarely utilize general crisis-prevention hotlines or seek mental health treatment. Life Crisis Services of St. Louis, Missouri, has instituted a Link-Plus component that receives referrals targeting depressed elderly in crisis from medical and mental health professionals (39). Case management and ongoing telephone contact is then provided. The Spokane Community Mental Health Center has developed the Gatekeepers Program, which casts a broader net by instructing community members who routinely have contact with older adults in the recognition of at-risk elderly. Once a referral is made, in-home assessment and comprehensive case management services are arranged (40). Similarly, the San Francisco Suicide Prevention Center has organized a Center for Elderly Suicide Prevention and Grief Related Services. The center provides 24-hr crisis intervention, home visits, networking within local agencies, and volunteer assistance with social services (39). The longitudinal impact and cost-effectiveness of these innovative programs on curbing late-life suicide rates awaits critical examination.

De Leo et al.'s intervention model, the Tele-Help/Tele-Check service, combines both telephone assistance and twice-a-week visits with clients to ascertain their needs and offer emotional support (41). In spite of the fact that the 12,135 participants in this program were "old-old" (mean age 79 years), only one suicide was completed over a 4-year span. In a previous study of the Tele-Check service, the same group reported improved mood scores, fewer general practitioner home visits, and fewer hospitalizations among those who had participated in the program for at least 6 months compared to those awaiting the service or who had just been enrolled (42).

Psychoeducational Interventions

The assumption that training primary care physicians to appropriately diagnose and treat geriatric depression will have a positive impact on late-life suicide rates lacks critical analysis and affirmation. Preliminary support for this assumption comes from an uncontrolled study from the Swedish island of Gotland, which reported notable declines in suicide rates in the year following a depression education program for primary care physicians (43). The result, however, was not sustained at 3-year follow-up, leading the authors to conclude that such educational activities must be offered at frequent intervals (44). Further concern regarding the primary care management of depression stems from the limited time allotted to patient visits and fiscal disincentives directed at nonprocedural care, particularly with the proliferation of managed care organizations. The extent to which primary care clinicians can address both physical and psychiatric issues under these constraints is a matter worthy of thoughtful debate.

Pratt et al. have developed a 3-hr educational program on depression and suicide that is appropriate for both professional and lay audiences (45). The workshop combines an 18-min slide show entitled *The Final Course*, a story of Mrs. Murphy, age 72, with didactics and discussions. Compared to controls, participants at postcourse examination demonstrated significant gains in knowledge about late-life depression and suicide and interventions that would be appropriate and applicable to older adults experiencing such distress. A host of psychoeducational curricula exist and should be used to train health care professionals, employees of social service agencies, those who interact with the elderly on a routine basis, and the American population in general (46,47).

CONCLUSION

Medical advances of the last century have had little impact on suicide rates of the general population of the United States. Suicide remains an all too common alternative to persistent suffering for the elderly, and demographers expect further increases in the rates of late-life suicide if current trends continue. While some optimism is engendered by the political and social activism of the "baby boom" generation, suicide rates are higher for this generation than for prior cohorts. The urgent need for biomedical, psychosocial, and health care delivery research cannot be overemphasized. Future research on late-life suicide should focus on [1] the neurobiology of the aging process and the mechanisms by which it contributes to affective vulnerability, [2] delineating the biological correlates of late-life suicidal behavior, [3] elucidating the complex bilateral interactions between physical and psychiatric illness, [4] identifying personality traits that may confer vulnerability or resistance to suicidal behavior, [5] developing therapeutic approaches that address hopelessness, [6] conducting controlled studies to ascertain the impact of psychoeducational programs for primary care clinicians, [7] examining the impact of various collaborative primary care/mental health treatment models targeting the elderly specifically, and, finally, [8] examining the effectiveness of innovative community outreach programs in reducing late-life suicide rates.

REFERENCES

1. Havens L. The anatomy of a suicide. N Engl J Med 1965; 272:401–406.
2. National Center for Health Statistics (NCHS) web site. http://www.cdc.gov/nchs/datawh/statab/unpubd/mortabs/gmwk291.htm
3. Murphy SL. Deaths: final data for 1998. Vol 48(11). National Vital Statistics Report. DHHS publication no. (PHS) 2000–1120. Hyattsville, MD: National Center for Health Statistics, 2000.
4. McIntosh JL, Santos JF, Hubbard RW, Overholser JC. Elder Suicide: Research, Theory, and Treatment. Washington, DC: American Psychological Association, 1994.
5. McIntosh JL. USA Suicide: 1992 Official Final Data. Washington, DC: American Association of Suicidology, 1995.
6. Parkin D, Stengel E: Incidence of suicidal attempts in an urban community. Br Med J 1965; 2:133–138.
7. Osgood NJ, Brant BA. Suicidal behavior in long-term care facilities. Suicide Life Threat Behav 1990; 20:113–122.
8. Carney SS, Rich CL, Burke PA. Suicide over 60: The San Diego Study. J Am Geriatr Soc 1994; 42:174–180.
9. Heikkinen ME, Lonnqvist JK. Recent life events in elderly suicide: a nationwide study in Finland. Int Psychogeriatr 1995; 7:287–300.
10. Lyness JM, Conwell Y, Nelson JC. Suicide attempts in elderly psychiatric inpatients. J Am Geriatr Soc 1992; 40:320–324.
11. Lester D, Beck AT. Age differences in patterns of attempted suicide. Omega 1974; 5:317–322.
12. Frasure-Smith N, Lesperance F, Talajic M. Depression following myocardial infarction: impact on 6-month survival. JAMA 1993; 270:1819–1825.
13. Mackenzie TB, Popkin MK. Suicide in the medical patient. Int J Psychiatry Med 1987; 17:3–22.
14. Conwell Y, Lyness JM, Duberstein P, Cox C, Seidlitz L, DiGiogio A, Caine ED. Completed suicide among older patients in primary care practices: a controlled study. J Am Geriatr Soc 2000; 48:23–29.
15. Conwell Y. Suicide in elderly patients. In: Schneider LS, Reynolds CF III, Lebowitz BD, Friedhoff AJ, eds. Diagnosis and Treatment of Depression in Late Life: Results of the NIH Consensus Development Conference. Washington DC: American Psychiatric Press, 1994:397–418.
16. Dorpat TL, Ripley HS. A study of suicide in the Seattle area. Comp Psychiatry 1960; 1:349–359.
17. Barraclough BM. Suicide in the elderly: recent developments in psychogeriatrics. Br J Psychiatry 1971; spec suppl no 6:87–97.

18. Conwell Y, Olsen K, Caine ED, Flannery C. Suicide in later life: psychological autopsy findings. Int Psychogeriatr 1991; 3:59–66.
19. Conwell Y, Duberstein PR, Cox C, Herrmann JH, Forbes NT, Caine ED. Relationships of Axis-I diagnoses in victims of completed suicide: a psychological autopsy study. Am J Psychiatry 1996; 153:1001–1008.
20. Conwell Y, Brent D. Suicide and aging I: patterns of psychiatric diagnosis. Int Psychogeriatr 1995; 7:149–164.
21. Duberstein PR. Openness to experience and completed suicide across the second half of life. Int Psychogeriatr 1995; 7:183–198.
22. Pitkala K, Isometsa ET, Henriksson MM, Lonnqvist JK. Elderly suicide in Finland. Int Psychogeriatr 2000; 12:209–220.
23. Beck AT, Schuyler D, Herman I. Development of suicide intent scales. In: Beck AT, Resnick HLP, Lettieri DJ, eds. The Prediction of Suicide. Bowie, MD: Charles, 1974:45–56.
24. Beck AT, Steer RA, Kovacs M, Garrison BS. Hopelessness and eventual suicide: ten year prospective study of patients hospitalized with suicidal ideation. Am J Psychiatry 1985; 142:559–563.
25. Beck AT, Brown G, Berchick RJ, Stewart BL, Steer RA. Relationship between hopelessness and ultimate suicide: a replication with psychiatric outpatients. Am J Psychiatry 1990; 147:190–195.
26. Hill RD, Gallagher D, Thompson LW, Ishida T. Hopelessness as a measure of suicide intent in the depressed elderly. Psychol Aging 1988; 3:230–232.
27. Ross RK, Bernstein L, Trent L, Henderson BE, Paganini-Hill A. A prospective study of risk factors for traumatic death in the retirement community. Prev Med 1990; 19:323–334.
28. Szanto K, Reynolds CF III, Conwell Y, Begley AE, Houck P. High levels of hopelessness persist in geriatric patients with remitted depression and a history of suicide attempt. J Am Geriatr Soc 1998; 46:1401–1406.
29. Breitbart W, Rosenfeld B, Pessin H, Kaim M, Funesti-Esch J, Galietta M, Nelson CJ, Brescia R. Depression, hopelessness and desire for hastened death in terminally ill patients with cancer. JAMA 2000; 284:2907–2911.
30. Felton BJ. The aged: settings, services and needs. In: Snowden LR, ed. Reaching the Underserved: Mental Health Needs of Neglected Populations. Beverly Hills, CA: Sage, 1982:23–42.
31. Gatz M, Smyer MA. The mental health system and older adults in the 1990s. Am Psychol 1992; 47:741–751.
32. Ben-Arie O, Welman M, Teggin AF. The depressed elderly living in the community: a follow-up study. Br J Psychiatry 1990; 157:425–427.
33. Diekstra RFW, Van Egmond M. Suicide and attempted suicide in general practice, 1979–1986. Acta Psychiatr Scand 1989; 79:268–275.
34. Johnson J, Weissman MM, Klerman GL. Service utilization and social morbidity associated with depressive symptoms in the community. JAMA 1992; 267:1478–1483.
35. Depression Guidelines Panel. Depression in Primary Care. Vol 1. Clinical Practices Guidelines. Pub #93-0550. Rockville, MD: US DHHS, PHS, AHCPR, 1993.

36. Sheikh A, Yesavage JA. Geriatric Depression Scale (GDS): recent evidence and development of a shorter version. Clin Gerontol 1986; 5:165–173.
37. Radloff, LS. The CES-D scale: a self-report depression scale for research in the general population. App Psychol Meas 1992; 7:343–351.
38. Katon W, Robinson P, von Korff M, Lin E, Bush T, Ludman E, Simon G, Walker E. A multifaceted intervention to improve treatment of depression in primary care. Arch Gen Psychiatry 1996; 53:924–932.
39. McIntosh JL. Suicide prevention in the elderly (age 65–99). Suicide Life Threat Behav 1995; 25:180–192.
40. Florio ER, Rockwood TH, Hendryx MS, Jensen JE, Raschko R, Dyck DG. A model gate-keeper program to find the at-risk elderly. J Case Manag 1996; 5:106–114.
41. De Leo D, Carollo G, Buono MD. Lower suicide rates associated with a tele-help/tele-check service for the elderly at home. Am J Psychiatry 1995; 152:632–634.
42. De Leo D, Rozzini R, Bernardini M, et al. Assessment of quality of life in the elderly assisted at home through a tele-check service. Qual Life Res 1992; 1:367–374.
43. Rutz W, Von Knorring L, Walinder J. Long-term effects of an educational program for general practitioners given by the Swedish Committee for the Prevention and Treatment of Depression. Acta Psychiatr Scand 1992:83–88.
44. Rutz W, Von Knorring L, Pihlgren H, Rihmer Z, Walinder J. Prevention of male suicides: lessons from the Gotland study. Lancet 1995; 345–524.
45. Pratt CC, Schmall VL, Wilson W, et al. A model community education program on depression and suicide in later life. Gerontologist 1991; 31:692–695.
46. Butler RN, Lewis MI. Late-life depression: when and how to intervene. Geriatrics 1995; 50:44–55.
47. Osgood NJ. Prevention of suicide in the elderly. J Geriatr Psychiatry 1991; 24: 293–306.

14

Factors Affecting Long-Term Prognosis and Maintenance Treatment Outcomes

Noah M. Meyers* and Charles F. Reynolds III
University of Pittsburgh School of Medicine, Pittsburgh, Pennsylvania, U.S.A.

INTRODUCTION: PUBLIC HEALTH SIGNIFICANCE OF DEPRESSION IN LATER LIFE

As the proportion of elderly persons in the world population grows, concerns about geriatric mental health become increasingly more pertinent to public health. According to a 1990 study conducted by the World Health Organization, unipolar major depression and suicide constituted the fourth most important cause of the global burden of illness-related disability, accounting for 5.1% of the total global burden of disease (WHO, 1996). In the United States alone, late-life major depression affects between 1 and 3% of the elderly living in the community (Mulsant and Ganguli, 1999). Prevalence rates of depression are higher in health care settings, where the illness affects approximately 10% of elderly patients in primary care settings and 15% of patients in nursing care facilities (Mulsant and Ganguli, 1999). Geriatric depression is projected to become even more widespread over the next decade, with the World Health Organization predicting that by the year 2010, the proportion of elderly as well as

**Current affiliation*: Cornell University, Ithaca, New York, U.S.A.

the number of elderly persons affected by depression will grow substantially (WHO, 1996).

Although late-life depression is prevalent, persistent, and disabling, it is not yet adequately recognized by many non–mental health primary care providers and continues to be underdiagnosed and undertreated. Data presented at the National Institutes of Health Consensus Development Conference indicate that while 1 in 6 elderly patients seen by their primary care provider is affected by depression, only 1 in 6 of those depressed patients is actually diagnosed and treated properly (NIH, 1992). Clinicians commonly attribute symptoms of depression like weight loss, sleep impairment, and fatigue to physical illness instead of depression. Even when a major depressive disorder is diagnosed correctly, primary care providers may not be inclined to inform their patient of the disease because they may be uncertain about correct treatment or even the validity of their own diagnosis. Even if diagnosed, late-life depression is often inadequately treated—by prescribing incorrect dosages of antidepressant medication, failing to consider possible drug interactions, or by discontinuing treatment at first signs of remission and thereby failing to prevent further relapse or recurrence.

The growing prevalence of geriatric depression is costly. Depression in old age is strongly linked to increased utilization of health care services. Depressed elderly patients require almost twice the number of medical visits, and the cost to the health care system is twice as much as for nondepressed patients (Unutzer et al., 1997).

Ultimately, if left untreated, geriatric depression can lead to additional health problems. The elderly (especially white males) have the highest rate of suicide of any age group, and most elderly suicides are strongly linked to depression. A study of suicide among elderly patients found that depression was a major predictor of suicides among the "old old" (Conwell et al., 1989). Among those 75 years of age and older, 60–75% of patients committing suicide had diagnosable depression. In fact, the majority of depressed patients had seen their primary care physician the month before committing suicide, and 39% had seen their physician the previous week (Conwell et al., 1989).

Depression contributes to the risk for death for causes other than suicide in elderly patients. In nursing home patients, major depression increases the likelihood of mortality by 59%, independent of previous physical health (Rovner et al., 1993). It can also lead to a variety of problems such as anxiolytic dependence and alcoholism, cognitive impairment, physical disabilities, and medical symptoms. One study found depression to be as debilitating as advanced coronary artery disease (Wells and Burnam, 1991).

Not only can depression trigger other problems and diseases, but chronic illness is also highly correlated to the onset of depression, demonstrated by the fact that while depression affects up to 1 in 10 of elderly residing in the community, chronic illness increases the ratio to 1 in 4 (for review, see Reynolds and Kupfer, 1999). When depression co-occurs with another illnesss, the negative effects of each are amplified.

MANAGING DEPRESSION IN OLD AGE: THE NEED FOR CONTINUATION AND MAINTENANCE TREATMENT

Though geriatric depression is both serious and widespread among the aging population, data on treatment success provide reason to be optimistic. In a recent study examining the efficacy of the antidepressant nortriptyline used in combination with interpersonal psychotherapy, 78% of the depressed elderly subjects achieved remission (Little et al., 1998). Another study found that the recovery rate of depressed elderly was comparable to the recovery rate of younger patients (Gildengers et al., 2002; Reynolds et al., 1996a). But while strategies for treating depression in the acute stage are effective in achieving remission, failure to provide continuation and maintenance treatments can often lead to relapse, recurrence, and chronicity. Many physicians fail to provide the necessary therapies and end treatment as soon as the patient first achieves remission (Alexopoulos et al., 1996). Without continuation or maintenance therapy, there is a high rate of relapse and recurrence (Reynolds et al., 2001).

Although a high rate of remission can be achieved when treating in the treatment of elderly patients who are experiencing acute depression, clinicians all too often lessen treatment intensity or terminate treatment once remission is achieved, thus diminishing patients' protection from future recurrences of depressive episodes. Therefore, recent research in the field of geriatric mental health has focused on how to prevent depression from following a chronic course (Reynolds et al., 2001).

One of the recent lines of research on preventing relapse and recurrence has focused on the use of interpersonal psychotherapy (IPT) in combination with antidepressant medication in maintenance treatment. In a study by Reynolds et al. (1999a), 180 depressed elderly patients treated with either IPT, the antidepressant nortriptyline, or both were examined over a period of 7 years. During the acute stage, all patients were treated with a combination of nortriptyline and weekly IPT sessions until remission was achieved. If acute treatment was successful, patients entered continuation therapy, consisting of the same dosage of nortriptyline and two monthly IPT sessions and lasting for 16 weeks. All patients completing continuation therapy without relapsing were then randomly assigned to one of four maintenance therapies: [1] medication clinic and nortriptyline; [2] medication clinic with placebo; [3] monthly maintenance IPT and nortriptyline; or [4] maintenance IPT with placebo. It was observed that the combination maintenance treatment of nortriptyline and monthly IPT sessions produced the best outcome, with only a 20% recurrence rate over the 3-year period of maintenance therapy.

Yet while tricyclic antidepressants (TCA) like nortriptyline are often successful in the acute and maintenance phases of treatment, they appear to lack certain advantages of the newer selective serotonin reuptake inhibitors (SSRIs). They are not as safe in overdose, not as well tolerated by some patients, and require monitoring of blood levels; moreover, their prescribing is considered more complicated by many primary care phisicians. Although it has been shown that SSRIs and TCAs are interchangeable in the acute phase of treatment (Schneider, 1999), until recently there have been no studies comparing the two in the maintenance phase of treatment. Preliminary data, however, are now available from an open trial compared the SSRI paroxetine with the TCA nortriptyline (NT) during 18 months of continuation and maintenance treatment. The study concluded that while subjects taking nortriptyline had a slightly lower rate of recurrence (10%, compared to 16% with paroxetine), the two were essentially equivalent (Bump et al., 2001). Further controlled assessment of the long-term or maintenance efficacy of SSRIs in late-life depression is needed.

Although it has been found that maintenance therapy consisting of the combination of antidepressant medication with IPT is effective in preventing recurrence, factors such as cost of combined treatment, patients' preferences, and other factors make this an unrealistic choice for many. Therefore it is important to ascertain whether some patients might respond just as well to monotherapy. A study by Dew et al. (2001) looked at the initial recovery patterns of depressed elderly patients and how this might predict which maintenance therapies would be best suited for each patient. Among patients with a rapid, durable response to acute treatment, the effectiveness of monotherapy (either NT or IPT) following recovery was very similar to that of combined therapy. Patients who took longer to recover but still made progress in the first 16 weeks of acute treatment had a better chance of staying well with combined therapy compared to monotherapy, while patients who had little evidence of change in the first 16 weeks had the same chance of remaining well with placebo as with any other maintenance therapy (Reynolds et al., 1999a).

DETERMINING THE PARAMETERS OF CONTINUATION AND MAINTENANCE TREATMENT

Continuation and maintenance therapy are key to achieving full and long-lasting remission and recovery. Though most agree that continuation therapy should containue for at least 6–12 months following remission, researchers have not yet reached a consensus regarding the amount of time that maintenance treatment should be continued after the initial 6–12 months. A recent survey of academic geriatric psychiatrists found that the majority of experts recommend continuing treatment for 1 year if the patient has had a single lifetime episode but 2 years or longer with a history of two or more episodes (Alexopoulos et al., 2001). For continuation and maintenance treatment, the experts surveyed strongly recommended using doses found effective during acute treatment (Reynolds et al., 1999b). Many believe that the clinical characteristics of the patients should guide the length and intensity of the maintenance treatments, and there have been several studies examining which characteristics make elderly patients more susceptible to relapse or recurrence. Important characteristics include the age at first onset of depression and the number of lifetime episodes, the current age of the depressed patient, the degree of cognitive impairment, and the quality of the patient's sleep. Each of these characteristics, either alone or in combination, affects the way that the depressed patient will respond to different forms of maintenance treatment.

One characteristic that has a strong correlation with chronicity is the age of the patient at the time of a first episode of depression. In one of the first major studies of the relationship between age at onset to subsequent illness course, Keller et al. (1983) found that the risk of developing chronic depression increased with each subsequent relapse. This would suggest that the chance of relapse and recurrence (and therefore chronicity) would be greater in patients whose first episode of depression occurs earlier in life, for there would be a longer period of time for the patients to experience a recurrence. A study by Brodaty et al. (1993) confirmed the finding by demonstrating that patients experiencing their first onset of depression before age 60 were more likely to relapse than those who had their first onset later in life. Both these studies came to the conclusion that early onset is more strongly associated with recurrences, which in turn leads to treatment resistance and chronicity.

Other recent studies, however, have found the opposite; namely, that a late age at onset of depression (which is generally considered to be at age 65 or older) was the best predictor of slow recovery or nonrecovery as well as chronicity in elderly patients (Alexopoulos et al., 1996). A study by Alexopoulos et al. (1996) also demonstrated a link between late onset of depression and greater medical morbidity and mortality. Even when compared to factors such as age, type of medication, and chronicity of episode, a late age at onset was still the strongest predictor of slow recovery. Compared to early-onset patients, late-onset patients were almost one-third less likely to recover from an acute episode after 2 years (Alexopoulos et al., 1996). Further, patients with cognitive impairment (specifically, executive dysfunction) were found to be at higher risk for relapse and recurrence during maintenance treatment with nortriptyline (Alexopoulos et al., 1999).

Other factors aside from slow recovery and chronicity have also been found to be predicted by late onset. For example, late onset was found to have a positive correlation with the appearance of residual symptoms (Conwell et al., 1989). This finding suggests that treatment for late-onset patients may not be as effective or long-lasting as for those with an early onset of depression. Late onset was correlated with a lower incidence of family history of depression as well (Conwell et al., 1989), implying that if depression first occurs later in life, the cause may be less related to genetic liability and more related to underlying psychosocial or medical factors.

It has been suggested that the differences in these findings can be explained by differences in the study methods used. Problems such as the varying definitions of "age of onset" as well as small control groups both contribute to the difficulty of comparing one study to the next, and differences between study samples are particularly noteworthy. Studies finding a correlation between late onset and chronicity, such as the 1996 Alexopoulos et al. study, tend to look at patients who were older at study entry and treatment tended to be naturalistic rather than controlled. Also, many subjects were found to have cognitive impairment or were psychotic, with 40% of the patients developing dementia after completing the study (Alexopoulos et al., 1996). It has been suggested that problems associated with aging might play an important role in the connection between late-onset and chronicity. Perhaps physical or cognitive problems might trigger or worsen depression, or latent medical or neurological disorders could serve to reduce the effect of antidepressant treatments (Alexopoulos et al., 1996). In contrast, many of the studies finding correlations between early onset and chronicity looked at younger patients who had little or no cognitive impairment, perhaps making it easier to look at the effects lifetime age at the onset of depression without attributing findings to underlying medical problems (Reynolds et al., 1998).

A recent study by Reynolds et al. (1998) suggested that age at first onset of depression does not play as big a role in chronicity as previously thought. This 1998 study compared early- with late-onset patients and found that the two groups were very similar in regard to the percentage who remitted, recovered, relapsed during continuation treatment, or experienced a recurrence in the first year. The only difference found was that the early-onset patients took an average of 5 to 6 weeks longer to achieve remission than their late-onset counterparts (Reynolds et al., 1998). Patients with earlier age at onset had a greater number of lifetime episodes of major depression, and a greater proportion had attempted suicide. One treatment implication of this observation is that elderly patients with early-onset depression require vigilance for suicidal behavior during the greater time required to achieve remission.

While there is still debate over the effects of the age at first onset of depression, there is no doubt that further research is needed in the field. It is necessary to understand further how the age at onset affects the course of the disease so that the most effective treatment can be prescribed. In particular, it will be important to understand how earlier onset increases the risk for suicidal behavior (Reynolds et al., 1998). One hypothesis is that early-onset elderly patients become discouraged when treatment does not rapidly produce improvement. Therefore, it is necessary for primary care physicians and other specialists to communicate with both the patient and the patient's family about what to expect during treatment. Patients and families need to understand that while the chances of remission in elderly patients are still high, depressive symptoms cannot be alleviated in just a few weeks, and that treatment may take months to be effective, especially if there are compounding medical problems.

It has long been believed that depression in the elderly, compared to that in younger patients, is harder to treat, and the ability to treat the illness successfully is inversely proportional to the patient's age. While it has been shown that the elderly as a whole take longer to get well and have higher rate of relapse during continuation than younger patients (Reynolds et al., 1996a), until recently there have been few studies examining the response rates of different subgroups among elderly depressed adults. For example, it was unknown whether a patient who was 65 years of age would respond to treatment the same way as an 85-year-old patient. And while more research is necessary, recent findings suggest that when comparing the "young old" (59–69), "middle old" (70–75), and "older old" (76–95), the older-old subjects are just as responsive to adequate antidepressant treatment as are the young-old (Gildengers et al., 2002).

Although many compounding mental and physical problems that increase with age may decrease the chances for treatment to be effective, when controlling for those other factors and concentrating solely on the age of the patient, data suggest that age plays an insignficant role in the patient's chances to respond well to acute treatment. In a recent study it was found that when comparing patients 60–69 years of age with those aged 70 and older, the differences in remission rates during acute therapy were not statistically significant (Reynolds et al., 1999c). With preliminary data finding that depressed elders of any age can respond well to treatment and with additional studies currently being run, the question now changes from "will elderly of all ages repond well to treatment" to the question of which treatment will be most effective for which patient.

Although elderly depressed patients of all ages have the potential to be treated, the most effective long-term treatment for each age group may vary. Once a patient has remitted from the acute stage, the major challenge becomes keeping the patient from experiencing a recurrence. Because it was found that patients aged 70 and older were twice as likely to have a recurrence during the first year of maintenance treatment (61% of patients experienced a recurrence compared to 30% of the 60–69 age group), it is necessary to find effective treatment strategies to prevent recurrence in the very old (Reynolds et al., 1999c). A recent long-term study examining the efficacy of the antidepressant nortriptyline and interpersonal psychotherapy in maintenance treatment found that when treating subjects 60–69 years of age, either nortriptyline or interpersonal psychotherapy were effective in preventing recurrence. However, because the response to antidepressant treatment in the middle old and older old is frequently more brittle, a combination of the two treatments was necessary to prevent recurrence more effectively in patients aged 70 and older (Miller et al., 2001; Reynolds et al., 1999a). Over half of these patients experienced a recurrence of depression when assigned to either monotherapy, compared to less than one-third of the patients assigned to combination therapy (Reynolds et al., 1999c).

Although age has not been linked to recovery rates, the quality of sleep of the depressed elderly patient has been. Five to ten percent of the elderly experience persistent insomnia, a known risk factor for the onset of depression (Ford and Kamerow, 1989). It has also been found that the presence of sleep disturbances predicts a less successful response to maintenance treatment. In a study of maintenance treatments for late-life depression, patients with poor subjective sleep quality had a poorer response to all treatment conditions than did patients with better sleep quality. When assigned to IPT, only 30% of subjects with poor sleep quality remained depression-free for 1 year compared to 90% of good sleepers (Reynolds et al., 1997a).

Although it is known that poor sleep quality is associated with poor maintenance treatment outcomes, the reasons for this link remain a matter of further research. Experts are questioning whether it is the actual quality of sleep that predicts a poor outcome or whether sleep quality is simply an indicator of residual depressive symptoms that would play a role in the outcome of maintenance treatment (Reynolds et al., 1997a). It would be important for future studies of geriatric depression to concentrate on the role that sleep disturbances or insomnia play in causing and treating depression. It is suggested that treating chronic insomnia early on might be a good primary preventive treatment for an onset of major depression (Reynolds et al., 2001), and studies are finding that cognitive behavioral therapy may be a good approach to treating the illness (Morin et al., 1999a).

SUMMARY

Depression in later life is often a relapsing and recurrent illness with a strong tendency to chronicity. Hence, patients, family members, and clinicians need to consider strategies that prevent a chronic illness course. This is particularly the case in patients with recurrent depression, with "double" depression (major depressive episodes superimposed upon chronic milder depressions), with severe index episodes associated with heightened suicidality or other comorbidity, and with a positive family history. The good news is that increasing evidence supports the conclusion that available treatments effectively prevent relapse, recurrence, and chronicity. The bad news is that patients often require more than simple monotherapy with medication to remain well and that the reimbursement for the best treatment is inadequate and discriminates against those with mental illness in later life. Additional research is needed to show the effectiveness of maintenance treatment in very old patients, especially through the long-term use of SSRIs and psychotherapeutic strategies adapted to those with cognitive impairment.

REFERENCES

Alexopoulos GS, Bruce ML, Hull J, Sirey JA, Kakuma T. Clinical determinants of suicidal ideation and behavior in geriatric depression. Arch Gen Psychiatry 56(11): 1048–1053, 1999.

Alexopoulos GS, Katz I, Reynolds CF, Carpenter D, Docherty JP, Ross RW. The Expert Consensus Guidelines Series: Pharmacotherapy of depression disorders in older patients. J Psychiatr Practice 7(6):361–376, 2001.

Alexopoulos GS, Meyers BS, Young RC, Kakuma T, Feder M, Einhorn A, Rosendahl E. Recovery in geriatric depression. Arch Gen Psychiatry 53:305–312, 1996.

Alexopoulos GS, Meyers BS, Young RC, Kalayam B, Kakuma T, Gabrielle M, Sirey J, Hull J. Executive dysfunction and long-term outcomes of geriatric depression. Arch Gen Psychiatry 57(3):285–290, 2000.

Brodaty H, Harris L, Peters K, Wilhelm K, Hickie I, Boyce P, Mitchell P, Parker G, Eyers K. Prognosis of depression in the elderly. A comparison with younger patients. Br J Psychiatry 163:589–596, 1993.

Bump GM, Mulsant BH, Pollock BG, Mazumdar S, Begley AE, Dew MA, Reynolds CF. Paroxetine versus nortriptyline in the continuation and maintenance treatment of depression in the elderly. Depress Anxiety 13:38–44, 2001.

Conwell Y, Nelson JC, Kim KM, Mazure CM. Depression in late life: age of onset as marker of a subtype. J Affect Disord 17(2):189–195, 1989.

Dew MA, Reynolds CF, Mulsant BH, Frank E, Houck PR, Mazumdar S, Begley AE, Kupfer DJ. Initial recovery patterns may predict which maintenance therapies for depression will keep older adults well. J Affect Disord 65:155–166, 2001.

Ford DE, Kamerow DB. Epidemiologic study of sleep disturbances and psychiatric disorders. JAMA 262:1479–1484, 1989.

Gildengers AG, Houck PR, Mulsant BH, Pollock BG, Mazumdar S, Miller MD, Dew MA, Frank E, Kupfer DJ, Reynolds CF. Course and rate of antidepressant response in the very old. J Affect Disord 69:177–184, 2002.

Keller MB, Lavori PW, Collins CE, Klerman GL. Predictors of relapse in major depressive disorder. JAMA 250:3299–3304, 1983.

Lebowitz BD, Pearson JL, Schneider LS, Reynolds CF, Alexopoulos GS, Bruce ML, Conwell Y, Katz IR, Meyers BS, Morrison MF, Mossey JF, Neiderehe G, Parmelee PA. Diagnosis and treatment of depression in late-life: consensus statement update. JAMA 278(14):1186–1190, 1997.

Little JT, Reynolds CF, Dew MA, Frank E, Begley AE, Miller MD, Cornes CL, Mazumdar S, Perel JM, Kupfer DJ. How common is resistance to treatment in recurrent, nonpsychotic geriatric depression? Am J Psychiatry 155(8):1035–1038, 1998.

Miller MD, Cornes C, Frank E, Ehrenpreis L, Silberman R, Schlernitzauer MA, Tracey B, Richards V, Wolfson L, Zaltman J, Bensasi S, Reynolds CF. Interpersonal psychotherapy for late-life depression: Past, present and future. J Psychother Pract Res 10(4):231–238, 2001.

Morin CM, Colecchi C, Stone J, Sood RK, Brink D. Behavioral and pharmacological therapies for late-life insomnia: a randomized controlled trial. JAMA 281(11): 991–999, 1999a.

Morin CM, Hauri PJ, Espie CA, Spielman AJ, Buysse DJ, Bootzin RR. Nonpharmacologic treatment of chronic insomnia. Sleep 22(8):1134–1156, 1999b.

Mulsant BH, Ganguli M. Epidemiology and diagnosis of depression in late-life. J Clin Psychiatry 60(suppl):9–15, 1999.

National Institutes of Health. NIH consensus conference. Diagnosis and treatment of depression in late life (review). JAMA 268(8):1018–1024, 1992.

Reynolds CF, Alexopoulos GS, Katz IR, Lebowitz BD. Chronic depression in the elderly: approaches for prevention. Drugs Aging 18(7):507–514, 2001.

Reynolds CF, Buysse DJ, Brunner D, Dew MA, Hoch CC, Hall M, Begley AE, Houck PR, Mazumdar S, Perel J. Maintenance nortriptyline effects on homeostatic control of sleep in elders with recurrent major depression: double-blind, placebo- and plasma-level controlled evaluation. Biol Psychiatry 42(7):560–567, 1997b.

Reynolds CF, Dew MA, Frank E, Begley AE, Miller MD, Cornes C, Mazumdar S, Perel JM, Kupfer DJ. Effects of age at onset of first lifetime episode of recurrent major depression on treatment response and illness course in elderly patients. Am J Psychiatry 155(6):795–799, 1998.

Reynolds CF, Frank E, Dew MA, Houck PR, Miller MD, Mazumdar S, Perel JM, Kupfer DJ. Treatment in 70+ year olds with major depression: excellent short-term but brittle long-term response. Am J Geriatr Psychiatry 7(1):64–69, 1999c.

Reynolds CF, Frank E, Houck PR, Mazumdar S, Dew MA, Cornes C, Buysse DJ, Kupfer DJ. Which elderly patients with remitted depression remain well with continued interpersonal psychotherapy after discontinuation of antidepressant medication? Am J Psychiatry 154(7):958–962, 1997a.

Reynolds CF, Frank E, Kupfer DJ, Thase ME, Perel JM, Mazumdar S, Houck PR. Treatment outcome in recurrent major depression: a post-hoc comparison of elderly ("young old") and mid-life patients. Am J Psychiatry 153(10):1288–1292, 1996a.

Reynolds CF, Frank E, Perel JM Imber SD, Cornes C, Miller MD, Mazumdar S, Houck PR, Dew MA, Stack JA, Pollock BG, Kupfer DJ. Nortriptyline and interpersonal psychotherapy as maintenance therapies for recurrent major depression: a randomized controlled trial in patients older than 59 years. JAMA 281(1):39–45, 1999a.

Reynolds CF, Frank E, Perel JM, Mazumdar S, Dew MA, Begley A, Houck PR, Hall M, Mulsant B, Shear MK, Miller MD, Cornes C, Kupfer DJ. High relapse rates after discontinuation of adjunctive medication in elderly patients with recurrent major depression. Am J Psychiatry 153(11):1418–1422, 1996b.

Reynolds CF, Kupfer DJ: Depression and aging: a look to the future. Psychiatr Serv 50(9):1167–1172, 1999.
Reynolds CF, Perel JM, Frank E, Cornes C, Miller MD, Houck PR, Mazumdar S, Stack JA, Pollock BG, Dew MA, Kupfer DJ. Three year outcomes of maintenance nortriptyline treatment in late-life depression: a study of two fixed plasma levels. Am J Psychiatry 156(8):1177–1181, 1999b.
Rovner BW. Depression and increased risk of mortality in the nursing home patient. Am J Med 94(suppl 5A):19S–22S, 1993.
Schneider LS. Treatment of depression in late life. Dialogues Clin Neurosci 1:113–124, 1999.
Schneider LS, Small GW, Hamilton SH, Bystritsky A, Nemeroff CB, Meyers BS, Fluoxetine Collaborative Study Group: Estrogen replacement and response to fluoxetine in a multicenter geriatric depression trial. Am J Geriatr Psychiatry 5:97–106, 1997.
Unutzer J, Patrick DL, Simon G, Grembowski D, Walker E, Rutter C, Katon W. Depressive symptoms and the cost of health services in HMO patients aged 65 years and older. A 4-year prospective study. JAMA 277(20):1618–1623, 1997.
Wells KB, Burnam MA. Caring for depression in America: lessons learned from early findings of the Medical Outcomes Study. Psychiat Med 9:503–519, 1991.
World Health Organization. Global Health Statistics: A compendium of incidence, prevalence and moratlity estimates for over 200 conditions. In: The Global Burden of Disease. Cambridge, MA: Harvard University Press, 1996.

Index

About the Editors

JAMES M. ELLISON is Clinical Director, Geriatric Psychiatric Program, McLean Hospital, Belmont, Massachusetts, and Associate Clinical Professor of Psychiatry, Harvard Medical School, Boston, Massachusetts. The author, coauthor, editor, or coeditor of numerous professional publications, he is a Distinguished Fellow of the American Psychiatric Association and a member of the American Society of Clinical Pharmacology, among other organizations. Dr. Ellison received the B.A. degree (1974) from Harvard College, Cambridge, Massachusetts, the M.D. degree (1978) from the University of California School of Medicine, San Francisco, and the M.P.H. degree (1993) from the Harvard School of Public Health, Boston, Massachusetts.

SUMER VERMA is Director, Geriatric Psychiatry Fellowship and Education Programs, McLean Hospital, Belmont, Massachusetts; Lecturer on Psychiatry, Harvard Medical School, Boston, Massachusetts; and Associate Professor of Psychiatry, Boston University School of Medicine, Massachusetts. The recipient of the Teacher of the Year Award from *Psychiatric Times*, he received the M.D. degree (1963) from Punjab University Medical School, Chandigarh, India.

ISBN 0-8247-4246-X
90000
9 780824 742461